The field of integrative oncology is exploding with new information, provocative testing, and truly creating precision medicine. Jenny has worked tirelessly, researching and connecting to these innovators and sharing the wealth of knowledge with all of us. Jenny's book is a valuable resource and, frankly, a lifesaver. This book needs to be on the shelf of every practitioner working with cancer and in the hands of their patients in order to create true prevention, monitoring, and maintenance. Blessings, Jenny, for releasing another gem!

—Dr. Nasha Winters, ND, FABNO, L.Ac
Founder and CEO, Optimal Terrain Consulting; coauthor, *The Metabolic Approach to Cancer: Integrating Deep Nutrition, the Ketogenic Diet, and Nontoxic Bio-Individualized Therapies*

Jenny gives you the understanding of *why* you need to be vigilant and then shows you the *how-to* from her many years of personal experience and education. This is a book that oncologists should take a tutorial from and every cancer survivor should assimilate into their lives—if they want to live.

—Ben Johnson, MD, DO, NMD, DSc
Best-selling author, *No Ma'am-ograms! Radical Rethink on Mammograms*; author, *Healing Waters*; coauthor, *The Healing Code and The Secret of Health: Breast Wisdom*

Jenny's book addresses a real need. Unfortunately when tumors are too small to be seen on a scan or the traditional blood markers are normal, patients are sent on their merry way, thinking that they are cancer-free. Then, a few years later, they wake up to the devastating news that the cancer has metastasized, and everyone seems surprised. The information in this book equips anyone who has been diagnosed or wants to prevent a cancer diagnosis with knowledge outside of the traditional cancer box. Awareness of these tests will save many, many lives.

—Véronique Desaulniers, DC
Founder, BreastCancerConqueror.com and
The 7 Essentials System

This is an outstanding book that fills a significant void in the cancer world. As an integrative oncologist, I see patients every day who are not aware of the many outstanding tests available to them for cancer detection as well as treatment monitoring. In her book *Cancer-Free! Are You Sure?*, Jenny Hrbacek provides us with excellent tools that should be an essential part of cancer treatment today. I use many of the tests mentioned in this book and have found them to be invaluable in my practice.

—Jonathan Stegall, MD
Founder, The Center for Advanced Medicine

Chasing the tumor has yet to produce the cure to cancer. This book reveals the origin of the illness while providing solutions. Jenny does a great job providing you with the latest in testing options, which can be warning signs and lead to the prevention of a formal diagnosis and assist in the development of a personalized targeted therapy plan. I invite you to learn how conventional chemotherapy, surgery, and radiation are quickly being replaced as we embrace new methods and technology to prevent, stop, and reverse the disease.

—Leigh Erin Connealy, MD
Author, The Cancer Revolution

In the past hundred years cancer incidence has skyrocketed. The way we are approaching cancer treatments today is incomplete. Jenny Hrbacek, RN, has put together a wonderful document and a step-by-step approach to understanding cancer, and has shown us the scientific approach to proper diagnostics and desirable treatments. The amazing compilation of scientific testing makes her book the most accurate compendium in cancer diagnostics. I recommend very highly that all oncologists and primary-care physicians study and implement the principles outlined in this book on all cancer patients.

—Constantine A. Kotsanis, MD
Medical director, the Kotsanis Institute

Jenny Hrbacek's book *Cancer-Free! Are You Sure?* leads the discussion on what it really means to be cancer-free. Her straightforward, well-researched, well-written, insightful book thoroughly explores the topic of—and provides valuable information for those individuals who might not be aware of—the myriad of cancer screenings currently available. I highly recommend Jenny's book as a guide for anyone at any stage of the journey, from diagnosis to treatment to remission and what lies beyond!

—Robert J. LaCava, MD, FACOG
Founder and medical director,
The LaCava Center for Integrative Medicine

When I first met Jenny, it was like a light from heaven came shining in my door. She is so full of life and zeal and was on a mission to find answers to the devastation that is caused by cancer. I can confidently say that those who combine conventional therapies with lifestyle and diet changes typically astound their doctors when test results come back improved. God created us to live an abundant life. This book will guide and empower you!

—STEVE STEEVES, CCN, ND
AUTHOR, *THE TRINITY DIET*

Cancer Patient Testimonies

I consider my friend Jenny Hrbacek one of the reasons I can call myself a cancer survivor, having had extensive treatment and recovery from HER2 triple-negative breast cancer.

I first met Jenny at a Survivors Offering Support (SOS) meeting. I had just been through the traditional medical treatment regime of discovering breast cancer through a biopsy, which led to chemo, then double-mastectomy surgery with reconstruction, followed by six weeks of radiation. Imagine my surprise when I heard Jenny speak at the SOS meeting and tell all assembled that what I had just experienced was no guarantee cancer would not return. And even more, there were many new alternative-medicine therapies available. Jenny challenged the audience that night with the question "Your doctor tells you your cancer is cured, but can you really be sure?" My first thought on hearing Jenny was that I chose to believe my doctors. I thought, "I have been assured by my doctors that I am cancer-free. I have already been through all of this. It would have been good to know about these new choices before I went through everything I've been through, but that is all past now." I kept all the information Jenny gave everyone that night, thinking I would never need it.

In September 2013 I felt a continuous pain in my sternum and left breast, the same breast where the original tumor was discovered and removed. Tests confirmed my breast cancer was back and had metastasized. After three years of educating myself about breast cancer and good health in general, I knew my first round of traditional treatment had failed me. It was time to link back up with Jenny.

Jenny has been a tireless advocate for my care and a fearless warrior on my behalf. As Jenny fights to win her own battle with breast cancer, she has dedicated considerable life energy to my fight and others' fights as well. Some people are closer than a sister. What Jenny discovered and brings to this book is the result of her dedication to our fight and to anyone who may get that dreaded call to announce, "You have cancer." Cancer is an evil thing. What Jenny reveals is invaluable when you have a big fight on your hands and a short time to figure out where to go and what to do. As you read through this well-researched book, I know you will be amazed at what the doctors never tell you. It takes a fighter like Jenny to dig it all out for us. I pray you will be as blessed by this book and Jenny Hrbacek as I am.

—DARNELL RICHARDS
SUGAR LAND, TEXAS

The question in the title, "Cancer-Free! Are You Sure?," could be the subject of many aspects of our life journey.

When faced with unknowns, what do we do with them? Some use curiosity and courage to dispel the unknown; many do not know what to do, and fear prevents them from going any further, so they wait it out and take their chances. For many, fear is based on our lack of knowledge about the situation.

Just imagine being able to address "Are you sure?" with the maximum peace and assurance possible. Imagine having someone to help you pursue the answer to this question—someone who has the wherewithal to provide the emotional support, curiosity, and courage to dispel the unknown.

Well, this is now available to you with Jenny Hrbacek, RN. Jenny has fought the battle of cancer and knows firsthand what the journey is about. In other words, "been there, done that, got that T-shirt."

With the work Jenny has done in providing tools to detect cancer early, you have the best possible resources one could have. She has gained the vitally important firsthand experience and knowledge to provide you with the support, encouragement, and expertise needed so you can address "Are you sure?" and move forward rather than living in fear. Consider the tragedy of those who have had cancer for years and didn't know it. I invite you to examine the information presented in this book.

Wouldn't it be worth taking the opportunity to see if you can move from "Are you sure?" to that peace-of-mind state, "I am sure!"

—PAUL BENNETT
DALLAS, TEXAS

My cancer journey began with my annual mammogram, which led to a sonogram, an MRI (magnetic resonance imaging), a biopsy, and finally the diagnosis: triple-negative, stage I. Stage I—good; triple-negative—not so good. It was rare and very aggressive, the doctor said.

My mom had gone through cancer seven years before, so I somewhat knew what would be in store for me.

I had the bilateral mastectomy surgery, and during my six-week recovery I found out Jenny Hrbacek had also been diagnosed with breast cancer and had the same surgery by my doctor and plastic surgeon. I had known Jenny and her husband through my work. Five weeks after my surgery I went to see Jenny, and that visit started our very special, friendship-filled, faith-filled, fight-filled, and even a little fun-filled walk together. I am so thankful I had Jenny on my cancer journey. (My husband called us "bosom buddies"!)

One day Jenny and I attended a cancer support group together, and I was overwhelmed and actually astonished to hear how many women in the room were there with a second or even third recurrence. There were only about five or six out of fifty women there who were going through cancer for the first time. After the meeting several of us talked in the parking lot. I decided that I was not coming back because this was not the "support" I needed.

I also remembered finishing my treatment and my doctor saying I could go back to my "normal life." Depression set in because I felt my "normal life" had resulted in cancer.

I remember Jenny bringing me a book one day, *Beating Cancer With Nutrition*. She was so excited! She told me, "This book empowers us! It's not just words but what we have to do."

I joined Jenny in visiting Dr. Ray in Rowlett, Texas. I took the Greek test and have been retested as well. Over the past three years, I have been "stable" and considered "in remission." At my last oncologist visit my numbers were better than ever! I continue to fight the fight with my changed diet, exercise, and supplements, as well as reducing my stress level. It's not always easy, and I'm definitely not perfect, but I do want my body and immune system to be strong enough to fight the cancer cells.

Jenny's medical knowledge as an RN was invaluable to me. She taught me to take control of my test results and challenged me to do my part. Her passion in wanting me and others to be healthy is terrific, and she stays on me even today, years later! I use the testing in this book to monitor my health.

I join Jenny Hrbacek in the cancer fight and in taking control of our health by good nutrition, supplements, and doing all we can do for this body God created for us so perfectly. This is all we can do, and our dear Lord will take care of the rest.

Thank you, Jenny and Dr. Hammon! You are truly a blessing to me. I am so grateful for your knowledge, passion, and loving care for me and so many others.

—Karen Glynn
Sugar Land, Texas

The doctor told me I had stage IV cancer that had metastasized from my breast to my bones and down my vertebrae to my ribs and into my pelvic and pubic areas, and even into some of my organs and lymph nodes. I had between three weeks and three months to live. Surely this was a mistake! How could this happen? I have never smoked. I have always been good to people. I cried out, "God, I have served You all my life. This can't be right!"

At the young age of forty-five, with one daughter married, one in college, and a son of fourteen, the doctors were telling me I was facing death.

For one year I fought the greatest battle of my life, both in the spiritual and the physical realms. Today I am standing whole, healthy, and cancer-free. This was accomplished without the use of chemo, surgery, or radiation.

I met Jenny in the fall of 2013, after my diagnosis and cancer battle, and we made an immediate personal connection. I felt her compassion and desire to help others, and I knew our meeting had not been by chance. Oh, how I wish I had the information she shares in this book many years ago. It is not necessary for cancer to go undetected, as mine did. Cancer is an awful disease, and this book contains instruments you can use to find it early and be victorious. I pray you will find enlightenment and direction within its pages.

—SHIRLEY WILLIAMS
MARATHON, TEXAS
AUTHOR, *STAGE 4 CANCER GONE*

CANCER-FREE!

CANCER-FREE!

JENNY **HRBACEK**, RN

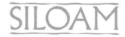

CANCER-FREE! by Jenny Hrbacek
Published by Siloam
Charisma Media/Charisma House Book Group
600 Rinehart Road
Lake Mary, Florida 32746
www.charismahouse.com

Cover photo by Michelle Deering

Visit the author's website at www.cancerfreeexperts.com.

Library of Congress Cataloging-in-Publication Data:
An application to register this book for cataloging has been submitted to the Library of Congress.

International Standard Book Number: 978-1-62999-553-3
E-book ISBN: 978-1-62999-554-0

18 19 20 21 22 — 987654321
Printed in the United States of America

This book is dedicated to the mission of creating a cancer-free revolution. Each word was written with the purpose of inspiring, educating, and equipping you with all you need to succeed.

Contents

PART III
ADDITIONAL INFORMATION TO CONSIDER

Foreword

AWORLD WITHOUT CANCER is possible. I collaborated for many years with Dr. Tsuneo Kobayashi in Japan. He is a molecular biologist who has shown us how, with early detection of cancer, the world could be nearly cancer-free. Many years ago Dr. Kobayashi realized the imaging method of detection was too coarse to detect tumors until they were well established. He achieved a major breakthrough in developing a new marker system that grades your cancer outlook on a scale of one to five. His rating of five is the equivalent to what in the United States is typically called a stage I cancer. In other words, when you top out on the Kobayashi scale, your problem is just now visible for the first time in the American system.

Dr. Kobayashi's patients undergo his annual cancer test, not because the doctor is trolling for business: Aha! A lump—sign this person up for chemotherapy and radiation. *Ka-ching!* No, Dr. Kobayashi wants his patients to avoid getting to that point.

Many of the tests described in this book are built on the foundation laid out by Dr. Kobayashi, and some of them are just as capable now of that kind of early detection. Early detection means you have to use the new tests Jenny Hrbacek describes in this book. She has done a marvelous, unparalleled job of finding and describing them. Your oncologist is most likely not able to tell you what Jenny tells you. Knowledge is expanding so rapidly that most doctors are unaware of the new tests.

After you have read Jenny's book and you move forward and use an early detection test, *do not* take the test to your oncologist, who may do harm to you with overly aggressive treatment. Early detection should not be used as a means to shuttle people into surgery, radiation, and chemotherapy. Most doctors don't know to offer much more than the standard toxic sixty-year-old therapies. Let Jenny tell you how to obtain personalized treatment that is proven to be more effective than the standard cookie-cutter treatment most cancer patients are told about.

Everyone who has been told his or her cancer has been treated needs to understand that cancer is seldom *cured* with standard therapies. Only by utilizing the tests Jenny describes will you be aware if your cancer is coming back while it is easier to treat.

Cancer cells and precancerous cells are so common that everyone, by middle age or old age, has them. If we have a strong immune system, we will have no problem because those cancer cells will be disposed of every day. But if our immune systems don't work right, we can have problems. And even then some of those cancers will go away on their own without any interference from modern medicine. As some researchers have said, it's interesting to know why we get cancer, but it is far more interesting to know why we *don't* get cancer!

The hero scientist who defeats cancer will likely never exist. Cancer is an intricate, potentially lethal collaboration of genes gone awry, of growth inhibitors gone missing, of hormones and epigenomes changing, of altered cellular respiration, and of rogue cells breaking free. Our world is full of heavy metals, devitalized foods, fungal infections, pollutants, endocrine-disrupting chemicals, carcinogens, and more factors that encourage cancer.

We must learn how to live cancer-free through the use of old-fashioned nutrition, targeted supplements, and therapeutic modalities such as homeopathy, acupuncture, microcurrent, lasers, pulsed electromagnetic fields, craniosacral therapy, and stress-reduction techniques.

If you want to avoid a cancer diagnosis, you need the knowledge in this book. This is a must-own book for you and your family. And give a copy to your doctor.

—GARRY F. GORDON, MD, DO, MD(H)

Dr. Gordon received his doctor of osteopathy in 1958 from the Chicago College of Osteopathy in Illinois. He received his honorary doctor of medicine from the University of California Irvine in 1962 and completed his radiology residency at Mount Zion in San Francisco in 1964. For many years he was the medical director of Mineral Lab in Hayward, California, a worldwide leading laboratory for trace-mineral analysis. Dr. Gordon is a cofounder of the American College for Advancement in Medicine (ACAM). He is the founder and a former president of the International College of Advanced Longevity, a board member of International Oxidative Medicine Association (IOMA), an advisor to the American Board of Clinical Metal Toxicology (ABCMT), and a full-time consultant for Longevity Plus, a nutritional supplement company. With Morton Walker, DPM, Dr. Gordon coauthored *The Chelation Answer: How to Prevent Hardening of the Arteries and Rejuvenate Your Cardiovascular System.*

Preface

Iᴛ's ᴛɪᴍᴇ ᴛʜᴀᴛ we take the fear out of cancer. In order to do that, we have to be willing to change. Today we have the tools, and the need is great. I'm going to ask you to set aside what you think you know about this disease and consider that we may have had the wrong approach. Within the pages of this book I will inspire you to reach for a greater future for humanity, one without the devastating effects of this disease. The information I share will educate and equip you to be part of the cancer-free revolution.

We've spent decades waiting for tumors to show up on scans and for people to get really sick. Today we have sensitive new tests that can detect cancer years before it becomes a big problem—so early that you won't qualify for chemotherapy, surgery, or radiation; in time for a multitude of health-building options to be implemented. You see, there are therapies and lifestyle adaptations that are proven in studies to stop cancer. Many of these are called metabolic therapies because they support healthy cells and stress the cancer cells. It's important that you're aware of these options, especially because it's well known that some cancers do not require toxic aggressive treatments, as they may never become life-threatening. I would have gladly used these strategies if I had known that I was on the path for a 2009 cancer diagnosis. Plus, the tests that I describe in this book would have provided a big warning, and the healing process could have started years earlier with no chemo or radical surgery. It's an unfortunate reality that most people are not aware of this new approach, and neither are their health care providers.

On the other side of the coin, for the most part we're still treating cancer with the same old methods. To be fair, we've made progress in the area of targeted drug therapies, but it's unclear as to whether they extend life more than a few months. These drugs should be used judiciously, and their use, validated through personalized genomic and chemosensitivity testing. These tests can identify the most powerful therapies for each individual. I'll teach how that's done so you can insist on a personalized approach.

The decisions you make concerning your health will have profound effects on how the remainder of your life will play out. If you've received a cancer diagnosis, I encourage you to curb your emotions and explore all your options. I know it's hard to slow down once you've been told you have cancer—you want it out immediately. However, the reality is that most cancers have been growing for years. In most cases it's absolutely worth your while to take a little time to look past the standard recommendations. I encourage you to explore beyond what is presented in this book. New discoveries are being made daily. I share what I found in my search; your journey may lead you down a different path. Be open, and consider your options. Your body was created to heal. Remember that broken bone or scraped knee. Those are perfect examples of the body's healing capability.

Join me, and let's learn:

+ The power of prevention
+ How to detect cancer really early and avoid harsh therapies
+ About the components of our current cancer system and what the future of a powerful approach to wiping out this disease should look like
+ If cancer is already well established, how to develop a personalized protocol and access the effectiveness of your therapies without invasive testing and radiation

I am so thankful you've picked up this text. May God bless our walk together. Now let's get started and learn how to live cancer-free!

Introduction

HOPE YOU'RE ENCOURAGED and enthusiastic to learn that we *can* take the fear out of cancer. We can do that by changing the way we deal with the disease. You see, prevention is the cure. However, knowing that we live in a "show-me" society, we need to look deeper at the issue. Over the last three to four years I've talked to hundreds of people who have been diagnosed with cancer. All of them wish they had known that they had the disease sooner. For example, if someone's tumor is 0.5 cm, she wishes she could have found it at 0.25 cm. This is a common desire because studies show that the sooner the cancer is discovered, the better the outcome. This information led to worldwide screening with mammograms and prostate-specific antigen (PSA) counts. The good news is that those tests are no longer the most sensitive. We can now detect cancer with a simple blood test when tumors are as small as 1–2 mm, long before they create a big problem and years before a formal cancer diagnosis would typically be made. You'll see how this is accomplished when you get to the testing section of the book.

Let's take a look at diabetes. History records that years ago we didn't find diabetes until the pancreas was in serious trouble. But in 1964 the Ames Company introduced the first strips for testing blood glucose by color code, and then in 1970 it introduced the first glucose meter.[1] Today people are routinely screened for early signs of diabetes, and if signs of the disease are found, lifestyle changes and medications can turn things around. Many times diet alone will correct the situation. We can apply the same process with different tools to cancer.

You might be saying to yourself, "We can't prevent cancer. It's a genetic disease." That's not true. Research has shown us that only about 5–10 percent of cancers come from a genetic origin.[2] That means we are doing something to cause the sharp increase in cancer that began in the early 1960s. A friend of mine uses the term PLDD. He says it like this: P-L-double D. The rapidly growing consensus is that cancer is a *preventable, lifestyle-driven disease*—hence a PLDD. Reports are that the average person has cancer many times in his or her life, but the person never knows it because the immune system takes care of it. In fact, the Harvard School of Public Health reports a study that an estimated 63 percent of male cancer cases could be prevented by lifestyle alone.[3] Imagine the

1

reduction in diagnoses if we added other cancer prevention strategies—such as compounds in superfoods that have been proved to kill the cancer stem cells that lie at the root of cancer malignancy.[4] All of this could happen before the discovery of a solid tumor.

The reality is that the immune system too often fails to beat the cancer. Today the National Cancer Institute reports that one out of every four deaths is caused by cancer. It's time for a change.

Here's what I want to do for YOU:

+ Inspire you to reach for victory and reject the fear that often accompanies cancer
+ Educate you on "cancer-free" strategies and testing options
+ Equip you to move forward with confidence
+ Connect you with the experts

So let's continue by imagining that you've been told you're cancer-free. Are you sure? Did you just have your annual physical with the standard lab work and receive a clean bill of health? Your doctor probably tested your cholesterol and maybe your white blood cell count to check for infection, but did he do any tests to look for signs of cancer? What if there were tests you could use to detect cancer before it was big enough to be felt? What if you could get scanned by a machine before a tumor was discovered and you found out it had been growing undetected for many years? What if there were steps you could take to see cancer coming early and knock it out before it becomes something really big and life-threatening? If you've had cancer, would you like to know about testing that will discover a recurrence early? And if you have cancer now, would you rather receive the one-size-fits-all, standard treatment approach or learn how to make sure you receive a personalized treatment plan?

Each of us deserves the very best, and that includes access to the most current testing and, if necessary, the best therapies available. I've made it easy for you and bundled up the information in this book. Read it carefully, and if you like, make notes.

Though I walked the path of a breast cancer patient, what I'll tell you applies to all types of cancer. So if you have cancer of the colon, lung, prostate, brain, or some other form, don't put this book down, because the information applies to you.

Cancer can be scary. I've been there, so I can tell you the fear of dying, or of losing life as you know it, can be irrevocably changing. Thoughts of enduring painful and expensive treatments, losing body parts and hair—all that and more instantly comes to mind. Those fears have a way of pushing out almost every other thought. You rush into surgery because you want the cancer removed from your body as fast as the nearest doctor can yank it out. You endure months of rigorous treatments. When all is said and done, you may ultimately find the cancer is back. And if it has spread, that is called a metastasis, and it kills 90 percent of cancer patients. The reality is that it was never gone; it simply could not be detected by the testing that was used. That does not have to be you. There is hope, and I believe we can beat this disease with a new approach. You are holding the keys to that approach in your hands.

For many cancer patients—and I am one—treatment of tumors is not the cure. Does that sound like a radical idea? I'll say it again: Cutting out a tumor does not cure cancer. Some people get lucky and live long enough to die of something else, but many do not.

Unless we embrace a new paradigm of prevention and personalized therapy, worldwide projections are that cancer cases will increase by 50 percent and that cancer deaths will increase by 60 percent from 2012 to 2030. The National Cancer Institute tells us that 67 percent of people diagnosed with cancer are "survivors," meaning they were still alive five years after their diagnosis.[5] An estimated 609,640 precious souls will die of cancer in 2018.[6] A report released by the World Health Organization (WHO) in early 2014 said the forthcoming rise in cancer worldwide is an imminent "human disaster." Christopher Wild, director of the International Agency for Research on Cancer, said to CNN:

> We cannot treat our way out of the cancer problem. More commitment to prevention and early detection is desperately needed in order to complement improved treatments and address the alarming rise in cancer burden globally.[7]

The first occurrence of cancer is generally easier to treat and more successfully treated than recurrences, especially when the cancer has metastasized. Once that happens, the outlook is often downright bleak. In the words of the National Cancer Institute:

> Although some types of metastatic cancer can be cured with current treatments, most cannot. Even so, there are treatments for all patients with metastatic cancer. The goal of these treatments is to stop or slow the growth of the cancer or to relieve symptoms caused by it. In some cases, treatments for metastatic cancer may help prolong life.[8]

Often cancer is not caught until it has spread into the lymph nodes, bones, or other organs, making recovery much more difficult. Did you realize that most oral, lung, and pancreatic cancers are not caught until a late stage because symptoms are often missed? And that lung cancer contributes to 25.9 percent of all cancer deaths? We can do better! You can check out loads of stats at https://seer.cancer.gov.

So if you've completed conventional cancer therapies, how do you know whether you really are as cancer-free as your doctor says you are? I learned the hard way that you usually don't know, and your doctor doesn't really know either. Standard cancer treatments may actually raise the odds significantly that the cancer will return. If you read the warnings on both radiation and chemotherapies, you will see that they can cause cancer. You can be in the dark as cancer cells gain a new foothold somewhere in your body. Eventually they build a fortress big enough to be seen on scans during routine cancer checkups. By then you have a *big* problem.

Or perhaps you've seen family, friends, and business associates spend time and money undergoing cancer treatments, and you don't want to go through that. If you could find out much sooner than when cancer is eventually detected with symptoms, tumor markers, standard scans, and biopsies that cancer was developing inside you, would you? A lot of people would. With an integrative physician you can learn to make lifestyle changes and greatly reduce the odds of hearing the words "Sorry, it's cancer, and we need to get you into surgery and begin chemo right away."

You need to know if cancer cells are hiding in your body. These cells can be identified, as can the substances they produce in the bloodstream. Most of the tests conventional doctors tell you about are designed to find cancer much later than the tests I'll tell you about.

I learned all this the hard way, but you can learn it the easy way—just keep reading.

My name is Jenny Hrbacek. I am a registered nurse from the big state of Texas. I was diagnosed with breast cancer using standard lab tests, biopsies, and scans used in the United States today. At the time of my diagnosis I seemed perfectly healthy and life was good. I had no idea how my life was about to change. As a patient, I was compliant and completed the recommended treatment protocol, and then I was congratulated and declared as having "no evidence of disease," meaning cancer-free for now.

I expected the treatments to cure me, as my cancer was caught fairly early according to the commonly accepted indicators. It seemed the candles were still warm on my celebratory cake when I discovered that, despite what my oncologists had told me, I was walking around with microscopic cancer cells still circulating quietly in my blood. Further, because of the initial cancer and the treatments I received, I was at a higher risk of having a recurrence of a more aggressive form of cancer. I was not cancer-free at all.

The familiar Big 3 approach of surgery, chemo, and radiation was developed after WWII and is still the norm. Conventional cancer treatment has become a big business offering a poor end product. To make things even worse, the American Cancer Society's Cancer Facts and Figures 2018 indicates that social inequality affects ethnic minority groups that are "substantially more likely to be diagnosed with cancer at a later stage, when treatment can be more extensive, costlier, and less successful."[9]

Today the "new kid on the block" treatment is immunotherapy. New drugs are coming to market that work with the immune system to kill cancer, although side effects can be severe. This is perhaps a promising addition to the Big 3. But early detection lags behind—they still wait for the lump, bump, or symptoms before engaging on any level. Data suggests that only 20–40 percent of patients respond to this new class of therapy, and the cost can be prohibitive.[10]

It is heartbreaking to witness the pain and suffering cancer brings, and I want to help.

I did several years of research and found many tests designed to detect the presence of cancer even before signs or symptoms develop. The science behind these tests is compelling. Today I use these tests to monitor my cancer status and the effectiveness of the therapies and lifestyle changes I have implemented to keep me on a path to health. This book tells you about detection tests that are more sensitive than what has become the standard of care. It is possible for you to have peace of mind, even if you have a family member or friend with cancer. Each test is broken down into easy-to-read sections providing information on the cost, how it works, what it tells you, benefits, limitations, and other important facts. Some tests are available without a physician and are simple enough to be performed at home. Others are more complex and require the guidance of a trained clinician. Several identify the best targeted therapies with which to formulate a personalized cancer treatment plan.

Most cancer patients finish their treatment and then are put in what I call the "wait, watch, and wonder program." Your physician *waits* a few months, then calls you in to *watch* for overt signs of cancer. Meanwhile, you are left to *wonder* if they will find more cancer and if you're really cancer-free. I don't recommend you wait, watch, and wonder unless you have a death wish.

In the search for solutions I found some exciting, simple, and great options. And we desperately need them because our lives are at stake—we haven't won the war on cancer. There is almost no national or global effort to prevent this disease. Oh yes, they tell us to stop smoking. The Centers for Disease Control and Prevention reports that 15 percent of Americans smoke—that leaves at least four out of five people with no prevention tools other than vague admonishments to eat better and exercise more. Good luck with that.

Cancer is a wily beast. It hides, but we have gotten better at finding it. Good early-detection tests are key. Such tests are available, legal, and sometimes even covered by insurance, but you won't usually hear about them at your local doctor's office. I will tell you where to find them.

And as a bonus, I will tell you some really important things—information I wish I'd known when I was diagnosed—about treatment side effects, the accuracy of scientific studies, what *survival* really means, how tiny tumors too small to be seen on a scan can begin the process of metastasis, why famous people don't fare any better than you and me with American cancer treatments, and why cancer cures can be toxic. I'll tell you what one food you never want to touch if you are serious about fighting cancer. Cancer is big business—you don't have to be caught up in it. Ask questions. Demand the best. Test early, and make sure you're cancer-free!

You'll discover there are some very good integrative oncologists out there, years ahead of their colleagues, who have impressive track records. Also, there are methods to rid the body of cancer without the risk of organ and immune system damage and other harmful side effects. And who knew there were cancer consultants who have been successfully guiding patients for years through the maze of conventional, complementary, and alternative options!

I invite you to go to my website's home page, www.cancerfreeexperts. com, and check out the "Resources List" within the "Free Downloads!" It includes information on helpful websites, books, videos, and reports you can access. You'll also find a link on how to find integrative physicians who can help you with testing, early intervention, and healing therapies.

In a cherished interview with Charlotte Gerson, daughter of Max Gerson, who pioneered the use of dietary therapy for the treatment of cancer and chronic diseases, Charlotte explained that cancer treatment must address toxicity and deficiencies to be successful.

You *can* take control of your health. Get tested and have peace of mind. If you've had cancer in the past, I encourage you to make sure with one or more of the tests that I talk about in this book. Patients who have chosen integrative therapies can use these tests to determine which treatments are working. Anyone whose previous therapy has failed him can use several of the tests to formulate a new targeted plan. And for those of you who want to avoid cancer, don't let it sneak up on you. Test and find it early, and then implement strategies to stop it—without the need for chemo, surgery, or radiation.

It's a big world out there! You have the right to choose, so choose well. Educate yourself. The decisions you make and the actions you take can save your life.

May God bless and direct you.

> Beloved, I wish above all things that thou mayest prosper and be
> in health, even as thy soul prospereth.
> —3 JOHN 2, KJV

Part I

Cancer 101

Chapter 1

My Story

I'LL SHARE MY story with you because, through all the fear and misery, I overcame! The Scriptures tell us that we will not be without tribulation in this life and instruct us to be overcomers. Please read on and learn. You can help bring about change. The hope for our future is great!

When I received the diagnosis of breast cancer in April 2009, I was forced to find time for six surgeries, four rounds of chemotherapy, a positron emission tomography (PET) scan, magnetic resonance imaging (MRI), a nuclear stress test, two computed tomography (CT) scans, a bone scan, and more doctors' appointments and lab tests than anyone should endure in a lifetime, all because of a little, 1.9 cm tumor, something as small as a penny.

At the time of my diagnosis, I felt great. I was a perfectly healthy forty-seven-year-old female, or so I thought. And I should know, right? I am a nurse.

I never had a problem with needles until they were aimed at me, and very quickly I began to feel like a walking pincushion. Today I can't even count the number of times I've been stuck for blood draws and infusions. And the whopping medical bills...I had insurance with a $10,000 deductible, plus a 20 percent co-pay. One hospital bill alone was roughly $35,000. I felt really bad about the amount of money that my family was spending on my treatment. That added to the stress of the situation.

The lack of control over my life was also a new experience. And with it came a pronounced loneliness. My husband, who loves me dearly, would leave for work, the kids would head off for school, and my dear friend Jacque would show up to take me to a doctor's appointment or help with dressing changes. Even with the multitude of cards and casseroles and support from family and friends, I felt so alone. I would lay my head on the pillow at night, and in the darkness it was just me, my prayers, my faith, and the cancer.

My official diagnosis was "invasive ductal carcinoma of the right breast with lobular features. Pathology staging of T1A N1A M0, Stage IIA, ER/PR positive, HER2 negative, and negative for BRCA1 and BRCA2 mutations."

From the moment I was told I had cancer, I felt an uncontrollable urgency to get rid of it—and quickly! I kept picturing myself on a train ride that I didn't remember buying a ticket for. I didn't understand that seven or eight years before, a ticket found its way into my back pocket with the words "All aboard—breast cancer, Jenny Hrbacek." I didn't know cancer starts developing almost a decade before it is usually discovered.

About a week after my diagnosis I had the double mastectomy, which I believed would get rid of the cancer. I chose a mastectomy because I wanted no possibility of having to deal with breast cancer again. Also, the breast and plastic surgeons said lumpectomies require radiation—that's protocol. They explained radiation damages the breast and makes any future reconstruction very difficult.

I selected a talented plastic surgeon who specialized in reconstruction at the time of the mastectomy. The thought of being bare-chested haunted me. My plastic surgeon showed me photos of his amazing work as well as let me interview several patients. I never thought of myself as a person who would have a plastic surgeon, but somehow the thought of replacing cancerous tissue with nice implants didn't seem so bad.

Upon waking up from the initial surgery, I was told the lab report said all my lymph nodes were clear. Unfortunately ten days later a revised report said one lymph node had a 2.4 mm seed of cancer cells. Suddenly the game plan changed. The National Comprehensive Cancer Network (NCCN) guidelines called for the immediate removal of all lymph nodes under my right arm, followed by chemotherapy. The NCCN also listed radiation as an option. Thank goodness, my breast surgeon, my plastic surgeon, and my heart said no to radiation. I questioned why it would be safe for me to have radiation while the radiation techs wear radiation exposure monitors and are protected by heavy aprons and steel-plated walls.

I agreed to four doses of chemotherapy. I received Taxotere® and Cytoxan®, which are broad-based drugs used for estrogen-positive breast cancers. *Broad-based* means that they target several of the anti-cancer receptors, pathways, or mechanisms. I have to interject—I should have insisted on chemosensitivity testing, but I had no idea it was available, so I proceeded without a personalized treatment plan. Chemosensitivity testing would have told my doctor the best drugs to use and also identified the ones that wouldn't work for me. The process was awful! My hair fell out on day fourteen, and I ended up in the hospital for five days in reverse isolation due to a fever and a low white blood cell count. One of the most shocking things about my hospital stay was the processed food—it was what they allowed. That meant no apples, cucumbers, or even lettuce on a hamburger.

Thank you to my husband and friends who were able to sneak contraband fruits and veggies past the nurses station. Four weeks later, after my next chemo infusion, I again had a spike in my temperature. Rather than call my oncologist and the hospital, I took two Tylenol and left it to the Lord. My temperature returned to normal the next day.

I read the side effects of the chemotherapy drugs I was given. Most of them sounded as bad as, if not worse than, having the original 1.9 cm tumor in my right breast. The possible heart, kidney, and liver damage, as well as the development of other cancers, didn't sound appealing. As I sat one day receiving a chemotherapy infusion, I looked around the room. The lady across the aisle from me was on oxygen due to heart damage caused by a listed side effect of her chemotherapy. The man to my left was so weak he needed a walker to stand—heart damage from his chemotherapy. I looked diagonally across the room and watched a young teenager with a brain tumor eating french fries and drinking a soda. He followed up with a bag of cookies. Believe me, I have nothing against cookies; I've eaten my fair share of them in my lifetime. However, in my new reality I looked at things from a cancer patient's perspective.

I knew that he and the other patients must want to live, or they wouldn't be subjecting themselves to these harsh treatments and suffering through the side effects. I decided to keep my mouth shut for the moment and reached for my IV pole and walked over to the patient snack area. There I found a vending machine full of cookies, crackers, candy, and so on. It's well known that sugar feeds cancer cells and compromises the immune system. If I could find this information after a few hours of internet research, why didn't the doctors and staff at this major cancer treatment facility know this? I couldn't understand why there were no educational posters around the room and no healthy snacks for patients receiving chemo.

My survival instinct kicked in. I gathered several medical studies, books, and supplements to take to my next appointment with my oncologist. I had a list of questions and felt armed with good data. I had barely made it through the waiting-room door when the nurse saw me carrying a container of dehydrated wheat grass powder, Essiac® tea, a few other supplements, and several books in preparation for my appointment with the doctor. She said, "You can't bring all of this stuff in here." I smiled and told her I felt certain that my doctor would want to know what I was taking and would be interested in my nutritional concerns during treatment. But I was wrong. My oncologist agreed that I couldn't bring in such material. He was more concerned with the report on my white blood cell count and the calendar to schedule my last chemo infusion. I was really taken aback by the response that I received, but I went ahead and handed him the copy of *Beating Cancer With Nutrition* by Patrick Quillin that I'd purchased for him. He actually tried to give the book back to me, saying I couldn't be giving him gifts. I was stunned. He seemed shocked I was trying to understand the disease process and told me most of his patients don't ask many questions. I continued, telling him it would be nice if they provided some healthy snack options in the vending machine. After a short pause he said, "Well, I am not in charge of the vending machine." I thought, "Well then, you are not in charge of me either." That was the end of oncologist number 1. I cringe every time I see one of the television commercials from this huge oncology facility promoting how much they "care."

So it was on to oncologist number 2. Even though I had completed my agreed-upon treatment protocol, I still felt I should have an oncologist, and I wasn't going back to oncologist number 1. Oncologist number 2 was at least willing to hear me out and added a few things to my protocol to counteract some of the side effects brought on by the chemotherapy. I was to see her every six months.

Moving on with my life, I joined a local breast cancer support group. We talked, had parties, and enjoyed monthly speakers. I was shocked to learn that approximately half of the women in the group had experienced a recurrence of their original breast cancer after being told they were cancer-free. They seemed satisfied with their medical care. They showed up wearing pink survivor caps and usually wigs. It seemed as if every month there was an announcement of another woman back in treatment with a recurrence. It was starting to make sense why oncologists want patients to come in for checkups every six months. They know completion of the NCCN treatment protocol leaves patients with a weakened immune system and a high risk of recurrence. They know the surgery, chemotherapy, and radiation they're offering are not a cure but only a treatment—which can be repeated for additional revenue.

That's when I set out to not be a statistic. I was determined to strengthen my damaged immune system. At one of the cancer support group meetings I met a new friend, who gave me the direction I had been praying for. After hearing her out, I made an appointment at the clinic where she was a patient. I was evaluated, and by the end of the day I was empowered and had taken the first steps toward regaining control of my health. Digging in my heels, I refused to live from oncologist appointment to oncologist appointment, praying for them to pronounce me cancer-free for a few more months.

My heart breaks for anyone living with the anxiety associated with regular "wait and wonder" cancer checkups. I receive several emails a month asking me to pray for someone who is going to one of those "cancer check appointments." Here is one:

> Pray for Neil tomorrow for a five-year cancer-free checkup. We won't know results until next week. Thanks for praying!
> Love, Kathy & Neil

This book is a result of the journey that started the day I drove four hours to meet with Dr. Ray Hammon of Integrative and Functional Health Center and RGCC USA labs (Research Genetic Cancer Center). It was now eight months after my surgery, and I was sporting two new beautifully reconstructed breasts. I was on a mission to strengthen my immune system. I had clean surgical margins and a clean scan, but after seeing that half the women in my breast cancer support group were experiencing a recurrence—some of them two or more recurrences—I wanted to be sure I would stay cancer-free.

Dr. Hammon said we should perform a blood test to see if I was really cancer-free. He explained that most people who have undergone conventional cancer therapies have cancer stem cells from the original tumor circulating in their blood, and those cells are the promoter of metastasis. The testing that I'd received wouldn't detect these cells.

He uses a lab in Greece where they utilize a patented process to harvest and grow in vitro (in a petri dish) any cancer stem cells that they isolate from the patient's blood sample. They are looking for cancer cells that have specific markers that identify them as cancer *stem* cells. If cancer stem cells are found, the test can move to the next level and measures the sensitivity of the cancer cells to specific chemotherapy drugs and many natural substances. In other words, the test creates a personalized treatment plan by identifying which drugs and natural substances would work for each patient's cancer and which ones would be a waste of time and money. My insurance company would not pay for anything that was not part of the NCCN cancer treatment protocol. This didn't matter to me. I recognize that the FDA only has regulatory authority in the United States, and it's a big world out there with many options. I got out my checkbook and paid for the test. I had to know if I had any cancer cells in my blood. I was determined not to have an oncologist order a PET scan—with its dose of sugar and radiation—and give me any more bad news.

When the RGCC results came back, I was shaken. "You have the highest level of breast cancer cells of anyone who has come through these doors," Dr. Hammon told me.

My hair had not even grown back yet from the chemo. What happened to the "clean surgical margins" and the "clean CT scan"?

I really thought the test would show I was cancer-free, with zero cancer cells in my blood. After all, I had completed surgery with clean margins and received four doses of very toxic chemotherapy and was on a six-month checkup program. But the test showed 14.2 cells per 7.5 cc's of my blood. It confirmed my biggest fear: I was just like the other women attending the cancer support group. Circulating cancer cells from the primary tumor were looking for a new place to set up shop.

Integrative and Functional Health Center immediately referred me to oncologist number 3, Dr. Jairo Olivares, MD, where I was told that with my high number of circulating tumor cells (CTCs) I needed to begin more chemotherapy immediately. I refused! I thought, "Why repeat a therapy that had failed?" He said he would give me ninety days to get my CTC count down below ten using nutrition, exercise, and the natural substance sensitivity testing results I'd received through Dr. Hammon and RGCC. If I was able to do it, he would support me. Dr. Olivares looked me sternly in the eyes and told me to do everything my sensitivity test had indicated and to make strict lifestyle changes—including a regimen of intravenous vitamin C and an extremely low-sugar, no-processed-food diet. I agreed and made an appointment to see him in a little over three months. I immediately started the program outlined on my RGCC test. I was grateful Dr. Olivares had the wisdom to consider the body's ability to heal when given the proper support.

The Father of Medicine, Hippocrates, said, "Let food be thy medicine and medicine be thy food." I did and found it really works for cancer. I came to see my standard American processed food diet was lacking so many of the herbs and nutrients proved to have anticancer properties. I learned I could take responsibility for my health and change my future.

Wow! Three months later it felt so good to walk into the next appointment holding a lab report that read "Jenny Hrbacek, CTC 5.5/7.5 cc of blood." Not only did I meet Dr. Olivares' goal of lowering my count below ten, but I was at 5.5! I continued with my protocol, and in another ninety days my CTC count was down to 2.9. Amazing! I did it without expensive and toxic chemotherapy. My hair was able to grow back, though, unfortunately, with a strange coarse texture. But I really didn't care; hair is hair!

I was beginning to understand how thousands of people have managed their cancer with natural therapies. The bookstores and internet are filled with testimonies. I had to learn more. I took every opportunity to attend integrative cancer conferences. I found myself in lecture halls sitting next to physicians who had dedicated their practices to combating cancer with less-toxic therapies, supporting the body so it can heal. I talked to every attendee who would speak with me, and I scoured the exhibit halls during the breaks. I took copious notes. I was able to interview doctors from across the United States and around the world. Wow, I have met some amazing physicians. I had read Suzanne Somers' book *Knockout*, but I never thought I would get to meet many of the doctors she interviewed. These people are more than just a chapter in a book; they are actively networking to learn as much as they can to help their patients. I have to tell you, I was like a kid in a candy store, like a sponge trying to soak up every detail I could absorb. These doctors spoke of terms and tools I didn't learn in nursing school and hadn't heard of during my personal cancer treatment. I had to learn what seemed like a new language and approach. I still have a hard time believing the average person doesn't have access to the information I learned. You have to work hard to find it.

During my research I discovered more about what cancer really is and how it can be detected early using many different tests. I wish I had known about them years before my diagnosis. When cancer cells duplicate or grow, they make errors in their DNA, creating resistance to the therapies being used. These mutating cancer cells require a multifaceted and targeted approach. They have an innate desire to survive and are always looking for ways to avoid being irradiated.

There are brilliant biologists, scientists, and doctors working far from the shores of the United States as well as right here in our country without the benefit of billions of dollars raised from groups such as the American Cancer Society and the Susan G. Komen foundation. These pioneers are providing excellent results with integrative approaches to cancer treatment. I am so excited to be able to share this knowledge on a larger scale.

In order to really wrap your head around the integrative side of cancer therapy, you should set aside the information you've learned from pharmaceutical marketing, the media, and the big money machine revolving around the cancer industry. Think outside the box. It doesn't matter what type of cancer you have; you need to be an educated consumer. Your health, or the health of someone you love, can benefit from what you learn.

I think back to when I got the initial diagnosis. I was in shock and scared. It all came at me so fast. I thought I was being given accurate and complete information about all my options. I let the surgeon remove my breast tissue because I had an overwhelming desire to get the cancer out of my body. I believed I was getting rid of the cancer and the possibility of any future breast cancer. I later learned that research shows there is no substantial increase in life expectancy in women who have had a lumpectomy with radiation versus a mastectomy.[1] Even with that well-established fact in the literature, women still ask for this surgery because they don't understand that removing the breasts does not make them cancer-free, only tumor-free. Before Dr. Hammon no one explained to me that removing my breast tissue did not mean breast cancer couldn't pop up somewhere else in the body. In fact, just the opposite, I was led to believe that removing my breasts would make me cancer-free.

I want to say a word about the lymph nodes. Just because lab reports say that they couldn't identify cancer in the lymph, it's not a cancer-free card! It only means they couldn't find it in the lymph. We want your entire body to be healthy and cancer-free. Years after my surgery the process of removing lymph nodes has been modified a bit. The American Society of Clinical Oncology now says that if only one or two of the sentinel nodes (the ones in the breast) are positive, you may not need the axillary nodes (the ones under the arm) removed. They've learned that removing them didn't really affect long-term survival.[2] This change in protocol came a little too late to help me. Even though I had only one sentinel node with a tiny, 2.4 mm, seed-sized positive area, they quickly scheduled more surgery to remove *all* the lymph nodes under my right arm. Guess what? They were clear—*no cancer*. What a wasted surgery. The surgical removal of my lymph nodes put me at risk for painful lymphedema. You may have seen people with swollen arms and legs wearing a tight stocking-like compression garment or sleeve. Usually the swelling was caused by the removal of lymph nodes. I pray quite often for the Lord to supernaturally replace my lymph nodes. Thank Heaven I've had no problem with swelling in my arm, as long as I stay out of the sauna. Here is a bit of information that might help someone: Heat causes the arteries to dump fluid into the tissues, and if the lymph system is not intact to drain the fluid back into the body for removal, swelling occurs. That means no hot tubs or saunas for cancer patients who have had a lot of their lymph nodes removed. I knew that heat can be very effective at fighting cancer and detoxing the body, so I didn't let this problem get in my way. I purchased a small tent-like sauna, the kind that you sit on a chair in, and it zips up around your neck so your head sticks out. My solution was to zip it up, with my right arm and shoulder sticking out. It looks a bit funny, but it works.

I look back on the decision process to have a double mastectomy with more clarity now. I based my surgical decision on incomplete information, at best. I'm still profoundly sad that no one corrected my false belief that removing all the breast tissue meant I would never have to deal with breast cancer again. In reality all I did was keep cancer from coming back in the breast tissue that went into the trash can. Tumors have a blood supply, which gives cancer cells a pathway to the bloodstream and the lymphatic system. So all I did was increase the chance a breast cancer cell would turn up later in someplace other than the breast. When doctors find the primary cancer in other organs, it is known as metastatic, often stage IV—not good. The information I had been given was that surgery with clean margins took care of the cancer—end of story. But it is not.

Throughout the entire treatment process, I kept asking about my immune system. If indeed every day the human body produces upwards of ten thousand cancer cells and the immune system routinely kills them, why did my immune system falter and let cancer cells multiply and grow into a tumor? I was repeatedly told it was "just bad luck" and there was no need for cleanses, vitamins, or a diet change.

All of my oncologists—remember that I had three because I kept firing them—told me that taking oral contraceptives had fueled the cancer. My pathology report was positive for estrogen receptors, and oral contraceptives contain synthetic estrogen. Every morning, I fed the breast cancer cells when I took the prescription given to me by my gynecologist to ease the side effects of menopause. I should have done my own research and not filled that prescription.

If you are wondering what happened to oncologist number 2, let me take a step back and fill you in. At a standard follow-up appointment she noticed my tumor markers were elevated somewhat. Tumor markers are seen in a blood test that looks for substances produced by cancer. The interesting thing was that my tumor markers were normal before my surgery, when I had the tumor. I was really concerned, because I had the breast tissue and the tumor removed. I went above and beyond! I didn't just have a lumpectomy; I had a mastectomy. But now I had elevations in my tumor markers! I thought, "What could be causing this elevation?"

Cancer, I feared. She wanted to order a blood test to look for cancer. I asked her what we would do if it was positive. She said, "The next step would be a PET scan to determine where the cancer had spread. Then we would start more chemotherapy." You can only imagine the thoughts going through my mind. I asked the Lord, "How can this be happening?" I felt as if I were trapped in a nightmare. The word *chemotherapy* rolled off her lips as if she was prescribing a couple of aspirin for a headache. In the confusion of the moment I said OK to her test. She handed me a lab slip and told me to have my blood drawn in the next few days at the lab. I did a bit of research and found that she would be sending my blood out for a CELLSEARCH® circulating tumor cell (CTC) test. Here is a description of the test:

> A simple, actionable blood test that helps oncologists assess the prognosis of patients with *metastatic* breast, prostate, or colorectal cancer... The first and only clinically validated, FDA-cleared blood test for enumerating circulating tumor cells (CTCs). CTCs are cancer cells that detach from a primary tumor and travel through the bloodstream or lymphatic system to other parts of the body.[3]

To give you a time reference, this happened about three months after I completed the chemotherapy. You can only imagine, I didn't sleep much, my mind was going in so many directions, and I was pleading with the Lord to heal me. The one bright thought was that the following day I had my first appointment with Dr. Hammon. He drew my blood and sent the vial to his laboratory in Greece to look for the presence of CTCs. I had never heard of CTCs, and now I had two doctors wanting to check me for them. You can only imagine my confusion. I was declared cancer-free a short three months earlier, and now this.

I spent several days in Rowlett, Texas, and had multiple IV infusions of high-dose vitamin C before returning home and having the CELLSEARCH test drawn.

About two weeks later I received the results from both CTC tests. The test result from CELLSEARCH found zero CTCs. And as I explained earlier, the results from the Greece lab reported a large number of cancer cells circulating in my blood, which would explain the elevation in my tumor markers.

I asked oncologist number 2 how the CELLSEARCH test she ordered showed I was cancer-free even though she suspected something was not right because of the increase in my tumor markers. And, of course, the other lab found a large number of cancer cells in my bloodstream. She said she was not familiar with the Greek test and dismissed its result. She did say there was no need for a PET scan because her test, the CELLSEARCH test, would not pick up cancer until it had metastasized to another organ, and she would continue to monitor my tumor marker labs. Let me say, this is no way to live, constantly being monitored for cancer!

Being a nurse, I was not satisfied with the dismissive answer. I wanted to understand the big discrepancy. I wanted to know what my CTC count was when I had the original, 1.9 cm tumor. To my surprise, she told me oncologists do not perform the CELLSEARCH CTC test at diagnosis because it will not pick up cancer cells *until the cancer has metastasized* to another organ. Basically the test is not very sensitive and will not pick up cells until the cancer has taken root in distant sites. So my next question was, "Are you telling me my CTC count was zero when I did have cancer, and it is zero now, and you're sure I do not have cancer?" She replied, "Yes, Jenny, you do not have cancer. Eat cupcakes, exercise, and take a multivitamin. Go enjoy your life."

I paused and thought, "Wow, I hope she's right because if she is wrong, I could be in really big trouble. I was educated enough to know a cancer cell does not jump from one area of the body to another area. It travels through the bloodstream. I was stunned to hear her explanation that standard practice in the United States is to test for CTCs only as a confirmation of cancer having metastasized, not to verify cancer-free status. I walked out and never went back. That was the end of oncologist number 2 for me.

I asked Dr. Hammon why the RGCC CTC test was able to find the cancer cells and the CELLSEARCH CTC test was not. He explained that the RGCC test was extremely sensitive and that I had had several intravenous infusions of high-dose vitamin C just before having my blood sample taken for the CELLSEARCH test. He further explained that the vitamin C effectively targets and kills cancer stem cells. I looked up the research and found him to be correct. The University of Kansas has done a great deal of research on this therapy and has produced an effective dosing protocol.[4]

I was still trying to wrap my head around all this, and here's what I discovered: according to the available data, a tumor has to be about 0.5 cm in size before it's detectable on a PET scan. There are new high-resolution

CT scanning machines that can find masses a bit smaller; however, you can't walk into your doctor's office and request one of these scans. You have to have signs and symptoms for the insurance company to approve it. If you are able to get one of these scans, you still wouldn't know much about the mass.

Something I found to be interesting is that some cells in a tumor are not cancerous. I learned at a conference of the International Organization of Integrative Cancer Physicians why doctors take multiple tumor tissue samples during a biopsy. It's because cancer cells might be found in just one or two of the samples. Some of the tumor can contain healthy cells.

Here's something else I discovered: a leading cancer researcher—Max Wicha, MD, professor of oncology and director of the University of Michigan Comprehensive Cancer Center—says standard cancer treatments can make things worse because when chemotherapy and radiation kill tumor cells, the dying cells send out inflammatory molecules that can summon more *cancer stem cells*.[5] These stem cells are like the wild card in a deck of cards. They can respond to the dying cells and essentially say, "Oh, we hear you are dying, and we can help you out by making more malignant cells like you." In other words, the chemo and radiation stimulated the production of more cancer stem cells.

The average oncologists never say one word about cancer stem cells to patients, much less provide treatments for them. It turns out that a large number of natural substances can help; we will learn more about those later.

After all this I have to admit that I felt betrayed by my surgeons and first two oncologists. I wanted to help others navigate this crazy cancer system and avoid the pitfalls that I found myself in. I put together a two-hour PowerPoint presentation, "Know Your Enemy and Win," and began speaking to groups. Through word of mouth newly diagnosed patients would get my phone number. Each call was a commitment of about three hours of my time, sharing what I had learned. Quite a few people were passionate about healing their bodies and not excited at the prospect of running out for surgical removal of body parts, toxic chemotherapy, and radiation. It was so encouraging to be helping people. At the same time, others chose to strictly follow traditional treatments. I was heartbroken to receive reports of nausea, hair loss, and the other side effects of harsh treatment protocols. I knew I needed a better way to get this information out. The outline of this book took shape.

During that time, with my improving CTC counts, I must confess I became a little complacent and stopped taking many of the elements in my personalized protocol. I indulged in dessert and an occasional glass of wine with dinner. I was confident I could manage the remaining cancer cells because I had the lab reports to prove it. My mistake was that I underestimated the tenacity of these cells to reproduce. After a two-year hiatus from strictly following my regimen, I decided to send my blood back to RGCC in Greece for a CTC count. I was disappointed to learn my numbers were up slightly to 3.3 from 2.9. Today I am back to managing those CTCs and giving my full attention to them. My goal is to get that number to zero. I understand now how important it is for any person who has had cancer to never let his or her guard down.

As time marched on, my phone rang often with calls from newly diagnosed cancer patients looking for answers to very serious questions. I received one such call from a woman named Angela. She asked if I was aware of any natural alternatives to the hormone-blocking drug tamoxifen.

Angela was forty-seven years old, just like me, when she was diagnosed with breast cancer. Her life was full and active. She was a busy single mom raising two teenagers, had a demanding career in medical case management, and was in her third season of triathlon participation.

It was very hard for her to say she had cancer. She was an avid hiker, once hiking sixteen hundred-plus miles along the Continental Divide testing sports equipment, the elements, and her endurance. She was a certified personal trainer and owner/operator of a sports training business for many years. She downed a green drink every day to make up for any shortfalls in her busy lifestyle and ate what she understood to be a healthy diet. People sought her out for health and fitness advice. For her, a cancer diagnosis was the ultimate insult because she considered herself an expert in health and fitness.

I share Angela's history because it helps to understand how cancer touches even the lives of those considered healthy and fit. Also, many of the calls I receive are from people in their twenties, thirties, and forties— people we would think are too young to get cancer.

Angela explained that in May 2012 she was feeling run-down and went to see her doctor. She also went for a regular 3-D mammogram and breast ultrasound to evaluate a lump in her breast—doctors had been "watching" it since 2008 because of her history of fibrocystic breasts. This time the radiologist wanted more samples, and the results turned out to be positive for invasive lobular carcinoma in her left breast.

Angela's surgeon told her it wasn't anything she did; it was just bad luck. She was urged not to put off surgery too long and was welcomed to "the club" with a pink bag full of brochures on breast cancer treatments and where to find wigs and such.

A few days later Angela saw the latest pathology report, indicating infiltrating ductile carcinoma in her other breast. She had two primary cancers, one in each breast. Her surgeon then felt a bilateral mastectomy was the best solution. Like most people at the start of a medical crisis, Angela looked to the authority of the white coat to help her make up her mind—certainly the doctor knows best. Angela was told that removal of all her breast tissue would take care of 90 percent of any future risk and that she would "have a greater chance of dying on the freeway on the way to work than from breast cancer."

The post-surgical recovery from a bilateral mastectomy is an experience for which no one can prepare herself. Angela's surgeon gave her the follow-up report. She had clean margins. However, they did find a micrometastasis in a lymph node but did not recommend treatment with chemotherapy. Her Breast Cancer Recurrence Score was 4, indicating an average distant recurrence of 5 percent.[6] With this score, she was not a candidate for chemotherapy or radiation, as the benefits did not outweigh the damaging effects the therapies would have on her health. Her oncologist suggested she take tamoxifen to suppress the estrogen hormones that were feeding her estrogen-positive cancer. He explained that she should take the drug for just the next five years because after five years the benefits no longer outweighed the side effects.

Did you catch that Angela had a confirmed micrometastasis? Her doctors knew the cancer had left the primary tumor, and all they offered her was a hormone blocker, even though it's known that hormone-receptor status can change.

Angela's research side kicked in, and she began looking into the side effects of tamoxifen: hot flashes, fatigue, depression, deep vein thrombosis, pulmonary emboli, and additional cancers. She learned the drug did not kill cancer cells; it only attempted to put any estrogen receptor-positive cell in remission by blocking estrogen receptor sites. The warning label states this drug is a known carcinogen.[7] It didn't make sense to her to take a substance that causes cancer.

She was beginning to understand the word *treatment* did not mean "cure" and that the treatment of symptoms was to be followed by more treatment of more symptoms. She felt guilty that she had temporarily given up her power and submitted to radical surgery. The importance of lifestyle and dietary choices, and their primary role in the development of cancer, was becoming clear. Most of all, she was feeling empowered and motivated to make changes and restore her health.

But friends and family were not happy to hear she was not buying into the full standard plan of care for post-surgical management. Feelings of guilt and doubt began to creep in.

Angela's unopened prescription bottle was still on her nightstand when she met with her breast surgeon one more time to discuss her concerns. The surgeon told her about another patient with similar ideas and concerns—a "bad patient" who was not following doctors' orders. This patient was even speaking on wellness and was eating kale chips, power berries, and other "nasty-tasting" things. The surgeon held out a business card with my name on it. Angela was pretty convinced she did not want to be a "good girl" and take the tamoxifen, so she grabbed that business card. When Angela made her first call to me, she said it was an answered prayer.

I applauded her research on less-toxic, supportive therapies. I explained to her the importance of getting confirmation of her cancer-free status. She made the same trek to Dr. Hammon at the Integrative and Functional Health Center that I had made. She learned about the RGCC test, often referred to as the "Greece test," and her subsequent test result of 4.2 CTCs per 7.5 cc of blood. She now knew why her doctors wanted her to take tamoxifen and come in for regular cancer checkups; she was not cancer-free at all.

The Greece test gave Angela a personalized list of the most effective chemotherapy drugs and natural substances indicated for her specific cancer. Angela began a program to detox her body and rebuild her immune system. She radically changed her diet, eliminating processed foods, carbs, and sugar. She bought a juicer and shopped for organic produce.

Both Angela and I were told our cancers had been developing seven to ten years before our initial diagnoses. We learned our high-carbohydrate diets were feeding our cancers. Carbohydrates break down into sugar, and cancer loves sugar—even the supposedly healthy "whole grains" we were eating. Plus, those grains were sprayed with glyphosate, an herbicide the World Health Organization has declared a probable human carcinogen.[8] The fox was in the henhouse wreaking havoc, and we had no idea.

Seven months later Angela received a call from Dr. Hammon regarding a follow-up CTC test from Greece to monitor the effectiveness of her lifestyle changes and treatment protocol. Her CTC count went down from 4.2/7.5 cc of blood to 2.0/7.5 cc of blood. This wonderful news gave her full confidence in the dietary and lifestyle changes she had made. A subsequent test showed her count dropped to 1.0/7.5 cc of blood. She did this without the use of tamoxifen; she did this with sincere motivation and a desire to stand up to cancer.

During the writing of this book I interviewed and worked with so many incredible clinicians. I only wish I had found them sooner. I often think about the pillow in my breast surgeon's office. It reads: "Yes, they are fake. My real ones tried to kill me." The sad truth is that even if the breasts are gone, they still may be trying to kill you.

Chapter 2

What Is Cancer?

CANCER WAS SOMETHING I simply hoped I would never get. I really never considered myself at risk, and if I was, I certainly didn't want to know it. Sound like a lot of people you know? Unfortunately around 1960, when the mechanization of farming exploded, along with the use of pesticides, herbicides, and fungicides, cancer rates began drastically rising.

Mention the term *cancer*, and the natural reaction of most people is a feeling of trepidation. And for some reason, possibly fear or denial, most people don't want to discuss it. However, the old saying "Out of sight, out of mind" doesn't work with cancer. Hiding from it doesn't make it go away. Today almost two of every five people will be diagnosed with the disease at some point in their lifetime.

I had no desire to investigate cancer. My first response to the diagnosis was to follow anyone who would help me make it go away. I walked the regimented path of procedures and appointments. It was comforting to have people take care of me. During those months I went along with the program, heaved a huge sigh of relief when my surgeries and treatments were over, and started to get back into my regular routine again—all without too much thought of what was going on in my body.

But once I realized I was likely to be one of those people back for a second or third round of treatment, I fervently researched the topic. I can honestly say that learning about cancer is not recreational reading, yet I knew my life was on the line. Ultimately it was my responsibility how my health would be restored. It wasn't something I could outsource to anyone in a white coat who offered the Big 3, as attractive as it might have seemed at the time.

It was important for me to understand the components of the disease. I found it difficult to define *cancer* in just a few words, so instead, I decided to tell you about its various names, its characteristics, its relationships, and how it acts in the body. I urge you to read this carefully so you too can become an informed advocate for your health.

CANCER

There's a growing number of scientists, researchers, and physicians who are redefining the mechanism that triggers the development of a cancer cell. It's been identified as a malfunction of mitochondrial energy metabolism in a healthy cell, thus causing the cell to become cancerous. Could it be that simple? Yet it's complicated. I explain the science behind this process in the metabolic section later in this chapter.

By another definition, *cancer* is uncontrolled cell growth.

It's generally given a name according to the area in the body where the tumor first appears—colon cancer, lung cancer, breast cancer, and so on.

A tumor can be benign, generally meaning that it doesn't have blood vessels to fuel its growth and it lacks the ability to invade neighboring tissue (metastasize). Benign tumors are usually surrounded by fibrous connective tissue and are not life-threatening.

The other type of tumor is a malignant tumor. Its main characteristic is uncontrolled cellular growth. The tumor produces its own blood supply system, pulling nutrients away from nearby healthy tissue. This overgrowth interferes with the body's normal functions. Malignant tumors can spread cancer cells to other parts of the body through blood vessels and the lymphatic system—the process of metastasis.

Cancer has many unique characteristics. Understanding the differences between a healthy cell and a cancer cell will help you make good decisions and understand why you're making those decisions. For instance, when you learn that your daily glass of orange juice, your vitamin-fortified breakfast bar, or your weekly Saturday morning doughnut contains an extraordinary amount of sugar that provides fuel for cancer growth, you come to understand why it pays to make better food selections. Your lifestyle, including daily diet and activity choices, is a huge factor in cancer progression and suppression.

The immune system is designed to jump into action and wipe out cancer cells; however, with the high rates of chronic health conditions and autoimmune disease, the system is often overburdened. It stops doing the job it was naturally designed to do, and cancer cells are allowed to flourish. Also, there are many conditions in the body that fuel cancer cell development and growth, especially toxins, nutrient deficiencies, processed foods, chronic inflammation, and hormone imbalances.

A typical tumor has billions of cancerous cells that contain genetic mutations. These cells are unregulated, and their sole function is reproduction and growth. If left unchecked, they can create a big problem.

The original tumor does not have to be life-threatening if caught early. It's the delayed detection and spread of aggressive cancer that makes the disease fatal.

Let's take a look at the characteristics of a healthy cell versus a cancer cell.

HEALTHY CELL	CANCER CELL
Has a predetermined life span Is programmed to die at the end of its life cycle—for example, red blood cells live about 120 days.	Has an unlimited life span resulting in continued growth and overgrowth
Reproduces only to replace a damaged or dead cell	Has uncontrolled growth that involves errors in DNA replication
Is aerobic (utilizes oxygen to create energy)	Is anaerobic (does not utilize oxygen as a primary source of energy) Uses fermentation, a metabolic process converting sugar to create energy (ATP)
Thrives in a pH-neutral environment	Thrives in an acidic environment
Needs a nutrient-dense environment—vitamins, minerals, enzymes, amino acids, etc.	Thrives on sugar and has increased amounts of insulin receptors to take in that sugar; reported to have up to fifteen times the insulin receptors of a healthy cell Readily metabolizes fructose for cell proliferation
Stays in its area of operation (i.e., kidney cells stay in the kidney—you would not find a kidney cell in the liver)	Has the ability to move around the body and invade other tissues (i.e., breast cancer often travels to the lung)
Has checks and balances in place to prevent it from growing in unregulated fashion	Grows faster than most of its healthy neighboring cells because it has lost its regulatory controls
Has the ability to use ketone bodies for energy	Is unable to use ketone bodies for energy
Has a regulated blood supply	Has an unregulated ability to create new blood vessels—resembling claw-like tentacles that invade and disrupt normal tissues, a process called angiogenesis

HEALTHY CELL	CANCER CELL
Is susceptible to chemotherapy-incurring cellular damage and possible death	Chemotherapy can cause tumor cell death as well as stimulate tumor cell mutations, making treatment more difficult. It can also stimulate cancer stem cell growth.
Works in unison with the immune system	Evades detection from the immune system due to a protective protein coating around each cell

THE DIFFERENT TYPES OF CANCER

Cancers are classified into five main categories, according to the kind of fluid or tissue from which they originate.

Carcinoma

A carcinoma is a cancer in the epithelial tissue that lines the surfaces of organs, glands, and other body structures. For example, a glandular cancer could be a breast carcinoma. Carcinomas account for the majority of all cancer cases.

Sarcoma

A sarcoma is a malignant tumor growing from connective tissue, such as muscle, tendons, cartilage, fat, or bones.

Lymphoma

Lymphoma is a form of blood cancer in which lymphocytes, the white blood cells that help protect the body from disease and infection, start to behave abnormally. Lymphoma may develop in areas such as the lymph nodes, blood, bone marrow, spleen, or other organs. Lymphomas are divided into two classifications: Hodgkin's lymphoma and non-Hodgkin's lymphoma.

Leukemia

Leukemia is a cancer of the blood cells. It generally starts in the bone marrow and results in high numbers of abnormal white blood cells. These cells eventually crowd out healthy blood cells.

Myeloma

Myeloma is a type of cancer that develops from plasma cells in the bone marrow. The plasma cells are protein-making cells that, when healthy, make different types of antibodies as part of the immune system. But when cells become malignant, they stop making the different types of proteins and make only a single type of abnormal protein. These abnormal proteins accumulate in the bone marrow and become a plasma-cytoma, which weakens bone integrity. If more than one area is involved, the diagnosis is multiple myeloma.

Two Categories of Cancer Cells

The two different categories of cancer cells that can be identified in the lab by their characteristics are tumor cells and stem cells. A common misconception is that cancer cells are located only in the tumor. This is almost always incorrect. A tumor as small as 2 mm—smaller than what is usually detected or operated on—has blood flow allowing cancer cells to be swept into the bloodstream. Some of these cells are tumor cells, and some are cancer stem cells (CSCs). Once the tumor cells are in the blood-stream, they are referred to as circulating tumor cells (CTCs). CTCs can respond to chemotherapy; however, the stem cells usually do not. They are the dangerous ones because they hold the DNA to begin producing more cancer cells that can lead to metastasis. Conventional therapies have repeatedly demonstrated an inability to eradicate the stem cells, which are estimated to be only a small percentage of cells in a tumor, less than 5 percent, according to most reports. Stanford Medicine Cancer Institute reports, "Only a small percentage of cells in tumors, the cancer stem or ini-tiating cells, drive the growth and metastatic capability of tumors. These cells must be eliminated to achieve a complete therapeutic response."[1]

This explains how a primary colon cancer can be surgically removed and the patient told he is cancer-free, yet the cancer reappears months or years later somewhere else in the body.

Dr. Hammon told me that a patient he had been following experienced a recurrence of cancer from a tumor that had been removed thirty-four years earlier. The hospital still had his original pathology slides and was able to confirm that his original cancer had metastasized.

Unfortunately these CTCs and CSCs are not detectable on scans. Specialized blood tests need to be ordered to find them. Cancer patients are told that they are cancer-free based on scans and basic tumor marker tests. I will tell you which tests to ask for.

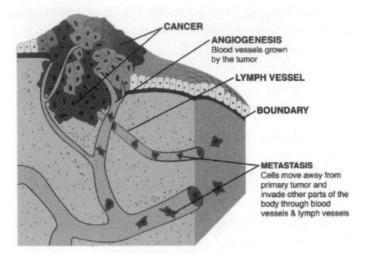

The process of cancer metastasis

CANCER SYMPTOMS

Why wait until you develop symptoms? We now have the ability to detect cancer really early—years before symptoms make its presence obvious. What a blessing it would be to find out you're in an early or precancerous stage. I keep saying that if I had known about the testing I tell you about, I could have saved myself a tremendous amount of anxiety, pain, suffering, time, and money. Don't wait for a tissue biopsy or PET scan to find out you have cancer. It takes many years for cancer cells to form a tumor large enough to be detected or cause symptoms. A 2009 study, for example, showed most early-stage ovarian tumors exist for years at a size two hundred times smaller than what standard, routine tests can detect reliably.[2]

The American Cancer Society defines *symptom* as a signal noticed by the person who has it, and that signal may not be easily seen by others. Symptoms such as fever, extreme tiredness, or weight loss are fairly common because cancer cells use much of the body's energy supply. Cancers of the pancreas usually do not cause symptoms until they are large enough to put pressure on nearby nerves and organs, causing back or abdominal pain. Cancer can cause many different symptoms, depending on where it is, its size, and how much it affects the organs or tissues. If a cancer has metastasized, symptoms may appear in other parts of the body.[3] Don't ignore even the smallest of signs. Better yet, get tested before symptoms develop.

I no longer subscribe to the philosophy that ignorance is bliss. Cancer is all too common today. Finding out sooner rather than later can make the difference between being able to live your life and pursue your dreams to the fullest, and struggling through an event that derails your career or, in the worst-case scenario, leads to an early and expensive death.

Here are a few reasons and/or symptoms that should prompt you to get tested:

+ Unexplained sudden weight loss
+ Fever
+ Fatigue
+ Pain
+ Yellow skin or eyes
+ Itching
+ Wounds that won't heal
+ Blood in the stool or urine
+ Diarrhea or constipation
+ Vomiting
+ Indigestion
+ Trouble swallowing
+ Shortness of breath
+ Mass in the breast or other part of the body
+ Chronic exposure to hazardous chemicals or low-level radiation
+ History of sun overexposure and sunburns
+ Undergoing treatment for an ongoing cancer
+ Taking medications with potential carcinogenic side effects
+ History of consuming known dietary carcinogens, e.g., large amounts of artificial sweeteners, colorings, flavorings, and preservative agents
+ Chronic exposure to drinking water containing high concentrations of chlorine, fluoride, pesticides, and other potentially carcinogenic chemicals
+ History of smoking or a non-smoker chronically exposed to secondhand smoke
+ Chronic stress
+ Depression
+ Emotional turmoil
+ Habitual caffeine or alcohol abuse
+ History of chronic viral infections such as herpes and HIV
+ Early detection of cancer
+ Diet consisting of a majority of processed food and cooked food
+ Family or past history of cancer

The most dangerous symptom is *no* symptom. This simply means that people with cancer don't always feel bad or have a physical symptom. Symptoms may not be present until the advanced stages of the disease. In the month leading up to this writing, I've had three precious people in my circle of friends diagnosed at stage IV—very progressed cancer. This could have been prevented with proper testing.

The integrative cancer world and I agree that cancer is a metabolic disease. It is helpful to understand the big picture because there are many interconnecting facets. Let's look closer at some of these.

THE SUGAR–LACTIC ACID CONNECTION

Cancer cells metabolize sugar for energy, and when they do, they produce a substance called lactic acid.

Otto Warburg, PhD, MD, documented decades ago that lactic acid levels increase in the blood if you have cancer because of a process now known as the Warburg Effect.

Dr. Warburg was a cancer researcher. He was awarded the Nobel Prize in 1931 for his work with cancer cell metabolism—how these cells find a way to survive in a low-oxygen environment by fermenting sugar for energy. When cells are deprived of a normal level of oxygen for a sufficient period of time, he said, cancer develops. Dr. Warburg found that cells become cancerous with only about one-third less oxygen transmission to the cells.[4] It has since been well documented that cancer cells display high rates of glycolysis—converting sugar for energy—whether they are well oxygenated or not.[5]

Life requires an intensive exertion of energy to operate muscles, remove wastes, make new cells, heal wounds, and fuel the brain. Oxygen has a powerful attraction for the body's workhorses—electrons. Cells use oxygen to turn food into fuel, an *aerobic* (with oxygen) process. But cancer cells thrive in an *anaerobic* (without oxygen) environment, meaning they do not utilize oxygen as their primary source of energy. They use sugar—glucose and fructose.

If you have ever worked out too hard in the gym and felt your muscles burning, that was lactic acid buildup at work—the muscles are fermenting glucose for energy, and lactic acid is the waste product.

The concern with a cancer patient is that lactic acid travels to the liver, where it is converted back to glucose—the cancer cells are cleverly participating in the production of their own fuel source. This merry-go-round of lactic acid and glucose is one reason cancer cells continue to grow in end-stage cancer patients even though the patient is too sick to eat.[6]

A diet high in sugar and starchy carbohydrates creates a bountiful buffet for cancer. That is why there is an old saying among cancer researchers: "Sugar feeds cancer." Healthy cells prefer fats for energy, but cancer cells primarily use sugar.

THE METABOLIC CONNECTION

Thomas Seyfried, PhD, is a biochemical geneticist and one of today's leading academic researchers promoting the treatment of cancer nutritionally. He is well versed in the Warburg Effect and published an extremely well-researched book in 2012 enticing the oncology field to revisit Warburg's work and rethink how we view cancer.

> We're not going to make major advances in the management of cancer until it becomes recognized as a metabolic disease. But in order to do that, you have to…present a massive counterargument against the gene theory of cancer.…
>
> If you transplant the nucleus of a cancer cell into a normal cell, you don't get cancer cells. You can actually get normal tissues and sometimes a whole normal organism from the nucleus of a cancer cell. Now, if the tumors are being driven by driver genes—all these kinds of mutations and things that we hear about—how is it possible that all of this is changed when you place this cancer nucleus into the cytoplasm of a cell with normal mitochondria? The gene theory cannot address this. It clearly…argues strongly against the concept that genes are driving this process.[7]

Seyfried argues convincingly that the traditional view of cancer as a genetic disease has been largely responsible for the failure to develop effective therapies and preventive strategies. The origin of the disease, he explains, is the malfunction of the mitochondrial energy metabolism and not of genetic source.

> Regardless of cell type or tissue origin, the vast majority of cancer cells share a singular problem involving abnormal energy metabolism.…the gene defects in cancer cells can arise following damage to respiration. … Many of the current cancer treatments exacerbate tumor cell energy metabolism, thus allowing the disease to progress and eventually become unmanageable.[8]
>
> Cancer growth and progression can be managed following a whole body transition from fermentable metabolites, primarily glucose and glutamine, to respiratory metabolites, primarily ketone bodies.[9]

In other words, gene mutations are not what cause cancer; gene mutations happen as a consequence of mitochondrial dysfunction. Seyfried's research reports that cancer starts when the "energy factories" inside the cell, called *mitochondria*, develop damaged cellular respiration. Identifying the causes of the damaged cellular respiration is believed to be the key to stopping or reversing the disease.

You could say that mitochondria are to human cells what the engine is to the automobile. Mitochondria are tiny energy factories inside each of our thirty-seven trillion or more cells. Seyfried says all cancer cells, regardless of their origin, have defective energy metabolism—dysfunctional mitochondria.

Seyfried's research documents the benefits of reduced caloric intake and a ketogenic diet as an alternate fuel source for a cell's respiratory function. Simply put, a ketogenic diet is high fat, moderate protein, and low carbohydrates. It has no sugars or starchy vegetables and grains that quickly turn into sugar in the body. Pastured eggs, butter and cream, coconut and olive oil, nuts, grass-fed meats, vegetables, and some fruits are high on the shopping list for ketogenic diets. It's a high-fat diet, and it's the opposite of what the USDA food pyramid preaches.

This fat-centric diet gets its name from ketones, substances made when the body breaks down fat for energy. The diet produces a high level of ketone bodies in the blood and low, stable blood sugar levels. It is a first-line therapy for treating epilepsy and is increasingly being considered in the treatment of many neurological diseases and injuries, including Parkinson's, Alzheimer's, stroke, traumatic brain injuries, and cancer.[10]

Seyfried says if we restrict sugar and provide fat for fuel, we can drastically reduce the growth rate of cancer. "Tumor cells cannot use...ketone bodies because of their respiratory insufficiency."[11] But, as he points out, few medical professionals are trained in the diet or understand how to tell patients to implement it.

There is more on the ketogenic diet in the chapter "Cancer—Beat It, Don't Feed It."

THE pH CONNECTION

A diet high in processed foods is acid-producing, creating an internal environment where cells struggle to get enough oxygen. Healthy cells need oxygen; cancerous cells—not so much. So, going back to the Warburg Effect, what causes cells to be deprived of oxygen? An acidic pH has a lot to do with it. The external microenvironment of a cancer cell is known to be acidic. Research in Cancer Cell International reports that "acidic pH increases not only the activation of some lysosomal enzymes with acidic optimal pH, but also the expression of some genes involved with pro-metastatic factors."[12]

I often wondered why cancer patients with significant tumors often appeared swollen and puffy. We now know the body will produce fluid in an attempt to neutralize the acidity around the cancer cells. The body is still trying to survive, even in end-stage situations. Another ongoing mechanism is that the cancer cells produce lactic acid, and the liver takes the lactic acid and converts it back into glucose, providing fuel for the cancer cells.[13] It seems to be a cycle of self-survival.

You're simply not going to have good health if your pH is out of whack. The body will constantly be struggling to balance it. This subject can be a bit complicated because cancer cells' intracellular and extracellular pH are both out of balance. That's why I strongly feel that any plan of action to assist the body in ridding itself of cancer must include a diet and lifestyle designed to promote a natural pH balance.

THE COLLAGEN CONNECTION

Research done by the late Nobel laureate Linus Pauling, PhD, and Matthias Rath, MD, suggests a collagen connection to cancer. Collagen is the fibrous, elastic connective tissue holding our bodies together. It makes up much of our tendons, ligaments, muscles, skin, hair, and other tissues.

Dr. Rath explains in his book *Cellular Health Series: Cancer* that cancer cells secrete a substance that helps them eat away at collagen, break out into the rest of the body, and invade healthy tissues. This is part of the process of metastasis. He says that if we provide the body with ample vitamin C, lysine, and proline—the building blocks of strong collagen production—aggressive disease can be controlled.[14]

THE NERVE CONNECTION

Holistic practitioners say it's important to get to the root of disease, not just treat symptoms. For the purpose of this discussion, the symptom is a tumor, and the root is the nerves. We know that for proper body function, the spinal column must be free of interference. With paralysis, for example, it's easy to understand there is a disruption in the nerves of the spinal column. But what if small compressions of this important body system interfere with the body's ability to heal? A 2010 study showed the direct response between a chiropractic adjustment and the body's immune fighting ability. After a spinal adjustment, IgG (immunoglobulin G) and IgM (immunoglobulin M) antibody levels were increased for the two-hour period studied.[15] IgG and IgM are immunoglobulin antibodies produced by the body's immune system in response to foreign substances such as bacteria, viruses, fungi, or cancer cells. These antibodies attach to foreign substances, causing them to be destroyed or neutralized.

THE HORMONE CONNECTION

The largest drop in breast cancer we have seen in the last fifty years came when women stopped using synthetic hormones. In 2002 the Women's Health Initiative Study showed a 26 percent increased risk of breast cancer for women using synthetic hormone replacement therapy— estrogen plus progestin.[16] The British Million Women Study and the French E3N Study also showed increased risk.[17] However, the Women's Health Initiative Study also showed the increased risk of breast cancer associated with the use of estrogen plus progestin declined markedly soon after discontinuation of combined hormone therapy.[18] Millions of women stopped using synthetic hormones. Breast cancer rates dropped.[19]

When we are not taking synthetic hormones to block pregnancy or dampen the effects of menopause, we are still awash in synthetic hormones. One source, for example, is bisphenol A (BPA), an artificial estrogenic compound widely used in cash register receipts, plastics for food containers, and children's toys. "Exposure of normal and cancerous human breast cells to low levels of BPA [leads] to altered expression of hundreds of genes including many involved in hormone-receptor-mediated processes, cell proliferation and apoptosis, and carcinogenesis."[20] About 80 percent of all breast cancers are estrogen receptor–positive, which means they grow in response to excess estrogen.

Other sources of synthetic hormones and estrogen mimickers include meat, dairy, and compounds in personal care products.

The human reproductive organs are particularly prone to cancer. Statistics tell us one in nine men will get a diagnosis of prostate cancer in his lifetime, one in eight women will get a diagnosis of breast cancer, and a woman's risk of getting invasive ovarian cancer is about one in seventy-nine.[21] All of these cancers are hormonally driven.

We usually think of sex hormones when we say "hormone," but our bodies use many different kinds of hormones as messengers. Melatonin, often called the anticancer or antiaging hormone, is produced in response to darkness; production peaks between 2:00 a.m. and 3:00 a.m. The body does most of its repair work at night—we replace about half a billion cells every night while we sleep. That energy-intensive process produces a lot of spare electrons called *free radicals*. The hormone melatonin is an extremely potent antioxidant that mops up those excess free radicals so they don't attack healthy cells. Studies have found that people who work night shifts are at increased risk for cancer, and women with breast cancer and men with prostate cancer tend to have lower levels of melatonin than those without the disease.[22] Melatonin "is a naturally produced cytotoxin, which can induce tumor cell death (apoptosis)."[23]

The thyroid gland makes thyroid hormones that regulate metabolism and support a strong immune system. Iodine is key to healthy functioning of the thyroid gland. Many people are deficient—check your levels.

THE ENZYME AND ANTIBODY CONNECTION

Cancer cells make systemic changes throughout the whole body. They produce specific identifiable enzymes and antibodies in the blood and urine that can be measured but often overlooked. Here are a few:

Nagalase

Nagalase (a-N-acetylgalactosaminidase) is an enzyme detectable in blood when cancer is present. This enzyme is secreted by cancer cells, pathogenic bacteria, and viruses. Nagalase suppresses macrophages, the fighter cells in the immune system. Too much nagalase and fighter cells never get the message to go into action and attack cancer cells. Nagalase is a tool that cancer cells cleverly use to ensure their own survival by allowing their continued growth to go unchecked.

ENOX2

Surface proteins called ENOX2 are produced only by cancer cells—healthy cells don't make them. ENOX2 proteins are shed into the bloodstream three to four years before most tumors reach detectable size. Finding these surface proteins early means we can detect cancer while it's still localized and potentially curable. These proteins also have molecular signatures that can be used to identify the source of the cancer.

Thymidine kinase (TK1)

Thymidine kinase (TK1) is another enzyme that can be measured when cancer cells are present. Its presence in blood serum is closely correlated to tumor development and progression. TK1 has been used in Europe for many years to monitor cancer cell proliferation/division and prognosis. Monitoring TK1 levels has been found to be quite useful for judging therapeutic success or failure.

Phosphohexose isomerase (PHI) and carcinoembryonic antigen (CEA)

PHI is an enzyme implicated in the spread of cancer, and CEA is an antigen present in the blood of many people with cancer.

THE MICROBE AND FUNGUS CONNECTION

There is a large body of evidence linking cancer with microbes and fungus. One school of thought says microbes are a causative factor in cancer; another says they take up residence in sick, cancerous cells only because a weakened body invites them.

The debate goes back to the nineteenth century, when Louis Pasteur (1822–1895) convincingly proposed that germs caused disease. But two of his contemporaries, Claude Bernard (1813–1878) and Antoine Béchamp (1816–1908), convincingly argued that the inner terrain of the body was more important because bacteria could not invade a healthy host and create disease on their own. It was only when the inner terrain was run-down that germs would find a hospitable-enough environment to set up housekeeping and do further damage. The argument basically goes like this: Bacteria are scavengers of nature. They do not cause disease, just as flies, maggots, and rats do not cause garbage—instead they feed on it. The debate still continues.

In any event, germs and fungus are part of cancer and need to be addressed and eliminated from the body for healing to take place. Microbes or parasites come in many forms, and studies show they are prevalent in cancer patients. The human body provides a perfect environment for their reproduction as well as a food source. Tapeworms, round-worms, flukes, yeast, mold, bacteria, and viruses all produce toxic waste, invade tissues, destroy cells, and steal nutrients from the body.

It is important to note that cancer cells have one big thing in common with fungus, yeast, and microbes. They all feed on sugar, and Americans have a huge appetite for sugar. Athlete's foot, nail fungus, vaginal irritation, constipation, itchy scalp, and skin rashes are all examples of probable fungal infections. These common occurrences have produced a prosperous industry dedicated to providing pharmaceuticals to address all our fungus and yeast flare-ups.

Microbes and fungus excrete waste by-products called mycotoxins that are carcinogenic and acidic and weaken the immune system. It is also known that fungus and microbes develop a sac to provide a shield to protect them from the immune system. Cancer cells do the same type of thing by producing proteins that make it hard for the immune system to recognize, penetrate, and destroy them.

Raphael d'Angelo, MD, of the ParaWellness Research program specializes in parasite testing. He says a cancer patient's recovery will plateau and not continue until all parasitic problems are uncovered.

> What we think is happening is that the parasites create tissue inflammation and destruction which bogs down the immune system and provides fuel for cancer growth and invasion by yeast. The yeast feed on the dying tissue and they secrete more toxins that further destroy tissue keeping the cycle of inflammation (which promotes cancer) going. By eliminating the parasites and the yeast the immune system is freed up to do its job of attacking and resolving the cancer.[24]

It is interesting to note that plants have built-in properties to protect them from fungi. Simply eating more fresh fruits and vegetables and good fats can transfer their protection to us. For example, coconut oil's medium-chain fatty acids exhibit antibacterial, antiviral, antifungal, and antiprotozoal properties.[25]

Many commonly eaten foods are contaminated with fungi and their by-product, mycotoxins. Peanuts, cashews, wheat, barley, cereal, corn, and alcohol have all been shown to be contaminated with fungal mycotoxins. It has been determined that the reaction so many schoolchildren have to peanuts is an allergy to aflatoxin, a natural toxin produced by certain strains of the mold growing on peanuts stored in humid silos. The highest risk of aflatoxin contamination comes from corn, peanuts, and cottonseed. Aflatoxin is a powerful carcinogen, known to cause liver tumors in laboratory animals.[26] Mycotoxins are carcinogenic.[27]

Diet modifications and natural antifungals such as oil of oregano and grape-seed extract can be helpful in the battle against fungus. Often the problem requires prescription drugs such as Diflucan, Nystatin, and Lamisil. Use careful consideration before consuming multiple rounds of antibiotics because most of them are made from fungi. Use antibiotics only when necessary, and be sure to replace the good bacteria that are killed off along with the bad.

Among the many books and websites I've researched about the fungus and cancer connection, Doug A. Kaufmann really made the light bulb go on for me. In his book *The Germ That Causes Cancer* he presents research implicating fungi as well as what role their harmful by-products—mycotoxins—play in the cause of cancer.[28] Doug has become a good friend and has invited me to be on his TV show many times. Check out www.knowthecause.com for more research on the fungal link.

Pasteur's rival, Dr. Antoine Béchamp, told us that a healthy inner terrain is the key to prevention and treatment of all diseases because germs thrive in unhealthy environments and not in healthy ones. Lifestyle elements such as wholesome nutrition and environmental and hygienic cleanliness, he said, were ignored in favor of "heroic" medical interventions that turned a profit for industry. He said this 150 years ago!

The smallest unit of life, Béchamp said, is not the cell but microzyma found inside the cell. Normally microzyma function harmoniously, but when the inner terrain shifts to favor disease, the microzyma change form into malevolent bacteria, fungi, and viruses. Then the microzyma themselves give off toxic by-products, further contributing to a weakened terrain.[29]

Béchamp's work lives on in physicians and researchers who think mainstream medicine is on the wrong track today because germs are first and foremost symptoms. Bernard Jensen and Mark Anderson, for example, said in their 1990 book, *Empty Harvest*:

> The germ theory is still believed to be the central cause of disease because around it exists a colossal supportive infrastructure of commercial interests that built multi-billion-dollar industries based upon this theory. To the scientific satisfaction of many in the health field, it has long been disproven as the primary cause of disease. Germs are, rather, an effect of disease.[30]

Another researcher who investigated the phenomenon of cancer bacteria for more than thirty years showed that "cancer microbes" were present in cancerous tissue and in the blood of cancer patients. He said it is a tragedy that modern medicine has refused to recognize and investigate the cancer microbe—the hidden killer in cancer, AIDS, and other immune diseases.[31]

THE INSULIN CONNECTION

Recent studies link obesity with the incidence and mortality of a number of cancers.

Insulin resistance—sometimes called metabolic syndrome—is when the insulin hormone is no longer able to efficiently lower blood sugar levels. Eating a lot of sugar over time calls for so much insulin that the mechanism becomes sluggish; cells don't bind with insulin, so glucose doesn't get into the cells very well. The pancreas is called upon to excrete more insulin, but it cannot maintain a high insulin output indefinitely. Then insulin levels begin to go down, and blood sugar levels go up. When the rise in blood sugar is severe enough, diabetes is diagnosed, and the door to cancer appears to swing open.

To quote Dr. Edward L. Giovannucci of the Harvard School of Public Health:

> Insulin may signal cells to increase rapidly in number through a variety of mechanisms. Insulin could directly signal growth, or it could do this by increasing the levels of other potent growth factors (insulin-like growth factors [IGF]), or it could make cells more sensitive to other growth factors. Although cancer is a complex, multifactorial disease, one of the consistent characteristics of cancer cells is their ability to grow uncontrollably and to be resistant to programmed death. Thus, growth factors are critical to the initial development of cancers, as well as to their progression. A number of studies now show that individuals with higher levels of circulating IGFs are at increased risk for developing colon, premenopausal breast, and aggressive prostate cancers than are individuals with lower levels.[32]

Obese people are more likely to have higher concentrations of both insulin and glucose, a situation that may promote cancer cells to grow, multiply, and spread rapidly. Whether the use of insulin by diabetics contributes to cancer or not is a debate raging among researchers right now.

THE GLUTEN CONNECTION

Many of us crave wheat because eating it releases feel-good chemicals, creating a drug-like effect on our central nervous system. That's the opioids in gluten, the protein contained in many grains, especially wheat, barley, and rye.

Opiates and opioids interfere with the body's natural killer cells, known as NK cells—specialized white blood cells dispatched by the immune system to defend the body. They are part of our first line of defense against cancer and virus-infected cells.

Also, the herbicide glyphosate, the key ingredient in the weed killer Roundup, sprayed on wheat is a probable human carcinogen and is linked to various health problems. A 2013 study, for example, concluded that "glyphosate exerted proliferative effects…in human hormone-dependent breast cancer."[33] The EPA raised the allowed residue levels of glyphosate on food crops in 2013. Although the American government maintains this herbicide is safe, the International Agency for Research on Cancer and the World Health Organization (WHO) call it a probable carcinogen.[34] It's the most heavily used agricultural chemical and is routinely found in the blood and urine of many Americans. It's sprayed not just on wheat but also on corn, canola, non-GMO soybeans, flax, potatoes, sugar beets, peas, lentils, millet, sunflowers, triticale, rye, and buckwheat.[35] Before my diagnosis of estrogen-positive breast cancer, I had been eating so-called "healthy whole grains." I wonder if my immune system could have defeated my cancer on its own had I not been feeding it the wrong fuel.

In 2017 California decided to add glyphosate to its list of chemicals that can cause cancer. Research shows that people with celiac disease and people with gluten sensitivities—which may be the majority of us—have a higher risk of cancer, heart disease, and death.[36]

Dr. William Davis' book *Wheat Belly*, Dr. David Perlmutter's book *Grain Brain*, Stephanie Seneff's book *Gut-Brain Secrets*, and Dr. Zach Bush's research and lectures have done a great deal to educate the public on this risk. Check out their work. I enjoy listening to Dr. Bush on YouTube lectures or at ZachBushMD.com.

THE INFLAMMATION CONNECTION

Inflammation is basically one of two types:

1. An immediate healing response—such as when you hit your thumb with a hammer and the skin puffs up. Your immune system sends white blood cells and other substances to the area to start the healing process.

2. Chronic inflammation—acting as a persistent and negative stimulus but falling below the threshold of perceived pain.

The source of the chronic stimulus might be pesticides, chemicals, heavy metals, gluten from wheat that inflames the gut, or a low-grade infection from a root canal. These persistent stimuli create a constant irritation, distorting the body's normal response.

Chronic inflammation can stimulate mutated cancer cells and enhance their survival and opportunity for metastasis.

> There is a clear relationship between certain chronic inflammatory conditions and the transformation of inflamed tissue into malignant tissue. For example, chronic gastritis (inflammation of

the stomach lining) and peptic ulcers may be a causative factor in 60–90% of stomach cancers. Chronic hepatitis (inflammation of the liver) and cirrhosis of the liver are believed to be responsible for about 80% of liver cancers. Colorectal cancer is 10 times more likely to occur in patients with chronic inflammatory diseases of the colon, such as ulcerative colitis and Crohn's disease.[37]

THE GENETIC CONNECTION

Most cancers do not occur because you inherited a "cancer-causing" gene. On that everyone agrees. Hereditary mutations, those passed on from parent to child, account for only about 5–10 percent of all cancers. Upwards of 90 percent of cancers are caused by life—the food we eat, the chemical exposures we struggle to process, and the stress we endure. Conventional oncology says those challenges trigger genetic mutations that cause cancer. According to the American Cancer Society:

> It is important to realize that mutations in our cells happen all the time. Usually, the cell detects the change and repairs it. If it can't be repaired, the cell will get a signal telling it to die in a process called *apoptosis*. But if the cell doesn't die and the mutation is not repaired, it may lead to a person developing cancer. This is more likely if the mutation affects a gene involved with cell division or a gene that normally causes a defective cell to die.[38]

But Warburg, Peter L. Pedersen, Seyfried, and others say that old school of thought is wrong—genetic mutations are just a downstream effect of the original problem. Cancer is really a "metabolic disease." The root cause, they say, is a defect in the cellular energy metabolism caused by a lack of sufficient fuel—oxygen. They point to the mitochondria, little power factories inside every cell that need oxygen to turn the food we eat into energy. When cells don't get enough oxygen, mitochondria struggle. Cells either die, or adapt like weeds to survive. If a cell adapts, it reverts to a more primitive anaerobic energy generation, meaning it burns sugar to stay alive, but it can't produce much energy for bodily functions. From there things start to spiral downward. Burning sugar for fuel instead of fat (ketones) generates far more reactive oxygen species (ROS) and lactic acid, which cause damage in large quantities. DNA changes follow, accelerating the progression of cancer.

Once gene defects come into play, there are two main types: oncogenes and tumor suppressor genes.

Oncogenes are a mutation of a "good" gene whose normal task is to control cell division properly. When oncogenes are present, cell division goes haywire. Cells have the potential to be turned on when they are not supposed to be, allowing cells to start the process of uncontrolled growth that can lead to cancer.

Tumor suppressor genes normally work to "slow down cell division, repair DNA mistakes, or tell cells when to die (a process known as *apoptosis* or *programmed cell death*). When tumor suppressor genes don't work properly, cells can grow out of control, which can lead to cancer."[39]

Most mutations involving oncogenes and tumor suppressor genes are acquired, not inherited.

THE ENERGY CONNECTION

Our trillions of cells communicate with tiny electrical signals. We see the body's electricity at work when we have an EKG to measure heart function or when someone is hooked up to a brain monitor in a hospital to measure ionic current flowing within the neurons of the brain. Remember all those TV shows where the monitor "flatlines"? The person is pronounced dead because his brain is no longer producing voltage.

Voltage is key to life. If you have a lot of it, that's good. If you have not so much, hello, disease.

Going back to Warburg, cancer is a failure of the mitochondria—the power factories inside each of our cells. If you have cancer, your mitochondria are not producing enough energy to do their job well.

We need the earth's protective magnetic field as much as we need food, water, air, and sunlight. The earth's pulsed electromagnetic frequencies (PEMFs) are of great importance to the internal regulation of every organism on the planet, including us. Prolonged weakening of the earth's magnetic field is associated with weakening of the immune system.[40] When the familiar pull of gravity is no longer present, muscles atrophy, bones lose their density, blood pressure shifts, and our ability to balance deteriorates.[41]

So if we are not getting our cellular batteries sufficiently charged from the earth, we can add energy with PEMF much the same way we add supplements to our diet because the soil in which our food is grown is not as nutritious as it was centuries ago. Everything that Otto Warburg said was bad about cancer is reversed with PEMF. PEMF acts as a "whole-body battery charger" by recharging all the cells in the body. Sick cells lose energy. Healthy cells run at about 70 mV. Cancer starts when you get down to 30 mV. "Cancer cells typically have a voltage of 20 mV and are in fermentation, meaning they need 10 times more energy from the environment. PEMF builds up energy within your cells, oxygenating and alkalizing the cells."[42] All metabolic processes are driven by this energy, including immune responses, oxygen and nutrient absorption, adenosine triphosphate (ATP) production, waste elimination, and reproduction. It takes an electromagnetic field to support the body's regenerative efforts.

THE LIFESTYLE CONNECTION

Smoking; obesity; sedentary lifestyles; too much alcohol; high consumption of sugar, pesticides, herbicides, and processed foods; and the questionable additives in our food and personal care products—some of which are suspected or known carcinogens—make up the short list of what is connected to an increased risk of cancer. Americans have tremendous opportunities and a bounty of daily choices that could nurture the strong immune system needed to fight and prevent cancer.

Unfortunately improving our lifestyle seems to be challenging in a society where we have been conditioned to depend on the so-called "easy fix" from a drug or medical procedure. It is not uncommon to see a lung cancer patient smoking or an obese person eating a slice of cheesecake. It is not uncommon for restaurants and food manufacturers to rely on refined salt for taste instead of health-promoting herbs and spices. It seems for most people the only successful motivation is crisis—such as getting a diagnosis of cancer or diabetes—and then it comes down to how strong their will to live is. Lifestyle change is where we get the biggest bang for the buck. Personal motivation is the key to making change, and I encourage you to find yours.

THE STRESS CONNECTION

Cancer and stress have been shown to go hand in hand, and stress is a known risk factor for cancer. The body responds to physical, mental, and emotional stress by releasing certain hormones; namely, epinephrine and norepinephrine. These hormones increase blood pressure, heart rate, and blood sugar levels. Studies have demonstrated that people who endure intense, chronic stress experience digestive and fertility problems as well as a weakened immune system. They also report increased problems from viral infections, colds, headaches, depression, anxiety, sleep problems, and cancer.[43]

In a 2013 study researchers at Ohio State University discovered a link between the activation of a stress gene and the spread of breast cancer to other parts of the body.[44] The gene, called activating transcription factor 3 (ATF3), is found in immune-system cells and may be a critical link between stress and cancer—enabling cancer to metastasize and cause death. Researchers already know the ATF3 gene is activated in response to stressful conditions in all types of cells. Normally "triggering ATF3 protects the body from harm by causing normal cells to commit suicide if there is a risk they have become permanently damaged by the stressful conditions."[45] However, in a cancerous situation, tumor cells communicate with immune cells and cause malfunction.

When doctors want to suppress the immune system to keep a patient from rejecting a transplant, they give stress hormones. When our daily lives stress us out, our body likewise produces stress hormones, and they are immunosuppressive. That's what is behind the axiom "Stress feeds cancer."

The doctors with whom I've spoken observed that patients who handle stress effectively have better outcomes, and in my interviews with cancer patients I noted that all of them had experienced a major emotional or physical trauma before their diagnosis. Stress is a major component of the cancer process and must be addressed. It can often be managed with exercise, counseling, support group involvement, forgiveness, learning to let go, and loving yourself.

A NEW LOOK AT CANCER METASTASIS

In 2017 I had the opportunity to attend an international conference at the Research Genetic Cancer Centers facility in Greece. During a lecture Dr. Ioannis Papasotiriou told everyone in attendance that they were able to capture a monocyte (a type of white blood cell) fusing with a cancer stem cell, creating a mutant new cancer cell. I think that the news made me stop breathing for a minute. I thought that white blood cells, part of our immune system, were supposed to gobble up cancer cells. Now we're learning that for some reason things can go really wrong, and these two can merge together and promote cancer metastasis.

Later, in November of 2017, at the Tripping Over the Truth retreat on metabolic cancer in Baltimore, Maryland, I was able to witness the process. During a presentation we watched a live-taped video of the process under a microscope. Dr. Papasotiriou explained that this fusion has been why the RGCC lab reports *no cancer stem cells* found in about 10–12 percent of late-stage cancer cases. These new mutant cells were escaping detection. He has worked to develop a method that will recognize these cells and plans to have it in place by late 2018, greatly reducing the small percentage of false negative results.

A Final Word on Cancer

I'm hopeful you no longer think of cancer as just a "tumor" to be cut out or bombed out of existence with chemo but rather as a complex systemic issue that has your body asking for help on many fronts.

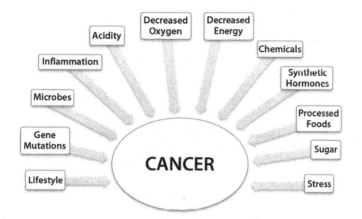

Factors contributing to cancer development.

Everything is permissible...but not all things are beneficial.

—1 Corinthians 6:12, amp

Chapter 3

Statistics—Misconceptions of Reality

I SPENT A GREAT deal of time questioning the statistical information I'd been given during my treatment and examining how misconceptions had affected the choices I made. As medical consumers, often in stressful situations, we place full trust in the information we receive, knowing that it affects the decisions we make. We assume it's factual, complete, and reliable.

Cancer statistics are often not what they seem and can be difficult to understand because of the way they're calculated and expressed. Numbers are manipulated to imply that patients who are counted as "cured" never experience cancer again and live a long life.

This chapter is not meant to criticize but to shed light on the truth and help you navigate through a very confusing trail of information.

THE FIVE-YEAR STATISTIC

Cancer survival rates are the first big manipulation you are likely to encounter. Survival rates are measured just five years out. They describe the percentage of people who are alive five years after a cancer diagnosis, excluding those who die from other diseases.[1] If a patient dies five years and one day after diagnosis, that patient is still counted in the five-year survival statistic. If the patient dies of a treatment-induced side effect—such as pneumonia due to a compromised immune system caused by the chemotherapy—the death is often reported as a death from pneumonia rather than being counted as a cancer death in the statistics. Consider cancer patients treated with radiation therapy who later die from a radiation-induced stroke. A study of cancer patients with head and neck tumors who received radiation therapy found stroke rates over their lifetimes were more than five times greater than expected. There was an average of 10.9 years between radiation treatment and stroke, and the increased risk of stroke persisted for fifteen years after radiation therapy.[2]

The cancer industry disguises important facts, such as that toxic therapies can themselves cause premature death. The death rate from cancer has barely changed since 1950.[3] It simply is not true to say we are winning the war on cancer. What we have is an effective way of manipulating data to sell harsh treatments that are profitable for those who make a diagnosis.

Meanwhile, cancer is striking earlier than ever before. It is not uncommon to see patients in their thirties with cancer. This was not the case fifty years ago. Cancer is now the second-highest cause of death in American children; only accidents take more lives.[4]

Clinical diagnosis at stage I or stage II also has a lot to do with the statistical manipulation. If the cancer is caught earlier, patients appear to be living longer. They reach the five-year survival date and are therefore counted among the survivors even though they later succumb to the disease. It is basically just a matter of moving the goalpost.

The five-year survival rate should be meaningless to you. What you want and should insist on is a treatment that will heal the body of cancer to the point where you live a normal life span and do not die a premature death from cancer. You want to die of something else—preferably old age.

PROBLEMS WITH OUR CURRENT PREVENTION METHODS

The good intentions of physicians and the media to promote the value of cancer screening does not equate to cancer prevention. Looking for a lump is not the same as working to prevent the lump. In some circles cancer screening is described as "trolling for business." If you have a lump, great! Bring on the biopsies and sign 'em up for the very profitable surgery/chemo/radiation.

We need to be leery of marketing campaigns advertising cancer screening and treatment under the guise of being helpful or increasing awareness. Where is the prevention factor? Could it be there are no revenues produced from prevention campaigns? But wait, couldn't a small portion of the billions of dollars raised for the cure be allocated for prevention? If it is, it's hard to see.

If you don't have a lump or a high PSA number or something else indicative of cancer, you are typically sent home with nothing—not even a pamphlet—about how to prevent cancer.

One good resource is the 2008–2009 President's Cancer Panel report, which contained a surprisingly candid discussion of the environmental contributions to cancer. At the very least, oncologists could be handing out copies of the executive summary to advise people to avoid known environmental carcinogens. Additionally many of the medical screening methods used today are ineffective or downright harmful. As the President's Cancer Panel report said:

The use of radiation-emitting medical tests is growing rapidly. Efforts are needed to eliminate unnecessary testing....No mechanism currently exists to enable individuals to estimate their personal cumulative radiation exposure, which would help patients and physicians weigh the benefits and potential harm of contemplated imaging and nuclear medicine tests.[5]

It is well known that radiation exposure can result in mutations or other genetic damage, feeding the cancer process. Medical devices that use radiation to screen or treat can add to the cancer burden. A 2010 study by researchers at the US Department of Energy's Lawrence Berkeley National Laboratory showed how exposure to ionizing radiation can alter the environment surrounding human breast cells, and then future cells are more likely to become cancerous.[6] "By getting normal cells to prematurely age and stop dividing, the radiation exposure created space for epigenetically altered cells that would otherwise have been filled by normal cells," said Paul Yaswen, a cell biologist and breast cancer research specialist with Berkeley Lab's Life Sciences Division. "In other words, the radiation promoted the growth of pre-cancerous cells by making the environment that surrounded the cells more hospitable to their continued growth."[7]

In recent years the US Preventive Services Task Force issued new guidelines calling for less screening with mammograms and PSA tests. Their goal was to reduce the significant harm from overtreatment. The move was met with protest from various groups that promote annual screenings. Yet these tests are far from perfect.

In the United States the risk of having a false-positive test within ten mammograms ranges from 58–77 percent.[8] A number of studies have concluded mammography's benefits fall far short of the advertising. A major study reported in the *British Medical Journal* in 2014 concluded that "the rationale for screening by mammography should be urgently reassessed by policy makers."[9] As Gina Kolata reported in the *New York Times*:

> One of the largest and most meticulous studies of mammography ever done, involving 90,000 women and lasting a quarter-century, has added powerful new doubts about the value of the screening test for women of any age.
>
> It found that the death rates from breast cancer and from all causes were the same in women who got mammograms and those who did not. And the screening had harms: One in five cancers found with mammography and treated was not a threat

to the woman's health and did not need treatment such as chemotherapy, surgery or radiation.[10]

Many cancers grow slowly, or not at all, and do not require treatment.
In fact, they may be best left alone, so let's monitor them with methods
that do no harm.

Studies find mammography detects essentially benign lesions in
women, but these lesions are termed "precancerous" and are then treated
preemptively at both a financial and emotional cost to women.

A study reported in 2012 looked at three decades of screening in the
United States and concluded:

> Our study raises serious questions about the value of screening
> mammography. It clarifies that the benefit of mortality reduc-
> tion is probably smaller, and the harm of overdiagnosis probably
> larger, than has been previously recognized. And although no
> one can say with certainty which women have cancers that are
> overdiagnosed, there is certainty about what happens to them:
> they undergo surgery, radiation therapy, hormonal therapy for 5
> years or more, chemotherapy, or (usually) a combination of these
> treatments for abnormalities that otherwise would not have
> caused illness.[11]

It was further reported by the 2014 study in the *British Medical Journal*
that "annual mammography does not result in a reduction in breast
cancer–specific mortality for women aged 40–59 beyond that of physical
examination alone or usual care in the community. The data suggest that
the value of mammography screening should be reassessed."[12]

In addition, a study of 1.8 million Norwegian women published in
2014 found much the same results—screening has a limited effect on the
discovery of serious and aggressive cancer cases and causes significant
overtreatment of conditions best left alone.[13]

In January 2013 the Swiss Medical Board conducted a global review of
mammography screening studies and recommended "no new systematic
mammography screening programs be introduced and that a time limit
be placed on existing programs."

> It is easy to promote mammography screening if the majority
> of women believe that it prevents or reduces the risk of get-
> ting breast cancer and saves many lives through early detection
> of aggressive tumors. We would be in favor of mammography

screening if these beliefs were valid. Unfortunately, they are not, and we believe that women need to be told so. From an ethical perspective, a public health program that does not clearly produce more benefits than harms is hard to justify.[14]

One option of many that I explain, breast thermography, which does not deliver an annual dose of radiation, has shown to be a better tool for early detection because it can see heat-producing tumor formations perhaps five years before a mammogram can pinpoint a possible tumor. Another option is the Videssa® Breast test, which detects breast cancer with a blood test.

Colonoscopy is another commonly recommended cancer screening. People assume colonoscopies save lives because it makes sense that removing precancerous polyps should reduce the incidence of cancer. But actually strong evidence for the concept was lacking. According to the National Cancer Institute, "Because there are no completed RCTs [random controlled trials] of colonoscopy, evidence of benefit is indirect."[15]

Finally, in 2014, a Yale Cancer Center study concluded an estimated half million cancers were prevented by colorectal cancer screening in the United States from 1976–2009.[16]

Arguments about effectiveness aside, one thing had never been in doubt about colonoscopy screenings: they are invasive and revenue generators. As the *New York Times* put it in a 2013 series on the high cost of American health care:

> [Colonoscopies] are the most expensive screening test that healthy Americans routinely undergo.... They are often prescribed and performed more frequently than medical guidelines recommend. The high price paid for colonoscopies mostly results not from top-notch patient care, according to interviews with health care experts and economists, but from business plans seeking to maximize revenue; haggling between hospitals and insurers that have no relation to the actual costs of performing the procedure; and lobbying, marketing and turf battles among specialists that increase patient fees.[17]

And the colonoscopy does not examine the small intestine. The American Cancer Society estimates 10,470 Americans will be diagnosed in 2018 with cancer of the small intestine.[18] Typically the diagnosis comes late, after there is blood in the stool or a blockage in the gastrointestinal tract.

Money often incentivizes motivations other than really good health care and puts the emphasis on revenue-generating procedures rather than prevention. *Efforts to look for cancer are not the same as efforts to prevent cancer.*

The BRCA1 and BRCA2 genetic testing is an example of money-dominating outcomes. If you are a carrier of the BRCA genes, you are perhaps more prone to develop cancer. The full test costs roughly $3,000 and is not always covered by insurance. A positive result will put a woman into a panic and often comes with the recommendation to remove the breasts, uterus, and/or ovaries. Those surgeries, and the reconstructive surgery that follows, are good revenue generators. We're learning that BRCA status doesn't affect long-term survival.[19] Keep an eye out for that ongoing research.

Doctors typically do not focus on the other side of the story—that of all the cases of breast cancer, the patients with a positive BRCA test are in the low single digits, about 5 percent. About 70 percent of the women with the BRCA1 gene mutation eventually develop breast cancer, and 17 percent of women with the BRCA2 mutation will develop ovarian cancer.[20]

Why don't all people with the BRCA mutation go on to develop cancer? This is the science of epigenetics—what causes some genes to express or not to express. We inherit two copies of each gene—one gene from our mother and one from our father. Usually we inherit at least one good gene, and that one keeps us healthy. But when we inactivate the good gene through smoking, environmental chemicals, stress, or a number of other factors still not completely understood, the "bad" gene can take over. Our genes are not our destiny. How we influence our genes is worthy of being developed into large educational and prevention programs from the government and the various cancer organizations.

Very often the BRCA test pushes women into the operating room. What doctors could be doing is giving people a choice by revealing the statistics and explaining what we know about how to affect genetic expression in favor of the "good" genes expressing. And how about monitoring patients for circulating tumor DNA or circulating tumor cells—simple blood tests able to find cancer years before the lump or bump? This seems like a much better option than the arbitrary removal of body parts. What of the other 95 percent of patients with breast cancer who have no genetic mutation? What caused their cancer? Most point the finger of blame primarily at environmental and emotional factors. Yet the medical establishment has not made it a priority to educate the public about non-drug and non-surgical interventions.

For example, there is a wealth of research—some five thousand peer-reviewed studies—on curcumin, the active compound in the herb turmeric. This is the spice that gives Indian food its yellow color. Curcumin is an anti-inflammatory, antioxidant, antimicrobial, and anticarcinogenic herb shown to reverse the tendency for bad genes to express. Research shows curcumin promotes apoptosis (cancer cell death), scavenges reactive oxidative species (ROS), and reduces the inflammatory cancer microenvironment.[21] Curcumin is not toxic, it is affordable, and you can find it in any grocery store. Did my doctors mention curcumin to me? Did they ever suggest it would be a good thing to add to my diet in terms of preventing a recurrence of cancer? Nope—not a word during my conventional treatment. I first heard about it a year later when I met Drs. Hammon and Olivares.

There is an urgent need to give patients information about proven, powerful prevention strategies to target cancer's multiple causative factors before they take hold. Curcumin is one very compelling intervention.

UNDERSTANDING DRUG CLAIMS

Drug companies, the FDA, the media, and many doctors use a numerical shell game to cleverly promote the limited benefits of many pharmaceuticals. By presenting only lucrative patented treatments and expensive insurance-approved tests, patients are rarely given all the information available with which to make a fully informed decision. Also, a very important factor left out of the statistics is the harmful and possibly deadly side effects of many of the recommended treatments.

Tamoxifen, the breast cancer treatment drug, is a classic case. It is classified by the WHO and the American Cancer Society as a human carcinogen, yet it is prescribed for cancer prevention.

In September 2000 *The Lancet* reported a study demonstrating that women who had taken tamoxifen and subsequently developed endometrial cancers had biologically aggressive endometrial cancers and therefore had a poor prognosis. In addition, "tamoxifen users were more likely to develop malignant mixed mesodermal tumours...and sarcomas of the endometrium, and had significantly reduced cancer-specific 3-year survival rates."[22]

According to a 2008 study, treatment of breast cancer with tamoxifen results in an increased risk of uterine cancer and higher chances of dying from it.[23]

It is a rare day when an oncologist takes the time to walk a breast cancer patient through the pros and cons of the research on the drugs—they just use them. Oncologists often do not tell cancer patients when they are being subjected to a one-size-fits-all therapy. For example, researchers determined that early-stage breast cancer patients who were HER2-negative derive no benefit from taking the commonly used anthracycline drugs in their chemotherapy.[24] Anthracyclines are a type of antibiotic derived from types of *Streptomyces* bacteria. However, approximately 80 percent of breast cancers are HER2-negative, meaning that only one out of five women with breast cancer will benefit from these drugs, and there is significant toxicity associated with their use. One study found that 7 percent of patients treated with Adriamycin® (doxorubicin), an anthracycline drug, developed congestive heart failure.[25] This is a serious side effect.

Chemotherapy drugs are toxic. It is a long-standing reality that oncologists hope the chemo will kill the cancer faster than it kills the patient. Why are we using drugs with serious side effects when the benefits are questionable at best?

Understand that patients bet their lives on statistics compiled by companies that make a lucrative profit from selling their pharmaceuticals. These companies are able to choose the sample group—who is included in the study—and control what data is included in the final report. Drug companies do not have to report all their studies, so the ones that didn't look good go in the trash can; the FDA and the public never see those. Details of clinical trials published in medical journals are too often written by authors with financial ties to the companies whose drugs they are writing about. As the *New York Times* reported:

> For years, researchers have talked about the problem of publication bias, or selectively publishing results of trials. Concern about such bias gathered force in the 1990s and early 2000s, when researchers documented how, time and again, positive results were published while negative ones were not. Taken together, studies have shown that results of only about half of clinical trials make their way into medical journals.
>
> …[GlaxoSmithKline in 2012] pleaded guilty to criminal charges and agreed to pay $3 billion in fines after the United States Justice Department accused the company, based in London, of failing to report safety data about its diabetes drug Avandia, and of publishing misleading information about Paxil, the antidepressant, in a medical journal.[26]

STANDARD OF CARE PRESENTED AS THE ONLY OPTION

Did you know drug companies are the only entities allowed to make health claims on their products? American law says drugs can make claims to cure, prevent, or treat a disease, but nothing else—not supplements, not food.[27]

The FDA has taken incredible steps to suppress information about foods that reduce the risk of disease. In 2005, for example, the FDA banned information about cherries' health benefits from appearing on websites and product labels, such as "tart cherries may reduce the risk of colon cancer because of the anthocyanins and cyanidin contained in the cherry," and that cherries may help with gout and arthritis pain. According to the FDA, when cherry companies disseminated this peer-reviewed scientific information, cherries became unapproved new drugs and were subject to seizure.[28]

Just the year before, researchers from Johns Hopkins Hospital reported phytonutrients in tart cherries suppress pain caused by inflammation about as well as the NSAID indomethacin.[29] Indomethacin is a powerful drug that can cause many side effects.

There is a long list of foods that have health benefits and are anti-cancer.[30] God created natural substances for us, such as vitamin C and mistletoe. These are not part of the American "standard of care," even though thousands of cancer patients have stepped out of the box and have chosen to use them with great success.

Conventional medicine presents its options for treating cancer confidently and offers little room for debate or flexibility. When you dig deeper and look at survival rates, it seems strange that patients and physicians place their confidence in protocols offering such poor outcomes. This reductionist and fear-based approach puts patients at a huge disadvantage when making decisions. The pharmaceutical compounds, surgeries, and radiation are not simple solutions and have major side effects.

During my cancer journey I was offered only the options of surgery, chemotherapy, and radiation. In fact, they were presented as an everyday activity, such as sitting down to a snack of milk and cookies. The ease at which these protocols are arranged is shocking. Get the diagnosis on Wednesday, be scheduled for surgery or chemo the following Monday. Sign here; get this lab work. Within a matter of days you're in the system—a very profitable system that may or may not do more than put a bandage on your problem. Many people spend more time shopping for a car than they do considering their options after a cancer diagnosis.

How many cancer patients read the paper inserts for the chemotherapy drugs before receiving them? You should ask to read those inserts before consenting to the first chemo session. You need to understand that the side effects and warnings in the small print can and often do occur. Organ damage, pain, and nausea top the list. Remember, you have time to do your homework. *There is almost always no need to be scheduled for treatment within days of the diagnosis.* The cancer likely has been growing for years. Although you may have an urge to yank it out tomorrow, step back, take a breath, and research. Discern what is salesmanship versus what is best for you.

UNDERSTANDING RISK

Oncologists often explain the benefits of chemotherapy in terms of "relative risk" rather than providing a straightforward assessment of chemotherapy's likely impact on the overall survival of the individual patient. Some of the commonly used terms are *relative risk reduction, absolute risk reduction and absolute survival benefit,* and the *number needed to treat* (abbreviated NNT). The whole statistic thing can get very confusing. But hang in here—this is vitally important to your ability to make an objective choice about treatment.

Remember the trouble with mammography screenings? Well, saving a life is great, yes. But at what price to hundreds of others who had benign anomalies, benign tumors, or cancerous tumors that would have spontaneously regressed or never presented a threat in a woman's lifetime? And what of the expense and emotional trauma endured by all those overdiagnosed and overtreated women? How many cancers are caused by the annual dose of carcinogenic radiation?

Relative risk is a statistic that expresses the benefit of receiving a medical intervention. While technically accurate, relative risk can have the effect of making the intervention look more beneficial than it truly is. For example, if receiving a treatment causes a patient's risk to drop from 6 percent to 3 percent, it is a relative risk reduction of 50 percent. Taken at face value, this sounds good. But another way of expressing this that is just as valid and perhaps more accurate is to say it offers a 3 percent reduction in *absolute risk*—but this statistical expression is less likely to convince patients to take the treatment. If a patient has a 97 percent probability of surviving ten years without chemotherapy and has a 98 percent probability with chemotherapy, the statistics would be reported as:

+ Absolute survival benefit = 1 percent
+ Relative risk reduction = 50 percent

It's unlikely many patients would choose to undergo chemotherapy because of the 1 percent absolute survival benefit. If the patient is given only the relative risk reduction statistic of 50 percent, along with a recommendation from her oncologist to take the therapy, most would likely agree and begin the protocol.

In any study where you want to exaggerate the benefits, use the concept of relative risk. Then minimize the side effects by reporting them in terms of absolute risk.

Many people would choose a drug claiming to improve their chances of killing cancer cells by 50 percent, rather than a drug claiming to eliminate cancer in one out of one hundred people. Both of these statistics are describing the same drug. They are just two different ways of looking at the same statistic. As a patient and chief decision maker, it's your job to look at the relative benefit in contrast to the absolute benefit.

In the award-winning video *Healing Cancer From Inside Out*, director Mike Anderson provides an illustration of how drug companies can use this mathematical sleight of hand to enhance their products.

> Say there were one hundred people involved in a clinical trial of a new chemotherapy drug. Out of the one hundred you expect two people to get breast cancer, but during the trial, after all one hundred people were put on the drug, only one person got breast cancer, meaning the reduction in breast cancer was one person out of one hundred. This is called the absolute benefit—one in one hundred, or 1 percent. This is not good news for the drug company because one in one hundred could happen by chance. But remember, two people were expected to get breast cancer, and only one got it—and one divided by two equals a 50 percent reduction. Through the magic of number manipulation this drug can all of a sudden reduce your chances of getting breast cancer by a whopping 50 percent. This is called the relative benefit. It magically turns the 1 percent absolute benefit into a 50 percent relative benefit.... There are other problems. Even though this drug may have helped only one person, its side effects greatly raised the risk of developing secondary cancers and other diseases in all one hundred people. In other words, everyone suffered harm from the drug, yet only one person may have been helped by the drug, and that could have been purely by chance.[31]

Drug advertisements boast about their latest "breakthrough" treatment. Pharmaceutical companies and cancer treatment centers advertise the relative risk to deceptively raise cure rates. Many media reports are not researched news reports but regurgitated press releases—marketing tools making the treatments appear more beneficial than they actually are. These reports present a study's findings in relative risk terms rather than absolute risk reduction.

The bottom line? Find out the following:

+ What is the absolute survivor benefit?
+ Out of one hundred people, how many benefited from this treatment?
+ Insist on clarification about how much time this treatment will buy you—is it days, months, or years?
+ If just days or months, what will your quality of life be like during that time?
+ Will the side effects of the treatment be worth it?

If your doctor won't tell you this information, look it up. Beware of what you read online from organizations that take sponsorship money from the pharmaceutical industry.

And most of all, remember that orthodox medicine does not have proven cures for cancer. *Effective* does not mean *cure*; it just means temporary tumor shrinkage.

Then you will know the truth, and the truth will set you free.

—JOHN 8:32, NIV

Chapter 4

Conventional Treatments and Testing

Today chemotherapy and radiation are still dominant as the go-to therapies. But did you know that they can promote new or secondary cancers? This is called collateral damage. Even the American Cancer Society acknowledges that chemotherapy and radiotherapy are carcinogenic.[1]

Over the last forty-five-plus years we have made progress in long-term survival of certain cancers such as testicular, Hodgkin's, and childhood leukemias.[2] However, challenges still exist with the majority of cancers. The public as a whole continues to tolerate and accept the weakness in mainstream therapies. Most patients reluctantly agree to a plan of care and hope for the best, having never sought out an alternative plan of care from an integrative oncologist. Cancer is a survivable disease, especially if you find it early and develop your attack plan wisely.

A major reason that chemotherapy, radiation, and surgery often fail to produce lifelong survival is that they don't eradicate the cancer stem cells. The public as a whole is not aware of this missing component of these therapies because they are not discussed and oftentimes scans will look clear. The reality is that chemotherapy and radiation can stimulate and increase the robustness of cancer stem cells.[3]

Drug Research Still Leads the Way

We are relentlessly flooded with drug advertising on television; we've been trained to expect a cure from the pharmaceutical industry. But it isn't happening. Headlines and articles tell the story:

- 2015—An article titled "How Much Cancer Costs" states that "the U.S. Food and Drug Administration approved a treatment for melanoma, a deadly skin cancer, which shrunk tumors in 60 percent of patients in a clinical trial. The drug's manufacturer, Bristol-Myers Squibb, will charge $141,000 for the first 12 weeks of treatment and $256,000 for a year of treatment, according to the Wall Street Journal. Experts fear the cost of the drug could keep some patients from receiving what could be the best care available."[4] These prices are out of reach for most uninsured and can have devastating effects on insurance companies.

+ 2013—An article titled "Study: Drug Given Routinely During Cancer Treatment Overused, Ineffective" stated the United States "wastes an estimated $6 billion annually on popular white blood cell–boosting drugs that have no medical benefits for most cancer patients using them."[5]

+ 2017—An article titled "Study Has Shown Chemotherapy Can Backfire and Make Cancer Worse" reports that chemotherapy actually does irreparable damage to healthy cells. This, in turn, causes them to release a protein (WNT16B) that hastens the rate at which the tumor grows and makes it more resistant to treatment in the future.[6]

+ 2011—The FDA declared the blockbuster pharmaceutical Avastin should no longer be prescribed for the treatment of breast cancer because the drug proved to be neither safe nor effective in treating the disease.[7]

The 2016 National Institute for Occupational Safety and Health list of antineoplastic (antitumor) and other hazardous drugs in the workplace warns health care workers about the serious risks of handling these substances, yet we are giving these drugs to people with cancer in the hopes of making them well.[8] And a 2013 paper, authored by Dr. Hagop Kantarjian, professor of medicine and chair of the Leukemia Department at MD Anderson, and signed by 120 leukemia specialists, shows the costs of leukemia drugs are actually harming patients. Call this one a case of financial toxicity.[9]

The pharmaceutical industry has come under scrutiny lately over the pricing issue. US President Donald Trump has pledged action to lower prescription drug costs. A study released in 2016 "found that the median monthly price of branded cancer medicines was nearly $8700 in the US, compared with roughly $3200 in China, $2700 in Australia, $2600 in the UK, $1700 in South Africa and $1500 in India."[10]

I point this out because I have spoken with so many people who max out their insurance, don't have insurance, or simply can't afford to be part of the system. Even the integrative approach limits access because insurance companies aren't anxious to pay for or promote true early detection, prevention, or healing therapies. We need to replace any legislators who won't fight for change. If we as a society demand more, our voice can be heard.

MARKETING VERSUS REALITY

Despite limited victories, the cancer industry in the United States has done a fantastic job at marketing. People see the Susan G. Komen races and the American Cancer Society's ads implying if you give a little more money, the cure is right around the corner. Most people do not research or read beyond the pamphlet their doctor may have given them until they are well into treatment.

The cancer industry's public relations machine keeps the public thinking that results of conventional cancer treatment are getting better all the time. The system works well for the research grant recipients and the pharmaceutical industry's shareholders, but it doesn't work nearly as well for most patients.

According to Dr. Guy B. Faguet, author of *The War on Cancer: An Anatomy of Failure, a Blueprint for the Future*, chemotherapy is just 2.1 percent effective in adult late-stage cancers after a five-year period.[11] He is citing the results of a study conducted by the Department of Radiation Oncology at Northern Sydney Cancer Centre and published in the December 2004 issue of Clinical Oncology.[12]

While 67 percent of newly diagnosed cancer patients are expected to survive, that is merely the five-year survival rate, meaning they are alive five years after their diagnosis. Moreover, fewer than 20 percent of patients with lung, pancreas, liver, or esophagus cancer are expected to live that long.[13] And if the disease has metastasized, about 90 percent of those cancer patients will die of their disease.[14] When I was diagnosed, I didn't know the standard of care for cancer had such a bad track record. I'd been a big believer in its effectiveness. After all, it's what the experts say we should do.

I didn't fully understand the impact of indiscriminately killing both cancerous and healthy cells with chemotherapy and radiation. I didn't understand the full impact of a weakened body trying to expel toxic drug treatments. I did not understand the importance of a healthy immune system. No one mentioned any of this as I was scheduled for surgery and chemo shortly after my diagnosis.

STILL FIGHTING THE SAME OLD WAR ON CANCER

I have firsthand experience from my diagnosis and journey through the halls of Houston's best hospitals. I watched as information on alternative, less-expensive, less-toxic, and less-invasive treatments was suppressed and even laughed at by those in the oncology business. Indeed, I was told to eat cupcakes after my initial treatment.

The American Medical Association (AMA), National Cancer Institute (NCI), and American Cancer Society regulate the protocols—the "gold standard" treatment regimens—for all official cancer treatments in the United States. Expensive drugs, invasive surgeries, and radiation are the primary components on the menu, and they're all I was offered. It's hard to resist the sales pitch when you're scared and you believe that these doctors have the best answers. You find yourself literally putting your life in the hands of persons or institutions unknown to you.

Physicians, like most people, don't feel comfortable discussing things they know very little about. Unfortunately our accredited medical schools don't offer courses on homeopathy and the wide array of natural therapies. Several physicians I interviewed told me they didn't learn about natural therapies in medical school and they had just one class on nutrition.

In 2010 a survey completed by 105 of the 127 accredited medical schools in the United States found that only 27 percent of the schools met the minimum twenty-five required nutritional hours set by the National Academy of Sciences.[15]

Our medical schools receive funding from pharmaceutical companies, and drug industry representatives are responsible for educating doctors on drug therapies. Deep-pocketed pharmaceutical companies sponsor destination medical conferences and events. Physicians need continuing education hours for their license renewals and gladly attend these events. Did you know some physicians receive research grants, perks, and gifts, as well as monetary payments for enrolling a patient in a research study?[16] I don't think that many will publicly admit to it, but my sources say it happens all the time.

Cancer is big money and big business. Don't let money and the insurance companies dictate your treatment. Keep in mind deductibles and co-pays. This money might be better spent on a healing therapy or on an early diagnostic test. Know that there are many options. Cancer is much easier and less expensive to deal with when it is caught early.

Unlike other kinds of doctors, cancer doctors are allowed to profit from the sale of drugs. Doctors in specialties other than cancer simply write prescriptions, but oncologists can make a significant part of their income by buying chemotherapy drugs wholesale and selling them to patients at marked-up prices—you don't go to a pharmacy and buy your chemo; the doctor has it.[17]

Also, keep in mind physicians have to deal with HMOs, insurance companies, and government agencies looking over their shoulders, and more doctors have become fearful of the legal ramifications of not "going with the flow." Stepping outside the box and recommending any treatments not blessed as being part of the standard of care—rules for treatment devised by state licensing boards and medical societies—can put doctors' licenses at grave risk.

So the old system changes very slowly. Cancer Treatment Centers of America is helping to bring meaningful change with the addition of organic food and holistic practitioners. Even with this, there is much more they could do.

CONVENTIONAL TREATMENT

Here are key things to know about the three commonly used modalities to treat cancer:

Surgery

Surgery is the oldest form of cancer treatment. It has a role in diagnosing cancer and finding out how far it has spread, a process called *staging*. Surgery can play a useful role by reducing the tumor burden—debulking the mass—and leaving the patient with less cancer to treat by other means.

However, surgery weakens the immune system and places great stress on the body of the patient. Also, we know cancer is not a localized disease; it is part of a systemic health problem. Surgical removal of the known tumor seems to make everyone feel better, but the elephant is still in the room.

Surgeons routinely tell cancer patients, "I got it all," but studies have shown that cancer cells are left behind in many patients, allowing malignant growths to recur.[18] I had successful surgery to remove my tumor, only to find plenty of cancer cells still circulating in my blood.

We've learned that a tumor as small as 1–2 mm has blood perfusion,[19] meaning it's connected to blood vessels, allowing cancer cells to flow from the tumor into the bloodstream and circulate throughout the body. The reality is that the size of the majority of surgically removed tumors is much greater than 2 mm. *Houston, we have a problem!* What about the

CTCs? We have the tests available to find and analyze them. Lifestyle, supplements, and integrative therapies can be used to clean up these stragglers.[20]

Don't be lulled into a false sense of security if you hear the term *clean surgical margins*, meaning that the pathology lab could not see any cancer cells in the tissue removed from the area surrounding the tumor. *Clean surgical margins* does not mean that you're cancer-free. You may even hear the term *no evidence of disease* (NED). This does not mean you are cancer-free either.

Surgery is not the curative treatment that so many people think it is; in fact, cutting into a tumor can release cancer cells into the patient's bloodstream.[21]

Here are a couple of interesting options to traditional surgery. Cryoablation uses extreme cold to freeze the tumors, reducing the need for surgery. Also, a pioneering surgeon, Vincent Ansanelli of New York, developed an FDA-approved surgical technique for breast cancer using a Co2 laser. Ansanelli uses the Co2 laser technique for every procedure, including the most extreme radical mastectomies with lymph node removal. All surgeries are done without general anesthesia, prescription medications, and hospitalization. Recovery is quick, enabling patients to resume their day normally.[22] I have personally spoken to a patient who had a left mastectomy in the morning and was walking around the streets of New York later that afternoon.

Chemotherapy

The cornerstone of a conventional treatment plan is chemotherapy, usually a "cocktail" of aggressive chemical cellular toxins. Chemo drugs kill both cancerous and healthy cells alike and wreak havoc on the body's immune system and organs. Dosages are set and accepted by organizations such as the National Comprehensive Cancer Network (NCCN), the American Society of Clinical Oncology in collaboration with the Oncology Nursing Society (ASCO/ONS), and the Cancer Therapy Evaluation Program (CTEP). All the while, a low-dose option, such as insulin potentiation therapy (see chapter 32, "Low-Dose Approach to Chemotherapy"), is rarely offered.

In the event that your doctor does not give you the package inserts from your chemo drugs so you can read the side effects for yourself, I'll list a few of them.

- Nausea and vomiting

+ Alopecia (hair loss)

+ Liver toxicity

+ Kidney toxicity

+ Cardiac toxicity (reducing heart function)

+ Fatigue

+ Hearing loss and damage

+ Bone marrow suppression

+ Immune suppression

+ Neutropenia (low white blood cell count)

+ Thrombocytopenia (low blood platelet count, clotting problems)

+ Anemia (low red blood cell count)

+ Inflammation of mucous membranes (ulcers)

+ Loss of appetite

+ Peripheral neuropathy

+ Vision damage

+ Skin and nail damage

+ Cognitive problems (memory)

+ Loss of libido (sex drive)

+ Infertility

+ Diarrhea and constipation

Chemo sessions are often spaced several weeks apart because the patient must have time to recover from the harsh effects of treatment. Particularly the white blood cell count needs to recover to keep the patient from acquiring a serious infection, and the red blood cell count needs to recover to carry oxygen throughout the body. Blood cells are made in the bone marrow, and bone marrow cells are rapidly dividing cells—the kind most susceptible to being killed by chemotherapy drugs. As the chemo kills the bone marrow cells, the body cannot rapidly make a generous supply of blood cells.

Some cancer cells will survive the pharmaceutical onslaught. During recovery time those surviving cancer cells get stronger.

Months or years later these surviving cells can result in a stronger cancer that is resistant to chemotherapy.[23] How does this happen? At least in a couple of ways.

The p53 gene is part of the body's machinery to prevent cancer in the first place. It was one of the first tumor suppressor genes ever discovered. It's on the lookout for cell damage and dispatches proteins to activate repair systems when DNA is damaged. If the damage is irreparable, it initiates cell death (apoptosis), which is a good thing because you want cancer cells to die. But when the p53 gene becomes mutated—part of its gene sequence is lost or deleted—it cannot manufacture the proper proteins. Most cancer patients have p53 protein mutations.[24]

It is unclear whether p53 mutations make tumors easier or harder to treat—you will find examples of both arguments in the medical literature. In any event, there is substantial agreement that a mutated p53 gene makes you resistant to chemotherapy.[25] Chemotherapeutic drugs cause DNA damage. If the p53 gene has a mutation and cannot repair or tell the cell to die, the cell lives on and becomes resistant to chemotherapy.[26]

Today it is estimated 90 percent of patients with metastatic breast, lung, prostate, or colon cancers will develop resistance to chemotherapy.[27]

What is missing in the literature is an emphasis on finding out why the p53 gene goes bad as we get older and what we can do to encourage our tumor suppressor genes to stay healthy.

In 2012 scientists led by the Fred Hutchinson Cancer Research Center reported that DNA-damaging chemotherapy treatment causes fibroblasts to make too much of a protein called WNT16B within the tumor's microenvironment. This protein is taken up by nearby cancer cells, causing them to grow and invade as well as resist subsequent therapy.[28] In other words, chemotherapy damages the DNA of healthy, noncancerous cells, causing them to produce molecules that, in turn, produce more cancer cells.

Then there is the problem of those pesky cancer stem cells—CSCs. As Max Wicha, MD, told us, standard cancer treatments are ineffective against CSCs, which are able to trigger a recurrence of cancer.[29]

Just about every doctor would agree that cancer is fundamentally a failure of the immune system. We all have cancer cells in us. If our immune system is working well, it cleans out those errant cells every day, long before they have a chance to take root and form a tumor.

Chemotherapy, unfortunately, does not strengthen the patient's immune system; it actually weakens it. Cells are most vulnerable to the drugs' killing effects when the cells are dividing. So rapidly dividing cells, such as your hair follicles, bone marrow, and gut lining, are most likely to die after a chemo session. Add to that list the rapidly dividing immune-system killer cells, which deal with fungi, bacteria, viruses, and damaged cells.

The late Bill Henderson, author, radio talk show host, and cancer coach, put it this way:

> Conventional cancer treatment (surgery, chemotherapy and radiation) destroys your immune system. Oncologists pay little attention to rebuilding it or changing your lifestyle. This is why patients with cancer treated with conventional treatment seem to get better, only to have the cancer recur in a few months or years in a more aggressive form. Additionally, the cancer that returns is usually resistant to the previous chemotherapeutic agents used. The weaker cancer cells have been killed off by the treatment and the stronger ones survive, only to reproduce themselves. Eventually, all are strong and treatment resistant.[30]

Throughout the decades of using chemotherapy, data has been collected that has linked certain types of chemotherapy agents to the development of specific secondary cancers. Alkylating agents interfere with a cell's DNA and are linked to leukemia. Platinum-based agents such as cisplatin or carboplatin are linked to leukemia, and the risk increases when combined with radiation. Topoisomerase II inhibitors stop cells from repairing their DNA and can cause leukemia. Targeted agents such as vemurafenib (Zelboraf®) and dabrafenib (Tafinlar®) target the BRAF protein, and they increase the risk of squamous cell carcinomas of the skin.[31]

I encourage you to insist on chemosensitivity and/or genomic testing before consenting to chemotherapy. Since chemotherapy drugs are extremely toxic to both cancer and healthy cells, it is critical that you receive a drug that has shown to be effective for your particular cancer.

Radiation

Radiation therapy is being promoted as quick and easy; however, using radiation is the equivalent to burning cancer cells to death while damaging healthy tissue in the area; collateral damage can be significant. Radiation has been documented to have caused secondary cancers in many patients exposed to it because radiation itself is carcinogenic.[32]

Radiation can produce scarring and reduce the blood flow to the treated area, leaving patients at risk for infection and delayed healing. This problem can become chronic and debilitating, requiring lifelong management.

Recently I was talking to a breast cancer patient who had undergone radiation. She was reporting chest soreness and pain, and her oncologist told her radiation can cause her ribs to fracture easily. I asked her if anyone had warned her about this possible side effect. She said no. It must have been in the tiny print on the forms she was told to sign.

The National Cancer Institute reports radiation therapy can cause new cancers many years after the completion of finished treatment. "In general, the lifetime risk of a second cancer is highest in people treated for cancer as children or adolescents."[33]

Depending on the part of your body being treated, immediate side effects can include:

+ Skin dryness, itching, peeling, or blistering
+ Fatigue
+ Diarrhea
+ Hair loss in the treatment area
+ Nausea and vomiting
+ Sexual changes
+ Swelling
+ Trouble swallowing
+ Urinary and bladder changes

In the past, standard practice was to aim an X-ray at cancerous tissue; it centered in a boxed-shaped area. That accounted for a lot of collateral damage. However, thanks in great part to computers, a new era is dawning when it comes to radiation. Today's computer algorithms, 3-D modeling, and very fine imaging can give specialists the ability to target a much more specific area—to be accurate to less than a millimeter. The concept of a cumulative, lifetime dose of radiation is shifting too. "More accurate delivery means the dead cells take the radiation with them," said Dr. Sean Devlin of the Institute of Integrative Medicine and Oncology in Santa Monica, California. "And in lymphomas, a cancer that starts in the cells of the immune system, there is what is called the abscopal effect. Basically when you treat one area of the body with radiation, it triggers an immune response cascade, meaning other areas of the body where there is cancer also respond even though they have not been treated directly."[34]

Additionally radiation can be combined with hyperthermia, Dr. Devlin explains:

> Many soft-tissue tumors are candidates for a combined therapy. A specific area of tissue is heated to 42°C (approximately 108°F). The heat does a number of good things. It dilates blood vessels

in and around the tumor, bringing more oxygen-rich blood and more medication directly into the tumor. Heat also stimulates the production and shedding of heat shock proteins (HSPs) which can activate an immune system response. HSPs are able to refold damaged proteins, part of the cellular repair mechanism, or mark irreversibly damaged proteins for destruction (apoptosis). And the heat itself kills many cancer cells.

Hyperthermia is done on the same day as a radiation treatment. In clinical trials, bladder cancer goes from a 15% response rate with radiation or chemo alone, to a 53% response rate when hyperthermia is added. Rectal cancer goes from a 20% response rate with radiation or chemo alone, to about 100% response with hyperthermia.[35]

The combination of radiation and hyperthermia may be available at large research institutes and universities, but it is often underutilized because many physicians and patients don't know about it. Some large hospitals or freestanding radiation centers have the newer guided radiation therapy systems.

Immunotherapies

These are "the new kids on the block." Former President Jimmy Carter made headlines in 2015 when his stage IV melanoma was treated with a new drug that targeted one of the proteins used by cancer cells to cloak themselves.[36] When cloaking proteins are inactivated, the body's own immune system can sometimes see the cancer and destroy it. Some think this new field of immunotherapeutic drugs may turn conventional treatment on its head because the cancer establishment is finally coming around to the idea of harnessing the power of the immune system. However, these drugs have demonstrated some serious side effects, and they are usually used in combination with chemotherapy. If these new drugs are not combined with diet and lifestyle changes, I suspect their effect is likely to be limited. Why? In part because our immune systems are not as robust as they were in, say, the 1950s. We have more chemicals, pathogens, and stress in our environment that compete for the immune system's attention on a daily basis. And the drugs themselves do nothing to nurture the long-term health of the immune system.

TERMS COMMONLY USED IN CONVENTIONAL TREATMENT

Remission

Let's define "remission." According to the American Cancer Society, there are two different types of remission:

1. "When a treatment completely gets rid of all tumors that could be measured or seen on a test, it's called a *complete response* or *complete remission*." (It's important to note the use of the words "could be measured.")

2. "A *partial response* or *partial remission* means the cancer partly responded to treatment, but still did not go away. A partial response is most often defined as at least a 50% reduction in measurable tumor."[37]

Wow! I thought remission meant the patient was successfully treated and is cancer-free for the time being. Unfortunately most people similarly have a distorted and incorrect understanding of *remission*. We now know the patient may still have microscopic cancer cells, but they're not clumped together in large enough numbers to be seen on a scan as prescribed by the cancer and insurance industries in the United States.

No evidence of disease

No evidence of disease (NED) is a term used when the oncologist can't detect cancer. NED is used more now than the word *remission*. I guess it's the best they have to offer. However, what is really wanted by the patient is a cure.

Survivor

Last, but not least, is the big "S" word: survivor. What does it really mean? You have lived five years beyond your diagnosis—so far.

TESTS COMMONLY USED IN CONVENTIONAL TREATMENT

Conventional cancer testing looks for cancer that usually has been around for years and has finally gotten large enough that it can be detected by these tests. Here is an overview:

PET scan

A positron emission tomography (PET) scan is not for early detection because the cancer must form a tumor large enough to absorb the radioactive glucose that is reflected on the computer images. We can learn a lot about the operation of a cancer cell by understanding how a PET scan works. Before a PET scan the patient receives an intravenous infusion of radioactive glucose. Cancer cells rapidly metabolize (take in and use) sugar and synthesize (absorb) the radioactive glucose. The body then is scanned, and areas with cancer cells will light up and be captured on the resulting images. Cancer cells take up sugar much faster than noncancerous cells. If the tumors are large enough, the scan can pinpoint the source of the cancer and detect whether it is isolated to one specific area or has spread to other organs, bones, or tissues. Small tumors under 1 cm may not show up on the scans; thus, the patient will be told she is fine.[38]

However, a clean or negative PET scan does not mean you don't have cancer. Patients are not told the technology has limits; the person could have microscopic tumors. Patients, or consumers, if you prefer, also are not informed there are steps they can take now to prevent cancer growth, such as consuming a low-sugar diet. And most oncologists don't warn patients about the danger of the injected radioactive sugar fueling their cancer, or about carcinogenic effects of the radiation.

A PET scan is often combined with a CT scan, which uses multiple X-ray images to produce detailed pictures of structures inside of the body, along with an MRI, which uses a magnetic field and pulses of radio wave energy to produce pictures. MRIs often provide different information about structures in the body than can be seen with an X-ray or CT scan. The downside of a CT is that it emits a hefty dose of radiation—"in some cases equivalent to about 200 chest X-rays, or the amount most people would be exposed to from natural sources over seven years." You hope your body can handle it. But if not, the damage can lead to cancer.[39]

My research shows that the most effective type of PET/CT is called a FDG-PET/CT for short. It "uses the tracer fluorine-18 fluorodeoxyglucose to highlight overactive cells, and scans the body with X-ray computed tomography, also called a CT or CAT scan."[40] Sounds complicated, but if you're going to get a scan, you want the best, right?

Tumor markers

According to the National Cancer Institute:

> Tumor markers are substances that are produced by cancer or by other cells of the body in response to cancer or certain benign (noncancerous) conditions. Most tumor markers are made by normal cells as well as by cancer cells; however, they are produced at much higher levels in cancerous conditions. These substances

can be found in the blood, urine, stool, tumor tissue, or other tissues or bodily fluids of some patients with cancer. Most tumor markers are proteins. However, more recently, patterns of gene expression and changes to DNA have also begun to be used as tumor markers.

Many different tumor markers have been characterized and are in clinical use. Some are associated with only one type of cancer, whereas others are associated with two or more cancer types. No "universal" tumor marker that can detect any type of cancer has been found.[41]

Looking at tumor markers is not an early-detection test because tumor markers are produced by cancer cells, and in most cases you must have a significant number of cancer cells for the tests to report as high. Monitoring tumor markers has become a standard of care that oncologists use at follow-up appointments. If a patient's labs show an increase in tumor markers, the oncologist most likely will order a PET and/or a CT scan. These tests have become common diagnostic tools physicians use to reveal the presence and severity of cancers.

It's important to know what is normal for you—what your personal baseline is. Do not feel safe just because your number is lower than the number considered high on the lab report. I didn't have elevated tumor markers when I was diagnosed with cancer.

By the time a patient has elevated tumor markers, the cancer may be well established. This information was a motivator for me to write this book to present other testing and early-detection methods. I caution you against relying solely upon these customary tumor marker blood tests.

Know too that tumor marker tests have major limitations as a diagnostic tool:

+ Noncancerous conditions at times may cause levels of certain tumor markers to rise.

+ Not all patients with a certain type of cancer have a higher level of a tumor marker associated with that particular cancer.

+ Tumor markers have not been identified for every form of cancer.[42]

Below is a list of some of the more common specific markers currently used in the clinical setting. Some are associated with only one type of cancer, while some are associated with multiple types of cancer. Remember, there is no universal tumor marker to detect any type of cancer.

CANCER TUMOR MARKERS[43]

MARKER	APPLICABLE CANCER(S)
Alpha-fetoprotein (AFP)	Liver cancer and germ cell tumors
Beta-2-microglobulin (B2M)	Multiple myeloma, chronic lymphocytic leukemia, and some lymphomas
Beta-human chorionic gonadotropin (Beta-HCG)	Choriocarcinoma and germ cell tumors
BCR-ABL fusion gene	Chronic myeloid leukemia, acute lymphoblastic leukemia, and acute myelogenous leukemia
CA15-3/CA27.29	Breast cancer
CA19-9	Pancreatic cancer, gallbladder cancer, bile duct cancer, and gastric cancer
CA-125	Ovarian cancer
Calcitonin	Medullary thyroid cancer
Carcinoembryonic antigen (CEA)	Colorectal cancer and some other cancers
CD20	Non-Hodgkin's lymphoma
Chromogranin A (CgA)	Neuroendocrine tumors
Chromosomes 3, 7, 17, and 9p21	Bladder cancer
Cytokeratin fragment 21-1	Lung cancer
Fibrin/fibrinogen	Bladder cancer
HE4	Ovarian cancer
Immunoglobulins	Multiple myeloma and Waldenström macroglobulinemia
Lactate dehydrogenase	Germ cell tumors, lymphoma, leukemia, melanoma, and neuroblastoma
Neuron-specific enolase (NSE)	Small cell lung cancer, neuroblastoma
Nuclear matrix protein 22	Bladder cancer

MARKER	APPLICABLE CANCER(S)
Prostate-specific antigen (PSA)	Prostate cancer
Thyroglobulin	Thyroid cancer
5-Protein signature (OVA1)	Ovarian cancer

Biopsy

The traditional biopsy is an invasive procedure to collect a tissue sample. It is not an early-detection test because a tumor large enough to be seen must be present. For the majority of cancers, a biopsy is used to make a definitive cancer diagnosis. It can sometimes be done in the doctor's office with a local anesthetic.

Often physicians recommend a biopsy for a patient when a physical exam or another test such as an ultrasound has identified a possible tumor. During a biopsy, a tumor may be punctured several times with a needle to retrieve an adequate amount of tissue to be examined under a microscope by a pathologist (a specialist in interpreting laboratory tests and evaluating tissues to diagnose disease). The pathologist will determine whether the tissue contains tumor cells and, if so, whether the tumor is benign (noncancerous) or malignant (cancerous).[11] But a tumor is not a solid mass of cancer cells. Imagine a slice of raisin bread. The scattered raisins are the cancerous cells, and the bread is the noncancerous cells. You would need to poke the piece of bread several times to find a raisin— maybe. Thus, there is a long-simmering debate about the safety of needle biopsies because of the number of insertions.

In some cases penetrating the tumor with a needle several times may inadvertently allow cancer cells to break away from a tumor and escape, thus spreading the cancer beyond the immediate tumor area. Several studies have found a higher incidence of cancer after biopsies.[45]

Biopsies became routine practice in the United States by the 1920s and were endorsed by both the American Cancer Society and the AMA. But as cancer researcher Ralph Moss tells us, many people have had strong reservations since the practice was developed.

> In 1940, the first American textbook on cancer treatment contained warnings on the dangers of biopsies. "The medical literature is full of pleas for and against biopsy of all types of tumors," wrote Cushman D. Haagensen, MD, of Columbia University, NY, in 1940. Some doctors are "inquisitive but afraid of doing harm with biopsy" (Haagensen 1940). Bradley Coley, MD, a

bone surgeon at Memorial Sloan-Kettering Cancer Center (and
son of the famous immunotherapy pioneer, William B. Coley,
MD), wrote that "there is some doubt as to the harmlessness of
needling such tumors. It may not be a wholly innocuous procedure" (Pack 1940). A survey taken at the time showed that most
surgeons agreed that the excision of suspect tissue was to be con-
demned and avoided.[46]

Disturbing a tumor by sticking a needle into it appears to leave an
opening and give cancer cells the opportunity to exit and travel to other
areas of the body. Since it is known that cancer cells attempt to move about
the body, be aware that a biopsy may just help them achieve that task.

Approximately 1.6 million breast biopsies are performed annually in
the United States, and only about 20 percent of them will result in a
cancer diagnosis. Some of the newer tests I tell you about are performed
with a simple, safer blood test, often referred to as a "liquid biopsy." No
raisin bread issues there because there are no punctures into the suspected malignant tumor.

ALTERNATIVE APPROACHES PUSHED ASIDE

Pioneers in healing cancer naturally, such as Harry Hoxsey, Royal
Raymond Rife, Dr. Nicholas Gonzalez, and Dr. Max Gerson, have presented patient records documenting the success of their treatments, yet
the evidence of their work has been dismissed or suppressed.

One has to question why the organizations that we believe are working
to help us are giving us such limited options to treat cancer. If surgery,
chemotherapy, and radiation fail, patients are sent home to die with no
mention of other proven therapies. Shouldn't the profession we trust with
our lives have a responsibility to give us *all* the options, not just the financially profitable ones?

Cancer is a wily beast. We need to be open to therapies other than just
those provided by the pharmaceutical industry. Half of the FDA's budget
is funded by drug companies, but that should not mean chemical assaults
are the only approach we take to treating cancer.

I toured several cancer clinics in Tijuana, Mexico, and was able to
speak with many of the doctors, staff, and patients. Like most people,
I thought a person must be desperate to go to one of these clinics on
the other side of the US border. After my firsthand experience, I completely changed my opinion. I learned that many of these doctors have
purposefully left the United States and set up clinics just fifteen minutes

inside the border of Mexico. With deep compassion and a desire to help patients heal from cancer, they refuse to be limited to the age-old trio of surgery, radiation, and chemo. I found they were using many protocols not allowed or accepted as cancer treatments in the United States, such as high-dose vitamin C, immune therapies, diet, insulin potentiation therapy (IPT), energy medicine, and detoxification. These clinics report they are healing 40 percent or more of the "terminal" patients who show up on their doorsteps.

Daniel Haley's *Politics in Healing: The Suppression and Manipulation of American Medicine* is an eye-opening book; it gave me a new perspective. Haley explains why we don't have effective nontoxic cancer cures and how the status quo prevents new ideas from entering medical research and practice. Here you can read about cancer cures that were, and still are, being relentlessly suppressed by the FDA and the AMA.[47]

IT IS TIME FOR CHANGE

We have twice as many cases of breast cancer as we did when the National Cancer Act was signed in 1971, kicking off the "war on cancer." That sounds like a failed agenda.

At the time, curing cancer looked like an easy task. It had taken America just a decade to successfully land a man on the moon. Surely in less time we could find a cure for cancer. We sequenced the entire human genome just sixteen years after the idea was born. But the cure for cancer has focused on treatment, not on root causes or prevention. We have not paid much attention to prevention, and we've pretty much ignored Warburg. We still don't have the *cure*; we only have *hope* for a cure and endless requests for more money.

"It's time to admit that our efforts have often targeted the wrong enemies and used the wrong weapons," said Devra Davis, PhD, MPH, founding director of the Center for Environmental Oncology.[48] The National Cancer Institute tells us that an estimated two-thirds of all cancers have environmental causes.[49] That, Devra Davis says, ought to make research into what causes cancer a high priority, but it does not.

> The war on cancer remains focused on commercially fueled efforts to develop drugs and technologies that can find and treat the disease—to the tune of more than $100 billion a year in the United States alone. Meanwhile, the struggle basically ignores most of the things known to cause cancer, such as tobacco, radiation, sunlight, benzene, asbestos, solvents, and some drugs and

hormones. Even now, modern cancer-causing agents such as gasoline exhaust, pesticides and other air pollutants are simply deemed the inevitable price of progress.

They're not. Scientists understand that most cancer isn't born but made....Of the nearly 80,000 chemicals regularly bought and sold today, according to the National Academy of Sciences, fewer than 10 percent have been tested for their capacity to cause cancer or do other damage....No matter how much our efforts to treat cancer may advance, the best way to reduce cancer's toll is to keep people from getting it.[50]

Statistics tell us that about 1.7 million Americans are diagnosed with cancer every year and over six hundred thousand die from it—a number about equal to the death toll from 9/11 happening every two days.[51] Yet the cancer industry spends very little of its multibillion-dollar resources on effective prevention strategies, such as dietary awareness, environmental toxins awareness, and immune system enhancements.

Dr. Kathleen T. Ruddy, a breast cancer surgeon in New Jersey, formed the Breast Health and Healing Foundation to focus public attention on the urgent obligation to discover the causes of breast cancer. Her question gets right to the point for women like me who have experienced breast cancer.

At least 30% of breast cancer is deemed preventable using known and proven risk reduction strategies. Yet less than 1% of all research funding is used toward this goal. If 30% of breast cancer is preventable, shouldn't we spend that portion of our research dollars trying to do so?[52]

It is preferable to prevent cancer rather than treat it. Isolated cancer cells are not threatening because they have no built-in support mechanisms. Kudos to the healthy immune system, able to sweep out those cells every day, just as we take out the household trash every night. But when the immune system is overwhelmed and those isolated cancer cells coalesce and take root, they build their own fortresses inside our bodies. They connect to the bloodstream and build their own highways—a network of blood vessels for ready access to food. Cancer cells are first at the feeding trough, robbing healthy cells of nutrition.

When you receive a cancer diagnosis, you are about to be sold something—a course of treatment. It really isn't much different from entering the marketplace to buy, say, cookware for your kitchen. You can buy Teflon-coated pans, or aluminum, or stainless steel, or glass, or several other options. The salespeople who sold the Teflon-coated pans talked a great story about the non-stick, easy clean-up features. But they didn't tell you the EPA identified a chemical compound used in the production of Teflon as a "likely carcinogen."[53] Aluminum pans don't come with warnings about the health hazards of aluminum leeching into your food. You can choose glass and stainless, but you have to ignore the salespeople pushing the toxic aluminum and nonstick options.

Likewise, when it comes to cancer treatments, there are options, and there is something to know about those options before you make your choice. Take time to educate yourself about the choices—look before you leap, as they say. Do not fall for the ploy that you absolutely must have surgery or start chemo within a few days of getting a cancer diagnosis. You owe it to yourself to do some homework.

Traditional cancer treatments are just that—treatments, not cures. After completion, patients begin the process that I call the "wait, watch, and wonder program."

DON'T WAIT, WATCH, AND WONDER

This program is offered to most cancer patients after completing their prescribed course of treatment. The patients are released to *wait* until their next oncology checkup, where the doctors will *watch* their lab and test results. All the while, the patients *wonder* if their cancer will come back.

Stop wondering, "Am I really cancer-free?" If you have already undergone treatment, choose one or more of the tests I describe in this book to confirm a cancer-free or survivor status.

Don't be an obedient patient and partake of this watch-and-see approach. Don't let cancer grow large enough to be seen on a mammogram or PET scan or detected via a biopsy. Detect it now. Deal with it now. Detox and support your body with the nutrients it requires. Cancer need not be a life-wrenching, life-threatening disease when found really early. Since the statistics tell us almost half of us will get a cancer diagnosis in our lifetime, it makes sense to look for cancer during a checkup, just as we look for diabetes and heart disease.

One final note: never lose faith in the body's own healing abilities. The body can reverse a cancer on its own—it's called *spontaneous remission*—and doctors see it happen often. Sometimes the body does it, and we only know it happened because tests showed the cancer "went away." I choose to call these occurrences *miracles*! Sometimes we can reverse a diagnosed cancer by giving the body tools to fight it—great nutrition, detoxification, and avoidance of carcinogens.

Get off of the revolving door of the cancer industry, and take control. Take your health back. Take time to do some research.

Chemotherapy and radiation are blunt, invasive instruments; there are other effective and more elegant ways to defeat cancer.

It is essential all options be considered, and I hope that someday the standard of care will include all that is truly available.

Chapter 5

Chemosensitivity, Genomic, and Natural-Agent Sensitivity Testing Overview

THIS EMERGING FIELD has great promise for improving patient outcomes. It takes us beyond the one-size-fits-all approach. The sad reality is, many patients are never offered these new approaches.

CHEMOSENSITIVITY TESTING

The National Cancer Institute describes a chemosensitivity assay as "a laboratory test that measures the number of tumor cells that are killed by a cancer drug. The test is done after the tumor cells are removed from the body. A chemosensitivity assay may help in choosing the best drug or drugs for the cancer being treated."[1]

Drug efficacy (or response) testing has been around since the late nineteenth century and early twentieth century through the work of Drs. Louis Pasteur and Paul Ehrlich and is used for determining which antimicrobial (antibiotic) will kill a certain strain of bacteria.[2]

Today, for example, patients with bladder infections give a urine sample to the lab, where it is tested with various antibiotics used for urinary tract infections. The doctor then writes a prescription for the antibiotic shown to do the best job of knocking out that particular infection.

Likewise, doctors can use the results of a chemosensitivity test to formulate the most effective and targeted cancer treatment plan.

If chemosensitivity testing is not done, you fall victim to the one-size-fits-all, broad-based approach of conventional oncology. Standard drugs from the National Comprehensive Cancer Network (NCCN) guidelines will be prescribed; a more effective drug may remain on the shelf. Chemosensitivity testing can prevent your exposure to a drug that not only would be ineffective at fighting your cancer but could be extremely damaging to your immune system.

Integrative oncologists have been using such testing for years. In my experience, many conventional oncologists are reluctant to embrace this new testing. It may be up to you to tell them about it. The one-size-fits-all testing and treatment plans are old-school—a thing of the past.

Suzanne Somers interviewed many cancer doctors and wrote several books on cancer therapy after her firsthand experience with breast cancer. She said, "Now that I realize chemosensitivity tests exist, it feels unconscionable that chemotherapy would ever, ever be administered without testing first to find out if the chemo is even compatible with the specific cancer."[3] She also asked, "If these tests could help us to take less chemo, or a better chemo for our specific cancer, why wouldn't we ALL be given these tests?"[4]

Somers is absolutely right. A personalized, targeted approach is a much better way to proceed.

The first method utilizes living tumor tissue or malignant fluid. The sample must arrive at the lab within twenty-four to thirty-six hours of collection; there living cells are exposed to different chemotherapy drugs and the best drug reactions are identified. Cell lines or genes are not evaluated. This type of test is not considered early detection because you must have a known tumor to get the test.

The second method falls a bit outside the National Cancer Institute's definition of chemosensitivity testing. This is because the laboratory, Research Genetic Cancer Center (RGCC), is based outside of the United States and uses the patient's individual cancer cells extracted from a blood sample, recently referred to as a liquid biopsy. These cells are exposed to different chemotherapy drugs, and the best reactions are identified. This changes things quite a bit because the test can be performed on cells extracted from a patient years *before* a tumor is located and biopsied. This test is a combination of chemosensitivity testing and genomic testing because the lab also looks at genetic markers on the cancer cells. RGCC is working with hundreds of integrative physicians in the United States and around the world who are treating cancer at its earliest stages.

Just as everyone's fingerprints are different, cancer cells are different too, and the information obtained from chemosensitivity testing can be invaluable. Also, tumors have the ability to develop drug resistance. This means patients need to repeat sensitivity testing and adjustments to the treatment plan. Fortunately insurance companies are beginning to pay for such testing.

GENOMIC TESTING

A new buzzword in oncology is *genomics*, which is advertised as the very best in personalized treatment. We hear terms such as *gene testing, genetic profiling, molecular testing, target profiling, whole cell cytometric profiling,* and *genomic testing*.

This method uses tumor tissue, blood, or other bodily fluids to identify chemo drugs that *should* produce the best potential treatment outcome. The goal of this type of test is to match known characteristics of a chemotherapy drug with the identified characteristics or "gene patterns" of the patient's cancer cells. In gene testing, chemotherapy drugs are not physically tested against the patient's cancer cells, as they are in chemosensitivity testing. Genomic testing provides a "theoretical potential" for the drug's success. Other biological mechanisms of the cancer cell, such as drug resistances, are often not considered.

I'll tell you about several labs that are offering this type of testing in the test chapters. This is a rapidly growing field, and new labs are joining the market every year.

ALTERNATIVE, NATURAL-AGENT SENSITIVITY TESTING

This testing can identify the most effective natural substances for treating cancer cells and boosting immune system function. Therapeutic doses of vitamin C, for example, have been proved to kill cancer cells.[5]

There are only two labs that I've identified that offer any type of testing for natural substances, even though there are increasing numbers of patients who are seeking natural therapies.

Many of the tested substances support the immune system while reducing the number of cancer cells through the process of antiangiogenesis or apoptosis.

Angiogenesis is the process the body uses to signal the growth of blood vessels to a tumor to provide it with nutrition for growth. The Angiogenesis Foundation in Cambridge, Massachusetts, reported that "cancerous tumors release angiogenic growth factor proteins that stimulate their blood vessel to grow" and that antiangiogenic therapies "literally starve the tumor of its blood supply" by interfering with this process.[6] This test identifies natural substances that are antiangiogenic to the individual patient's tumor cells.

Apoptosis is the process of inducing cell death. However, cancer cells have lost their natural programming to die—they keep duplicating endlessly. This test identifies natural substances that cause cell death to the individual patient's tumor cells.

Consider these headlines:

+ 25 Cancer Stem Cell Killing Foods Smarter Than Chemo & Radiation[7]

+ Better Than Chemo: Turmeric Kills Cancer Not Patients[8]

+ Anticancer Potential of Plants and Natural Products: A Review[9]

+ Science Proves That Garlic Kills Cancer Cells[10]

+ 5 Ayurvedic Herbs That Have Been Shown to Destroy Cancer Cells[11]

RGCC in Greece tests for roughly fifty natural substances ranging from mistletoe to curcumin, and new ones are added periodically. Biofocus in Germany tests a smaller list of different natural substances.

CONCLUSION

If you've chosen the chemotherapy route, identifying the most powerful drugs for *you* in the beginning is much better than starting with the standard, generic rounds of chemo. There's not much worse than finding out that a course of chemotherapy didn't work for you.

The up-front costs may seem high, but it's a much better approach in the long run. Please do not retreat if your insurance company or Medicare will not pay for chemosensitivity or genomic testing. Many labs offer financial assistance. I'm pleased to report that some insurance companies are succumbing to the pressure and are offering full or partial coverage.

Part II

Tests

I N THIS SECTION you will learn about tests that are revolutionizing the way we think about cancer and how we can deal with it in a new, powerful way. Examine each one carefully, as each provides different information. This is a rapidly expanding field, and new companies will be joining in. The future is great if we embrace these new tools.

Learn:

- How to detect cancer years before standard imaging tests.

- How to detect cancer years before you discover a lump.

- How to detect cancer years before symptoms appear.

- How to avoid chemotherapy, surgery, and radiation by utilizing "ultra-early detection."

- How to avoid a tissue biopsy.

- How to confirm that you are really cancer-free.

- How a blood sample can provide unique characteristics of cancer CTCs.

- How to identify which natural substances have anticancer effects.

- How to identify which agents will be effective hormone blockers.

- How to identify which drug and immune therapies have the best anticancer effects.

- How to identify the drug and immune therapies that will *not* work well.

- How to develop a personalized blueprint for therapy with genomic and chemosensitivity tests.

- How to identify drug resistance.

- How to identify cancer metastasis.

- How to determine if your treatments are working.

+   How to see a recurrence coming early.

+   How to assess the immune system.

+   How to identify the site of origin of cancer.

Chapter 6

AMAS Test

Oncolab Inc.
36 The Fenway
Boston, MA 02215
Phone: 800-922-8378;
    617-536-0850
Fax: 617-536-0657
www.Oncolabinc.com
info@oncolabinc.com

THIS CHAPTER IS based on information provided by Oncolab Inc. and David Getoff, CCN, CTN, FAAIM, as well as research done by the author. Check the Oncolab website for updates.

SUMMARY AND EXPLANATION

This test is an aid in early cancer detection and follow-up. AMAS stands for *anti-malignin antibody in serum*, and it is a blood test. It measures levels of the anti-malignin antibody whose levels rise early in the course of malignant cell growth during rapid replication. The antibody is produced in response to a substance called malignin, which is found to be present in most malignant cells.

The test does not indicate where cancer may be located, so other diagnostic tests will be needed to identify the location. The test is less accurate late in the disease, when the antibody response is less robust or is blocked by antigen excess.

The AMAS blood test was developed by Samuel Bogoch, MD, PhD, and his wife, Elenore Bogoch, MD, DMD. Dr. Samuel Bogoch is a neurochemist who received his PhD in biochemistry from Harvard University. He discovered and researched the anti-malignin antibody. The AMAS test is patented and Medicare-approved.

INTERPRETATION

AMA levels of 0–99 micrograms per ml serum are normal, levels of 100–134 are borderline, and a level of 135 or above indicates cancer may be present.

HOW TO OBTAIN THE TEST

The test must be ordered by a physician. Visit www.oncolabinc.com and do a physician search. Physicians may register by calling Oncolab at 800-922-8378, and test kits will be shipped at no charge.

Follow instructions included in the kit. Blood must be spun down to acquire serum. Tests must be shipped back to Oncolab with either FedEx or UPS overnight. Dry ice is required in packing. The requisition to order the AMAS test must contain specific requested medical information and must be signed by both the patient and physician.

ACCURACY

False positives are 5 percent, and false negatives are 7 percent. "Antimalignin antibody is elevated in 93 to 100 percent of cases in which active nonterminal malignancy is the clinical-pathological diagnosis."[1] In studies of more than eight thousand patients and controls, the AMAS test was found to be 95 percent accurate. Over seventy thousand determinations have been performed. Oncolab Inc. reports 99 percent specificity and 95 percent sensitivity.[2]

In terminal cancer where the immune response is poor, AMA levels will fall, but that is not indicative of the cancer burden. Test results have been shown to be elevated up to nineteen months before clinical detection. "AMA is normal in 96 percent of cancer patients who no longer have evidence of disease."[3] Go to www.oncolabinc.com to learn more about publications, case studies, peer reviews, and references.

COST

The cost is $249. Practitioner fees are extra. Overnight UPS or FedEx shipping, the blood-draw fee (usually $25–$50), and dry ice are extra.

Oncolab does not accept any insurance other than Medicare. Medicare patients should include a copy of their Medicare card and be sure to include the physician's NPI number on the requisition form. Other patients should check with their insurance companies to determine if they reimburse for the AMAS test. Receipts are provided, and you can file a claim for insurance reimbursement.

PROCESS TIME

Results are sent out within five business days of Oncolab receiving the serum sample. The results are sent directly to the doctor. After the physician has received the results, you can contact Oncolab and request a HIPAA medical release, and Oncolab will send you your results.

BENEFITS

+ The test identifies the presence of cancer.
+ "AMAS test may be useful in indicating disease progression and prognosis."[4]
+ This is a tool to monitor patients who are at a "high risk for cancer, and for follow-up purposes on patients already diagnosed and/or treated for cancer."[5]

LIMITATIONS

The test identifies only the presence of cancer, not the origin or type of cancer cells. "A low AMA level can occur in non-cancer, in advanced and terminal cancer, and in successfully treated cancer in which there is no further evidence of disease; clinical status must be used to distinguish these states."[6] Also, "the AMAS test is not by itself diagnostic of the presence or absence of disease, and its results can only be assessed as an aid to diagnosis, detection or monitoring of disease in relation to the history, medical signs, and symptoms and the overall condition of the patient."[7]

NOTE TO THE READER FROM DAVID GETOFF, CCN, CTN, FAAIM, NATUROPATH, AND BOARD-CERTIFIED CLINICAL NUTRITIONIST

I have been utilizing the AMAS test with my patients and family members for about 20 years. I find it to be an exceptional but often misunderstood test. In advanced cancer or in those with extremely poor immune function the test may show a normal level of circulating anti-malignin due to the inability of the body to react to its cancer cells. This IS NOT a false negative. In fact, it gives me important information. When a currently diagnosed cancer patient shows a normal AMAS test, it increases my worry and gives me a phenomenal indicator to follow. After I teach them how to change their diet and we add in missing nutrients and many immune-boosting or modulating supplements, I am looking for the next AMAS, in

3 to 4 months, to come back as elevated. This would indicate we have succeeded in ramping up the body's immune system. On the other hand, if the first test comes back elevated, as it should in a patient with active cancer, then as we accomplish all the required support, I am looking to have the AMAS numbers slowly decrease as the body destroys more and more of the malignant cells.

The other way I use this test is with my non-cancer patients. I even included myself in this group. Here, I run the AMAS test to take a preventive glimpse at the amount of anti-malignin in the person's serum. Since the test seems quite able to identify people, who, if nothing changes in their lives, may be diagnosed with cancer over the next 5–10 years, as indicated by a borderline or elevated AMAS result, I gain the opportunity to work to prevent this occurrence. I have helped many individuals improve their immune function through diet and supplementation, thereby giving their body the tools required to better attack cancer cells and bring the AMAS number back to normal. I recently did this in 2016 with my own AMAS results. Although I was quite surprised to find an elevated AMAS when I had the test run, with how well I eat and the supplements I take daily, it did not cause me to worry. Through energetic testing, I determined which immune supplements my body required, and I took them daily for the next 9 months. My three-month AMAS dropped down to borderline and in nine months was down to normal. I will rerun my AMAS in a year to take a look, and I have decreased my doses of these added products.

It is my belief, if AMAS tests were run every 3 years as a part of any good preventive testing program, and if the practitioner is well versed in how to support the immune system, we could prevent thousands of cancer deaths every month. Mainstream will likely never embrace this test for the following reasons. First, they were not taught about it in medical school and don't even know it exists. Second, they don't understand what I have just taught you and so they may feel it gives false positives and negatives rather than simply testing the amount of anti-malignin antibody in your serum. Third, it will find elevated results in many who have no tumors yet, and so they feel it is wrong. Fourth, it cannot tell them where these [cells] may be, so it does not help them aim their radiation, determine what chemo to use, or indicate where to operate.

For me the test is fantastic. I do not care where the cells are. My job is to help my patient's body to eradicate these cells, and the body does know where they are.

For more information on my practice, go to www.DavidGetoff.com and look for the two cancer buttons and the initial consultation button.

THOUGHTS

I did not include this test in the first editions of the book because I had heard so much conflicting information about it. Then I met David Getoff, who is passionate about the benefits of it and thinks it's misunderstood. You be the judge.

My word of caution with this test is that patients with advanced cancer or extremely poor immune function may get a *normal* result. Knowing this up front, it is important to consider all the data and each patient carefully. I would refer you to David Getoff's letter here, as he explains this phenomenon and how he uses it to develop a plan to build and support the body's immune system.

I caution you about relying solely on any one test. This test and others should be used in conjunction with other methods to develop a broader clinical picture. See www.Oncolabinc.com for more information and additional references.

Chapter 7

Biocept

CIRCULATING TUMOR CELL COUNT AND BIOMARKER IDENTIFICATION

Biocept Inc.
5810 Nancy Ridge Drive, Suite 150
San Diego, CA 92121
888-332-7729
www.biocept.com
customerservice@biocept.com

THIS CHAPTER IS based on information provided by Biocept and research done by the author. Please refer to Biocept's website for updates.

SUMMARY AND EXPLANATION

Biocept performs a simple, noninvasive blood test. It's sometimes referred to as a liquid biopsy, meaning that instead of a traditional, tissue biopsy, this lab can test the cancer from a blood sample. When cancer metastasizes, or spreads, it sheds cells and DNA fragments into the blood. The capture and detection of circulating tumor cells (CTCs) is used in identification of early cancer, in early detection of relapse, and in monitoring the response to treatment. The test can provide information on the number of CTCs, as well as specific biomarkers on the CTCs and circulating tumor DNA fragments (ctDNA).[1]

CTCs detach from a primary tumor and flow into the bloodstream, where they can be captured and analyzed. Elevated CTCs at any time in the course of clinical treatment can be indicators of disease progression. ctDNA can find its way into the blood through either apoptosis (cancer cell death) or necrosis of the solid tumor tissue.[2]

Biocept testing can detect specific biomarkers from both ctDNA and CTCs—which are characteristics of your individual cancer cells—which can help guide your doctor in determining appropriate therapy options. Many different cancer biomarkers have been identified, and targeted therapies are in clinical use. Some of the common biomarkers tested by Biocept are HER2, ER, EGFR, BRAF, ALK, PD-L1, KRAS, NRAS,

PR, AR, ROS1, RET, MET, and FGFR1. The biomarker information provided can be utilized in both conventional and integrative therapies.

Your results are provided in two parts: One is the number of CTCs found. The other is a report on the biomarkers identified. This result assists physicians in understanding the characteristics of your disease and building a responsive, personalized, and effective treatment plan.

Biocept offers testing for breast cancer, prostate cancer, colorectal cancer, lung cancer, melanoma, and gastric cancer tumors.

INTERPRETATION

Test results will provide the number of CTCs. Biomarkers will be reported as "Detected" or "Not detected."

HOW TO OBTAIN THE TEST

The test must be ordered by a physician, and he or she will need to contact Biocept directly to order the test. The blood sample may be drawn at your doctor's office, or you may use an outside lab. An overnight courier service is used to ship the sample to Biocept. You do not need to fast before the test. Biocept recommends you wait two weeks after treatments to have your blood drawn.

ACCURACY

+ Biocept is a CLIA-certified and CAP-accredited lab.
+ Individually validated biomarkers with 83–90 percent sensitivity and 92–99 percent specificity.[3]

COST

Biocept's test has two parts, which are priced separately. There is a fee for the CTC detection and enumeration and a fee for the specific biomarker identification.

Many health plans cover Biocept's services. Some plans only offer coverage for the biomarker identification portion of the test. Insurance information can be submitted with the test, and Biocept will bill you for any unpaid balance. If you do not have insurance, the cash price was less than $700 at the time of this publication.

Biocept offers a Financial Assistance Program "designed to aid...patients who have unique financial situations based upon income, expenses, or financial hardship....It is possible to reduce or eliminate the patient's financial responsibility."[4] Contact Biocept at 888-332-7410 for information on the application process. It may be possible to reduce or eliminate the patient's financial responsibility.

PROCESS TIME

Biocept normally provides your physician with the results of the tests within three to seven days of when the sample is received by Biocept.

BENEFITS

+ Assists as a diagnostic tool for selecting the appropriate agents to be used for therapy

+ Detects the presence of a resistance biomarker upon disease progression

+ May be used to evaluate patient prognosis as well as response to therapy

+ Used as a noninvasive alternative to traditional tissue biopsies

+ Assists in the confirmation of remission and patient monitoring

LIMITATIONS

Testing is limited to NCCN guideline–driven biomarkers and does not include research-related mutations. The test is only effective on solid tumors and can only be used for breast, prostate, colorectal, lung, gastric, and melanoma cancers.

THOUGHTS

In the past a tissue biopsy procedure was required for testing. Liquid biopsy is so much easier. I love that Biocept offers this noninvasive option for CTC detection and can tell you the quantity of cells detected while also providing specific biomarkers of the cells. The information obtained can be used in conventional oncology by your physician to decide which drugs to use, while an integrative physician can use the same information to apply natural therapies. Remember, biomarker results may predict the best potential treatments. There is no reason to do the cookie-cutter treatment plans when this personalized testing can be used. My hope is alternatives such as this will make traditional tissue biopsies a thing of the past. Moreover, the high probability of insurance coverage makes a liquid biopsy something to consider. Always confirm a negative result with other testing, as you could possibly have a type of cancer that this test does not detect.

References are available at www.biocept.com under the "Our Technology" tab in the "Publications" section.

SAMPLE TEST RESULTS

Biocept
Completing the Answer™

Biocept, Inc.
5810 Nancy Ridge Drive, Suite 150
San Diego, CA 92121

Target Selector™

Patient Information

Patient Name:	
Patient MRN:	
Address:	
Date of Birth:	Sex: F
Diagnosis:	Breast Cancer

Client Information

Ordering Physician:
Order Location:
Address:
Account Number:
Phone:
Fax:

Specimen Information

Accession#:		Collected Date/Time:	02/16/2018 10:30 AM
Client Accn#:		Received Date/Time:	02/17/2018 10:00 AM
Specimen Type:	Peripheral Blood	Reported Date/Time:	02/26/2018 03:57 PM
Volume (mL):	27	Test(s) Ordered:	TARGET SELECTOR ™

Results

CTCs : DETECTED

HER2 Gene Amplification by FISH : DETECTED (1 CTC / 27 mL)

ER Analysis of CTCs by ICC : NOT DETECTED

AR Analysis of CTCs by ICC : NOT DETECTED

PR Analysis of CTCs by ICC : NOT DETECTED

Supporting Data

Enumeration of Circulating Tumor Cells by OncoCEE™: 5

Number of Cytokeratin+ CTCs	3
Number of Cytokeratin- CTCs	2
CD45 negative Cells of Unknown Significance (CUS)	0

*A CTC is defined as a cell with the following staining pattern : CD45 negative, DAPI positive, Cytokeratin positive or Cytokeratin negative. These cells are captured from blood samples with antibodies targeting cell surface proteins (EPCAM, HER2, EGFR, MUC1, CMET, MSC, CD318, NCAD, MOV18, and TROP2).

This assay does not determine malignancy. All results should be interpreted by a qualified physician in conjunction with all other pertinent clinical, pathological and radiological findings. Clinical investigators believe that presence of circulating tumor cells (CTCs) in blood is an indicator of metastasis. Metastasis is a complex multistep process that includes epithelial-mesenchymal transition (EMT), in which tumor cells are characterized by loss of cell adhesion, repression of E-cadherin, acquisition of mesenchymal markers, increased cell motility, and invasiveness.(1) The cells of unknown significance (CUS) may represent damaged circulating tumor cells. AR is a therapeutic target for treatment of prostate cancer and more recently of estrogen receptor- negative breast cancer. AR expression in patients tumor cells indicates that patients with prostate cancer or estrogen receptor negative breast cancer might respond to therapeutic treatment with antagonists against AR or drugs affecting AR expression.(13,14) Approximately 80% of breast cancer patients have tumors expressing the estrogen receptor (ER), with majority also expressing the progesterone receptor (PR).(18) These tumors are classified as hormonal receptor positive and tend to respond to treatments that either lower estrogen levels (aromatase inhibitors) or block estrogen from binding to breast cells (e.g., tamoxifen) to support their growth. (19) HER2 is recognized as an

Customer Service 888-332-7729
FAX 877-300-1761

www.biocept.com
© 2017 Biocept, Inc. All rights reserved.
Page 1 of 2

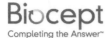
Completing the Answer™

Target Selector™

Biocept, Inc.
5810 Nancy Ridge Drive, Suite 150
San Diego, CA 92121

Patient Information

Patient Name:		Accession #:	
Patient MRN:		Received Date/Time:	02/17/2018 10:00 AM
Date of Birth:	Sex: F	Reported Date/Time:	02/26/2018 03:57 PM
Diagnosis:	Breast Cancer		

important predictive and prognostic factor in breast cancer.(2) HER2 status is predictive of a potential response to HER2 targeted agents such as tykerb and trastuzumab.(3)

CTC Image   HER2 FISH Image

(Blue=DAPI, Green=CK)   (Orange=HER2, Green=CEP17)

Method: Target Selector™ by Biocept

Positive and negative controls were run and reacted in an appropriate manner. Target Selector(TM) uses antibody based capture and detection to analyze circulating tumor cells (CTCs) in a micro-fluidic channel. Immunofluorescence (IF) is utilized by Biocept to detect Estrogen receptor (ER) status (antibody clone SP1). Immunofluorescence (IF) is utilized by Biocept to detect Androgen receptor (AR) status (antibody clone D6F11). FISH analysis is performed using Pathvysion(TM) DNA probe kit. Immunofluorescence (IF) is utilized by Biocept to detect Progesterone receptor (PR) status (antibody clone YR85). This test was developed and its performance characteristics determined by Biocept Laboratories. It has not been cleared or approved by the US Food & Drug Administration (FDA). This test is used for clinical purposes. This Laboratory is certified by the Clinical Laboratory Improvement Amendments of 1988 (CLIA-88) to perform high complexity testing.

References:
Thiery, J. P., Acloque, H., Huang, R. Y., and Nieto, M. A. (2009) Epithelial-mesenchymal transitions in development and disease, Cell 139, 871-890. Efficient capture of circulating tumor cells with a novel immunocytochemical microfluidic device. Biomicrofluidics 5, 034119 (2011). Detection of EpCAM-Negative and Cytokeratin-Negative Circulating Tumor Cells in Peripheral Blood. Journal of Oncology, Volume 2011(2011). A Novel Platform for Detection of CK+ and CK- CTCs. Cancer Discovery December 2011 1:580-586. Correlation of hormone receptor status between circulating tumor cells, primary tumor, and metastasis in breast cancer patients. Clin Transl Oncol 2015 Jan. Ahmed, A., Ali, S., and Sarkar, F. H. (2014) Advances in androgen receptor targeted therapy for prostate cancer, J Cell Physiol 229, 271-276. Ni, M., Chen, Y., Lim, E., Wimberly, H., Bailey, S. T., Imai, Y., Rimm, D. L., Liu, X. S., and Brown, M. (2011) Targeting androgen receptor in estrogen receptor-negative breast cancer, Cancer Cell 20, 119-131. Gusterson, B. A., Gelber, R. D., Goldhirsch, A., Price, K. N., Save-Soderborgh, J., Anbazhagan, R., Styles, J., Rudenstam, C. M., Golouh, R., Reed, R., and et al. (1992) Prognostic importance of c-erbB-2 expression in breast cancer. International (Ludwig) Breast Cancer Study Group, J Clin Oncol 10, 1049-1056. Prescribing information for lapatinib (TYKERB®), Novartis Pharmaceuticals Corp., April 2017. Prescribing Information for trastuzumab (HERCEPTIN®), Genentech, Inc., April 2017. Kohler, B. A., Sherman, R. L., Howlader, N., Jemal, A., Ryerson, A. B., Henry, K. A., Boscoe, F. P., Cronin, K. A., Lake, A., Noone, A. M., Henley, S. J., Eheman, C. R., Anderson, R. N., and Penberthy, L. (2015) Annual Report to the Nation on the Status of Cancer, 1975-2011, Featuring Incidence of Breast Cancer Subtypes by Race/Ethnicity, Poverty, and State, J Natl Cancer Inst 107, djv048.

Electronically Signed by: 02/26/2018
Example M.D., Pathologist

Technical component for CTC Enumeration, ICC Stains and FISH Markers were performed at Biocept Laboratory, 5810 Nancy Ridge Drive, San Diego, CA 92121. CLIA ID 05D1029526.

Customer Service 888-332-7729
FAX 877-300-1761

www.biocept.com
© 2017 Biocept, Inc. All rights reserved.
Page 2 of 2

Chapter 8

BreastSentry™

Innovative Diagnostic Laboratory
8751 Park Central Drive, Suite 200
Richmond, VA 23227
855-420-7140
www.myinnovativelab.com/breastsentry/
customerservice@myinnovativelab.com

THIS CHAPTER IS based on information provided by Innovative Diagnostic Laboratory and research done by the author. Check the Innovative Diagnostic Laboratory website for updates.

SUMMARY AND EXPLANATION

BreastSentry is a blood test that is used for breast cancer screening. The test can be performed at your yearly exam during a routine blood draw. Unlike other tests that identify cancer in its later stages, the BreastSentry test can help identify early cancer indicators.

INTERPRETATION

"BreastSentry is a sophisticated blood test that measures the levels of two bio-markers, proneurotensin (pro-NT) and proenkephalin (pro-ENK), which are highly predictive of a woman's risk for developing breast cancer.... Clinical studies have shown that elevated levels of pro-NT and decreased levels of pro-ENK are strong, independent risk factors for the development of breast cancer."[1] Elevated risk scores can help your physician determine if further screening is necessary.

Results are reported on a predetermined scale. A physician will provide interpretation.

HOW TO OBTAIN THE TEST

The test must be prescribed by a physician or clinician. Test kits can be obtained by contacting the lab.

ACCURACY

Studies completed by the American Society of Clinical Oncology and the American Association for Cancer Research confirm that elevated pro-NT and decreased levels of pro-ENK are relevant indicators of breast cancer progression.[2]

COST

Some insurance carriers are providing coverage. Innovative Diagnostic Laboratory will verify coverage. The cash price is approximately $300. This does not include the cost of the blood draw or the physician fee.

PROCESS TIME

Patient test results will be reported to the ordering physician within approximately ten business days of the receipt of the sample.

BENEFITS

+ Is processed with a small blood sample
+ Is noninvasive
+ Provides early cancer detection
+ Screens for indicators of breast cancer irrespective of breast density

LIMITATIONS

+ Does not provide the stage of cancer

THOUGHTS

I would love to see this test offered at annual physicals. It's a great early screening with no radiation as with a mammogram. With really early indicators, you have time to look at things such as hormones, immune function, vitamin D levels, and more, avoiding toxic therapies. References are available at www.myinnovativelab.com/scientific-papers/.

Sample Test Results

Innovative
DIAGNOSTIC LABORATORY

BreastSentry™
LABORATORY RESULTS

Patient	Name:	Phone #:	Patient ID #:	Specimen	Collection Time:	Specimen ID:	Provider	Requesting Provider
	Fasting Status:	Gender	Birthdate:	Age:	Collection Date:	Report Type:		
	Height:	Weight:	BMI:	Prev. BMI:	Received Date:	Report Date:		Client ID:

Test Results and Interpretation

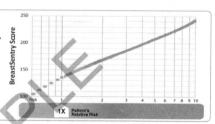

The patient has an **Average** risk score.

Increased levels of pro-NT and decreased levels of pro-ENK are predictive of a woman's risk for development of breast cancer.

| | 1X | Patient's Relative Risk |

Test Description

Test results are reported with a 95% CI (Confidence Interval).

The BreastSentry™ test measures the levels of pro-NT and pro-ENK biomarkers in fasting plasma to help determine a patient's Risk for developing breast cancer relative to the risk in an average risk population.

Biomarker Levels

Biomarker	Levels	Normal Range
Proneurotensin pro-NT (pmol/L)	81	< 100pmol/L
Proenkephalin pro-ENK (pmol/L)	43	> 44pmol/L

Clinical Recommendations

If the BreastSentry score is elevated, the patient should discuss with their physician whether advanced imaging is indicated.

Average risk scores for the BreastSentry test do not rule out breast cancer. When caught early, breast cancer may be treatable and beatable.

The BreastSentry risk score is determined by interrelating fasting plasma levels of proneurotensin (pro-NT) and proenkephalin (pro-ENK). These neuropeptides have been found to be highly predictive of breast cancer risk [1,2,3,4].
Published studies suggest that lifestyle changes such as exercise, diet and reduced opioid use may result in a change in pro-NT and/or pro-ENK values over time [5,6]. These changes may be associated with a reduction in breast cancer risk.
Annual testing with BreastSentry can assist patients in tracking their progress with lifestyle changes and updating their future risk of breast cancer.

Reference

1. Melander O, et al, Plasma proneurotensin and incidence of diabetes, cardiovascular disease, breast cancer, and mortality. JAMA. 2012; 308(14):1469-75
2. Melander O, et al, Validation of plasma proneurotensin as a novel biomarker for the prediction of incident breast cancer. Cancer Epidemiol Biomarkers Prev. 2014; 23(8):1672-6
3. Melander O, et al, Stable Peptide of the Endogenous Opioid Enkephalin Precursor and Breast Cancer Risk. J Clin Oncol. 2015 Aug 20;33(24):2632-8
4. Oeffinger KC, Fontham EH, Etzioni R, et al. Breast Cancer Screening for Women at Average Risk: 2015 Guideline Update From the American Cancer Society. JAMA.2015;314(15):1599-1614
5. Michael Schäfer, Shaaban A. Mousa. Opioid therapy and tumor progression. Advances in Palliative Medicine. 2009. 8:53-56
6. Go, Vay Liang W. and Demol, Pierre. Role of nutrients in the gastrointestinal release of immunoreactive neurotensin. Peptides. 1981. 2(Suppl 2): 267-9

Disclaimer

The BreastSentry Test is intended for use in average risk women. Average risk is defined as women without any of the following: a personal history of breast cancer, a confirmed or suspected genetic mutation known to increase risk of breast cancer (eg, BRCA), or a history of previous radiotherapy to the chest at a young age. Patients with a known history of impaired renal function or heart failure are not candidates for BreastSentry Test.

Laboratory Director | CLIA No. 49D2059683 | NPI No. 1962846790   Test Report ©2017 IDL   Rpt ver: IDL 2.1
©2018 Innovative Diagnostic Laboratory | 8751 Park Central Drive, Suite 200 | Richmond, VA 23227 | www.MyInnovativeLab.com   Ref ver: 2.0
Source:

Chapter 9

The Cancer Profile©

American Metabolic Laboratories
1818 Sheridan Street, Suite 102
Hollywood, FL 33020
954-929-4814
www.americanmetaboliclaboratories.net
cs@americanmetaboliclaboratories.net

THIS CHAPTER IS based on information provided by Emil Schandl, PhD, at American Metabolic Laboratories. Please refer to the American Metabolic Laboratories website for additional information and updates.

SUMMARY AND EXPLANATION

The Cancer Profile© is an early-screening test for cancer. It is also an effective tool for monitoring regression or progression of disease. It was developed by Emil Schandl.

The Cancer Profile comprises seven tests:

Human chorionic gonadotropin (HCG—Blood and Urine)

Also called the pregnancy hormone, or the malignancy hormone by Emil Schandl, HCG is an autocrine-proliferating factor and is tested two ways:

+ HCG (IMM)—tests for intact and molecular forms of HCG except the alpha subunit in the blood.

+ HCG Urine—a highly sensitive quantitative test for HCG in the urine. American Metabolic Laboratories uses an exclusive method of performing this test.

Phosphohexose isomerase (PHI)

The PHI enzyme has been called the human autocrine motility factor (AMF) and has been an implicating factor in the metastasis, or spread, of cancer. It regulates and channels cells into anaerobic metabolism (i.e., sugar metabolism).

Carcinoembryonic antigen (CEA)

CEA is an antigen present in the blood of many people with cancer.

Gamma-glutamyltranspeptidase (GGTP)

GGTP is an enzyme present when the liver, pancreas, or biliary system has been damaged due to therapy or disease. It is also affected by heart, lung, and kidney disease.

Thyroid-stimulating hormone (TSH)

Detects high or low thyroid activity. Many cancer patients and those who are developing cancer or receiving chemotherapy are hypothyroid.

Dehydroepiandrosterone sulfate (DHEA-S)

DHEA is often referred to as the adrenal "anti-stress, pro-immunity, longevity hormone."[1] Most cancer patients, as well as those who are developing cancer, have low serum DHEA-S levels. This hormone is needed for T-lymphocyte production as part of the immune cellular response system against cancer, bacterial infections, and viral infections.

INTERPRETATION

Tests ordered by a personal physician for a patient will have the results mailed to the ordering physician. The doctor can authorize the release of the results directly to the patient. Tests ordered directly with American Metabolic Laboratories will have the result mailed directly to the person tested.

The test includes a ten-minute phone consult. Positive test results may warrant a lifestyle change through metabolic therapy. An absolute final diagnosis is done with tissue pathology. The following are a few factors related to specific components of the test.

HCG may be elevated in existing cancer, in stress that is leading to cancer, or in a developing cancer in some cases as early as ten to twelve years before an actual tumor could be detected by other methods. HCG is also elevated during pregnancy. Normal results are less than 1.0 mIU/mL; the gray zone, i.e., a less-certainty zone, is 1.0–3.0 mIU/mL. Results that should be seriously considered are those above 3.0 mIU/mL. Keep in mind that a positive result does not necessarily mean there is an existing cancer. Positive results may indicate a developing cancer, as it may take seven to ten years for cancer to develop to the point where it can be detected by other means.

PHI can be elevated in a developing cancer or existing cancer. It also can be elevated in patients with many other conditions, such as disease of the heart, liver, or muscles; AIDS; hypothyroidism; or an acute viral infection. If acute conditions can be eliminated as the cause of elevated PHI, the result may indicate cancer is in the developmental stage. Normal results are less than 34.0 U/L; the gray zone is from 34.1–40 U/L. However, in patients with existing cancer, a change within even the normal range could be significant. Dr. Emil Schandl of American Metabolic Laboratories told me he feels that the PHI is the driving force behind cancer stem cell proliferation.[2]

The CEA test was initially "developed to monitor colorectal cancers. It is actually an excellent non-organ-specific cancer marker. It can be elevated in most types of cancers."[3] Normal results are less than 3.0 ng/mL; the gray zone is 3.1–5.0 ng/mL.

GGTP levels are considered normal when they are less than 29 IU/L in females and 35 IU/L in males.

TSH levels are normal when in the range of 0.4–4.0 micro IU/L.

DHEA-S levels are low or zero in most cancer patients. Normal is 35–430 mcg/dL for females and 80–560 mcg/dL for males.[4]

How to Obtain the Test

Individuals and physicians can obtain the test. Call 954-929-4814 to order and have a test kit shipped to you.

Accuracy

CA Profile reports 87–97 percent of positive test results were confirmed by biopsy in diagnosed cancer cases.

Cost

The Cancer Profile costs $549. Credit cards are accepted. There is an additional fee for the blood-drawing service to be paid to the laboratory you use (typically $25–$50). If you need a doctor to order your blood draw, American Metabolic Laboratories can provide this service for an additional fee of $25.

All insurance claims are considered out of network and require your own physician's prescription, which must be written by a licensed MD or DO for consideration by your insurance company. Medicare and Medicaid are not accepted by American Metabolic Laboratories. Inquire about shipping charges when ordering.

American Metabolic Laboratories offers an additional test called the

Longevity Profile, which includes the CA Profile. This test costs approximately $1,386. See its website for details.

PROCESS TIME

Tests are run every Wednesday. Results are mailed out via USPS First Class mail on the Friday of that week.

Special Instructions

For shipping domestic or international orders, no ice is required. Test kits must reach American Metabolic Laboratories within seven days. Be sure to collect the first morning urine and transfer it to the collection vial before going to the laboratory to have blood drawn. International orders should be shipped using Global Express.

BENEFITS

The tests are designed to detect malignancies at their earliest stages. The Cancer Profile has been proved to be an excellent resource for early detection when producing abnormal clinical laboratory results, sometimes even years before an actual diagnosis by other methods. It is valuable in monitoring the progress of cancer patients as well. It is able to detect brain tumors. (Note: Some tests are not able to detect brain cancer due to limitations of the blood-brain barrier.)

LIMITATIONS

+ You must have a physician's prescription if filing an insurance claim.
+ The Cancer Profile is neither organ- nor site-specific.
+ This test does not stage cancers; however, retesting allows comparison with prior results to monitor progress while in treatment, while at the end of treatment, and for early detection of recurrence.

NOTE FROM EMIL K. SCHANDL, PHD, AMERICAN METABOLIC LABORATORIES:

I have personally designed these profiles and many years of experience have shown success as high as 97 percent. This means that if there are 100 cancer cases diagnosed by biopsy, 97 may yield positive results. These observations were generated by examining some 40,000-plus patients. I can assure you these series of clinical laboratory tests are very useful for early detection of biochemical changes leading to cancer. The panels are also very productive in monitoring an individual's progress while receiving therapies, metabolic, conventional or the judicious combination of both. A positive result is a warning sign that may warrant a complete change of lifestyle risk factors through evaluation and implementation of metabolic therapy. It is much easier to prevent cancer than to cure it. I strongly recommend the Cancer Profile, and even more so the Longevity Profile, on an annual basis as part of your most comprehensive health watch. In the event of abnormal cancer marker/s results, it is wise to also perform the TK1 test for additional confirmation and follow-up of those findings.

Cordially yours,

E. K. Schandl, MS, PhD, FACB, CC (NRCC), SC (ASCP), Oncobiologist, Clinical and Nutritional Biochemist, Clinical Laboratory Director (States of FL, NY, CA)

THOUGHTS

The Cancer Profile test can be lifesaving. Not only can it be used to monitor known disease, but it can identify precancerous conditions.

The seven tests included provide a multifaceted result, and each test can be used to validate the other results. For example, the Cancer Profile provides multiple indicators, and if more than one of the seven test results returns positive, there is a stronger body of evidence to suggest a problem.

Just as Emil Schandl stated in his note to the reader, this test can be used as a proactive part of your annual physical exam. It can be utilized to identify a new cancer or a cancer recurrence at its earliest stages. For example, I received a phone call from a patient who was treated for breast cancer two and a half years ago. She was declared as having no evidence of disease (NED) at the time. She said her MRI and PET scan last month indicated a lesion on her chest wall, in her liver, and in the lymph nodes. Had she been monitoring her health status with a test such as the Cancer Profile, she may have been able to intervene long before the tumors were large enough to appear on the scans.

The longer I work with these tests, the more I see occasions where people have used a true early-detection test like this one, then followed up with a more conventional test. The second test tells them they don't have cancer, leaving them not knowing what to make of the apparent contradiction. But it's not conflicting information—it is affirmation. The first test is a true early-detection test, able to "see" cancer forming much earlier than the second test, which likely can't detect cancer until it has been growing long enough to form a lump or bump.

Through the years Emil Schandl has tested thousands of people who were thought to be healthy. Approximately 40 percent of them got a "false" positive with the Cancer Profile. In other words, a conventional cancer test did not confirm the presence of cancer. Let's think about that for a moment: According to national statistics, one out of every 2.5 individuals will develop cancer in America—that's 40 percent of the population. Are these 40 percent of "false" positives individuals in the early stages of developing cancer? Are their cancers too early to be picked up by more conventional and late diagnostic tests? It makes sense to me that they are.

See   www.americanmetaboliclaboratories.net/ca-profile.html   for references.

Chapter 10

Cologuard®

Exact Sciences Corporation
441 Charmany Drive
Madison, WI 53719
844-870-8870
www.cologuardtest.com

THIS CHAPTER IS based on information provided by Exact Sciences Corporation and research done by the author. Please refer to the Exact Sciences website for more information and updates.

SUMMARY AND EXPLANATION

Colorectal cancer is the fourth–most commonly diagnosed cancer and the second-leading cause of cancer deaths in men and women combined in the United States. Unfortunately most cases are not found early or before it has spread beyond the tissues of the colon or rectum. Cologuard® was approved by the FDA in August of 2014. It requires a prescription and can be done in the privacy of your home.

This cancer screening test looks for blood in the stool and altered DNA. The wall of the colon naturally sheds cells daily; abnormal cells will be picked up by stool as it passes through. Cologuard uses advanced stool DNA technology to find altered DNA from these abnormal cells, which could be associated with either cancer or precancer.

Any positive result should be discussed with your doctor and followed by a diagnostic colonoscopy.

INTERPRETATION

The test result is reported as "positive" or "negative." Information from the DNA analysis and blood test are combined to reach the test result. A positive result must be followed by a diagnostic colonoscopy. Individuals with negative results should consult with their doctor to determine when and how repeat screening should occur.

How to Obtain the Test

Ask your doctor for the test. There is a discussion guide to help you talk to your doctor available at www.cologuardtest.com/how-to-get-cologuard. The test must be ordered by prescription through a licensed clinician.

Cologuard is shipped directly to your home. Instructions for collecting a stool sample are included and easy to understand. The kit includes a prepaid UPS return shipping label. Please note the sample must be shipped within twenty-four hours of collection and received by Exact Sciences Labs within seventy-two hours of collection. For this reason, it is recommended collected samples be shipped Monday through Thursday.

Accuracy

In a ten thousand–patient clinical study, Cologuard found 92 percent of colon cancers and 42 percent of high-risk precancers with 87 percent specificity.

Both false positives and false negatives can occur. In a clinical study of Cologuard, 13 percent of people without cancer or precancer tested positive. Patients with positive results should have a follow-up diagnostic colonoscopy. Patients with negative results should continue with an appropriate screening program. Cologuard results, when used for repeat testing, have not yet been evaluated.[1]

Cost

Cologuard is covered by Medicare. Traditional Medicare (Part B) patients do not have any co-pays, deductible amounts, or coinsurance. Medicare covers Cologuard once every three years as long as you are between fifty and eighty-five years of age and you are at average risk for developing colon cancer.[2]

Medicare will not cover the test if you have symptoms your doctor thinks may be related to colon cancer, if you previously had a positive colonoscopy that found polyps or cancer, or if your doctor determines you have a high-risk family history of colon cancer.

The test is also covered by a variety of private insurers. Check with your provider to confirm coverage. Co-pays and/or deductibles may apply. If you have private insurance coverage, Cologuard will bill your insurance company on your behalf. Please note, if your insurance coverage is denied, you will be responsible for the unpaid balance. The maximum out-of-pocket cost of Cologuard is $649, and the cost depends on the covered benefits of your specific insurance plan.

PROCESS TIME

Test results are typically delivered to your doctor within about two weeks of the lab receiving the completed test kit.

BENEFITS

+ The test can identify the presence of cancer and precancerous cells.
+ The test is available for Medicare coverage for adults fifty to eighty-five years of age who are at average risk for colon cancer.
+ No special bowel preparation or dietary restrictions are required before taking the test.
+ The test is done in the privacy of your home.
+ The test is less invasive than a colonoscopy.

LIMITATIONS

Results should be interpreted with caution for individuals over age seventy-five, as the rate of false positives increases with age.

Cologuard is *not* approved for people with a high risk of colon cancer. These may include:

+ People with a personal history of colon cancer, polyps, or other related cancers.
+ People with a family history of colon cancer.
+ People with a positive result from another screening method within the last six months.
+ Patients who have been diagnosed with a condition associated with high risk for colorectal cancer, including inflammatory bowel disease (IBD), chronic ulcerative colitis (CUC), and Crohn's disease.

Cologuard should not be used by those who have or may have blood in their stool due to actively bleeding hemorrhoids, menstruation, or other existing conditions, as this may result in a false positive. Cologuard is not a replacement for diagnostic colonoscopy or surveillance colonoscopy in high-risk individuals. Cologuard may produce false positive or false negative results.

THOUGHTS

Research tells us that once colon cancer metastasizes, approximately 87 percent of people will not be alive in five years. Thus, early screening for colon cancer is critical.

This test looks for the presence of blood in the stool and also at the DNA. I like the added component of the DNA analysis, which is not available in other home test kits. CellMax is another company that is offering a similar test.[3] References are available at www.cologuardtest .com and https://academy.cologuardtest.com/data-publications.

Chapter 11

Colon Health Screening for Occult Blood in Stool

COLORECTAL CANCER IS often called the "silent killer." Excluding skin cancers, colorectal cancer is the fourth–most common cancer diagnosed in both men and women in the United States.

Cancer that begins in the colon is called colon cancer. Cancer that begins in the last six inches of the large intestine (the rectum) is called rectal cancer. Cancer that begins in either of these areas is called colorectal cancer (CRC). About 70 percent of patients with CRC have no family history of the disease, so it does not appear to be primarily inherited.[1] Deaths from CRC could be nearly eliminated if most people learn the basics and get tested.

SUMMARY AND EXPLANATION

A home test kit, available at specialty drugstores or online, can be used to detect "occult," or invisible, blood in the stool. Fecal occult blood is an indicator of a problem in your digestive system.

If blood is detected, it is important for your doctor to determine the source of the bleeding in order to properly diagnose and effectively treat the problem. Blood may be seen as red or black tar-like feces and may appear in the stool because there are:

+ Benign or malignant growths or polyps in the colon
+ Hemorrhoids (swollen blood vessels near the anus and lower rectum that can rupture and cause bleeding)
+ Anal fissures (splits in the lining of the anal opening)
+ Intestinal infections
+ Ulcers
+ Possible bowel conditions, such as colitis, Crohn's disease, celiac disease, or diverticular disease[2]

+ Bacterial infections
+ Food allergies to items such as dairy and wheat that have irritated the colon wall and caused bleeding

INTERPRETATION

Stool samples are collected in a clean container and evaluated by detecting color changes on the test card. Some test kits instruct you to simply drop the test card into the toilet after a bowel movement. Follow instructions included in your kit.

HOW TO OBTAIN THE TEST

You can purchase fecal occult blood test kits at specialty pharmacies or order them online. Each test kit provides specific instructions, and most offer a toll-free number to call if you have questions. Since colon cancers may only bleed from time to time, rather than continually, you will need to collect three different stool samples. The stool samples should be taken one day apart. Be sure to purchase a kit that includes at least three separate test cards.

Do not perform the test if you have one of the conditions in the bulleted list above, if you have diarrhea, or if you are menstruating.

ACCURACY

Negative test results mean there was no blood found in the stool sample. Patients with negative results should continue to follow their doctors' recommendations for regular cancer screening.

COST

Most test kits are priced at $10–$80.

PROCESS TIME

Usually results are read in two minutes. Follow test kit instructions.

BENEFITS

+ The test can detect the presence of unknown colon cancer so treatment can be started earlier.
+ Cost is low compared with a colonoscopy.
+ The test is noninvasive.

+ The test is convenient, quick, and easy and can be done at home.

+ No cleansing of the colon is necessary.

LIMITATIONS

+ Positive results may be due to a condition other than cancer.

+ The test requires further testing to determine the cause of the bleeding.

+ The test fails to detect non-bleeding polyps.

+ False positives can occur.

THOUGHTS

Many people don't want to do a colonoscopy or don't have the funds or insurance available to get one. A home fecal blood test kit provides a more affordable option. It is my belief that everyone, beginning in their thirties, should do this test for the early detection of colorectal cancer.

Regular screening can often find colorectal cancer early, when it is most likely to be curable.

When relying on colonoscopies for colon cancer testing, it is important to remember a colonoscopy is done on the large intestine and can miss a lesion in the small intestine. More information is available at http://stopcoloncancernow.com/colon-cancer-prevention/screening-methods/fecal-occult-blood-test-fobt.

Chapter 12

ColonSentry®

Innovative Diagnostic Laboratory
8751 Park Central Drive, Suite 200
Richmond, VA 23227
855-420-7140
www.myinnovativelab.com/colonsentry
customerservice@myinnovativelab.com

THIS CHAPTER IS based on information provided by Innovative Diagnostic Laboratory and research done by the author. Check the Innovative Diagnostic Laboratory website for updates.

SUMMARY AND EXPLANATION

Colorectal cancer is the second-leading cause of cancer deaths in both men and women in the United States and is preventable and easily treated if caught early. ColonSentry is a simple blood test that gives an early warning of colorectal cancer. It measures the expression of seven gene biomarkers in the blood. The test can be done along with other blood work at your annual exam.[1]

INTERPRETATION

Results are reported on a predetermined scale. The physician will provide the interpretation.

HOW TO OBTAIN THE TEST

The test must be prescribed by a physician or clinician. Test kits can be obtained by contacting the lab.

ACCURACY

Reported sensitivity is 72 percent; specificity is 70 percent.

COST

Innovative Diagnostic Laboratory will verify possible insurance or Medicare coverage. The cash price is approximately $350. This does not include the cost of the blood draw or the physician fee.

PROCESS TIME

Test results will be reported to the ordering physician in approximately ten business days from the receipt of the sample.

BENEFITS

+ The test is processed with a blood sample.

+ The test is noninvasive.

+ The test provides early detection.

+ There is no need to handle stool.

+ There is no fasting, dietary instructions, or special preparation.

LIMITATIONS

+ This test does not provide the stage of cancer.

+ The test should not be used as a stand-alone diagnostic tool.

THOUGHTS

Screening for colon cancer is getting easier and easier. Unfortunately most people avoid getting tested until symptoms appear. A blood test makes the process very easy. Don't wait too long. References are available at www.myinnovativelab.com/scientific-papers/.

SAMPLE TEST RESULTS

Innovative
DIAGNOSTIC LABORATORY

ColonSentry®
LABORATORY RESULTS

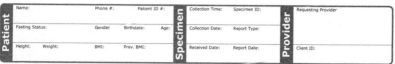

Patient						Specimen			Provider	
Name:		Phone #:	Patient ID #:			Collection Time:	Specimen ID:		Requesting Provider	
Fasting Status:		Gender	Birthdate:	Age:		Collection Date:	Report Type:			
Height:	Weight:	BMI:	Prev. BMI:			Received Date:	Report Date:		Client ID:	

Test Results and Interpretation

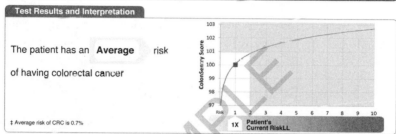

The patient has an **Average** risk

of having colorectal cancer

‡ Average risk of CRC is 0.7%

ColonSentry Score — 97, 98, 99, 100, 101, 102, 103

Risk 1 2 3 4 5 6 7 8 9 10

1X   **Patient's Current RiskLL**

Test Description

Test results are reported with a 95% CI (Confidence Interval).

The ColonSentry® test measures the expression of 7 gene biomarkers in whole blood to help determine a patient's **Current Risk** for having colorectal cancer (CRC) relative to the current risk in an average risk population.

Gene Expression

Gene	Cycle Threshold
ANXA3* (ΔCt)	1.9
CLEC4D* (ΔCt)	2.5
TNFAIP6* (ΔCt)	1.8
LMNB1* (ΔCt)	1.8
PRRG4* (ΔCt)	0.9
VNN1* (ΔCt)	1.5
IL2RB (Ct)	24.6

* Difference with respect to IL2RB

Clinical Recommendations

If the results indicate that the patient's current risk is elevated (2X or more), the patient should be referred for further evaluation with procedures such as colonoscopy. Average risk scores for the ColonSentry® test do not rule out colon cancer. When caught early, colon cancer is both treatable and beatable.

Average Risk: recommendation** for FIT, FIT-DNA, flexible sigmoidoscopy, CT colonography, or colonoscopy.
Elevated Risk: recommendation** for colonoscopy.

** Screening for Colorectal Cancer US Preventive Services Task Force Recommendation Statement. JAMA Jun 21, 2016; 315(23):2564-2575

What to do next?

According to USPSTF*, an average risk patient is a man or woman who is at least 50 years old, is asymptomatic for CRC, has no personal history of benign colorectal polyps, colorectal adenomas, CRC or inflammatory bowel disease, and does not have a first degree relative with CRC. The presence of conditions such as pancreatic cancer, systemic sclerosis or CLL might affect the risk score.

Screening for colorectal cancer reduces mortality through detection and treatment of early-stage cancer and detection and removal of adenomatous polyps. The degree to which each of these mechanisms contributes to a reduction in mortality is unknown, although it is likely that the largest reduction in colorectal cancer mortality during the 10 years after initial screening comes from the detection and removal of early-stage cancer. Colonoscopy is a necessary step in any screening program that reduces mortality from colorectal cancer.***

*** Screening for Colorectal Cancer US Preventive Services Task Force Recommendation Statement. JAMA Jun 21, 2016; 315(23):2564-2575

Disclaimer

This test is not recommended for patients that have previous history of colorectal cancer, or pre-cancerous (e.g. adenomatous) polyps, or familial or inherited colon polyp syndromes, or inflammatory bowel disease, or have received chemotherapy and/or radiation.

Laboratory Director | CLIA No. 49D2059683 | NPI No. 1962846790   Test Report ©2017 IDL   Rpt ver: IDL 2.1
©2018 Innovative Diagnostic Laboratory | 8751 Park Central Drive, Suite 200 | Richmond, VA 23227 | www.MyInnovativeLab.com   Ref ver: 2.0
Source:

Chapter 13

EarlyCDT-Lung Test

Oncimmune (USA) LLC
8960 Commerce Drive, Building #6
De Soto, KS 66018
888-583-9030; 913-583-9000
www.oncimmune.com
ClientServices@oncimmune.com

THIS CHAPTER IS based on information provided by Oncimmune and research done by the author. Please refer to the Oncimmune website for updates.

SUMMARY AND EXPLANATION

Lung cancer is the leading cause of cancer deaths. The EarlyCDT-Lung is a simple blood test that detects the presence of seven different autoantibodies against specific lung cancer–associated antigens. These autoantibodies may be detectable up to four years before a tumor is visible. Oncimmune reports it is effective in detecting all stages of lung cancer, including the earliest stages. Oncimmune's goal is to advance early lung cancer detection to the greatest extent possible using the autoantibody assay technology utilized in the EarlyCDT-Lung test. The test works by evaluating a known process: When a tumor is present in the lung, it produces abnormal proteins, or antigens, not normally found in the blood. The body reacts rapidly to the abnormal proteins/antigens by producing the related antibodies. If preset levels are exceeded, the test will be positive.

Testing is currently only recommended for individuals with a pulmonary nodule. The test may be used as part of the physician's assessment of the risk of a nodule being malignant and also to detect cancer earlier in nodules that are being monitored by repeat CT scanning, or "watchful waiting." Nodules in watchful waiting have a 7–10 percent risk of being cancer, and the test can help find many of these cancers faster. Anyone with a history of cancer, except basal cell carcinoma, is not eligible for this test. Lingering antibodies from a previous diagnosis could cause a false positive result.

INTERPRETATION

Test results are reported as no significant level of autoantibodies detected, a moderate level detected, or a high level detected. A no-significant-level-of-autoantibodies detected result indicates a lower likelihood of having lung cancer than a moderate or high level but does not mean cancer is not present or will not develop; continued monitoring is recommended. A moderate-level result adds more than 25 percent risk to a nodule's risk of cancer and indicates you are at increased risk of having a lung cancer. A high-level result greatly increases your risk of having a lung cancer, and this result shifts all nodules classified as intermediate risk into the high, "intervention" risk category (greater than 65 percent risk).[1]

How to Obtain the Test

The test must be ordered by your treating physician. EarlyCDT-Lung is available through many affiliated laboratories as a send-out test. Your physician can inquire whether the test is available through his or her laboratory of choice. If not, then your physician can contact Oncimmune's Client Services department at 888-583-9030 or ClientServices@oncimmune.com to request a blood collection kit. Oncimmune will send a test kit upon request, which includes the materials for FedEx prepaid overnight return shipping to the lab. The test kit includes a simple finger stick collection system that allows the patient to collect the blood with a pinprick to a finger, if that is preferred over the standard blood draw.[2]

Accuracy

For patients with a pulmonary nodule(s), Oncimmune reports 98 percent specificity for high-level results, meaning only 2 percent of patients without lung cancer will get a false positive high-level result, and 78 percent of patients with a high-level result will have a lung cancer. For a moderate-level result, the false positive rate is only 7 percent, and 59 percent of patients with a moderate-level result will have a lung cancer. The accuracy of the test in the target population is 83 percent for a moderate level and 84 percent for a high level.[3]

Cost

Oncimmune will bill Medicare Part B or your primary insurance carrier for the cost of the test. The test requisition form (included in blood collection kit) must be completed and signed, and photocopies of the front and back of your insurance card or cards are required to be returned with the blood sample. Your out-of-pocket cost will be limited to copays, deductibles, and coinsurance, as determined by your health care plan. Oncimmune offers a Financial Assistance Plan for patients who are underinsured or uninsured. Oncimmune encourages patients to call or email Oncimmune's Client Services department for additional information and eligibility for financial assistance. Out-of-pocket expenses may be reimbursable through flexible spending accounts or health savings accounts.

PROCESS TIME

Results take less than one week and will be sent directly to the ordering physician.

BENEFITS

+ Early detection
+ Increased survival rates. (The five-year survival rate of 18.1 percent more than triples to 55.6 percent with early detection.)[4]

LIMITATIONS

The test is not effective on individuals with previous cancer. The body will have produced antibodies to previous cancers, and those lingering antibodies can produce a positive result on this lung cancer test.

This test is only available for individuals who qualify as part of the target population.

THOUGHTS

Considering approximately 80 percent of lung cancers are found late in the disease process and only 18.6 percent of patients survive five years,[5] this is a very needed test. Cancers caught early translate to quicker intervention and higher survival rates. References are available at http://oncimmune.com/lung-cancer-test/earlycdt-lung-papers-publications/.

Another lab offering the EarlyCDT-Lung test is Innovative Diagnostic Laboratory. Its website is www.myinnovativelab.com.

This chapter is dedicated to my uncles, Don Behrend and Clarence Herzog. Both died after being diagnosed with very advanced lung cancer. This early-detection test could have saved their lives.

SAMPLE TEST RESULTS

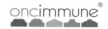
Leading early cancer detection

*Early*CDT®–Lung
Nodule Risk Assessment

8960 Commerce Drive, Bldg. 6, De Soto, KS 66018
888-583-9030

*PDF version of the test result available through our results
portal. Call 888-583-9030 to set up results portal.*

Patient Report

Patient	Specimen Information	Physician
PATIENT 5 **Sex:** F **DOB:** 7/4/1962 **Age:** 55	**TRF ID:** 08312017-HL **Collection Date:** 1/3/2018 **Received Date:** 1/5/2018 **Report Date:** 1/6/2018	Example HL7 Physician Example HL7 Clinic 123 Sesame St. De Soto, KS 66018

EarlyCDT-Lung Test Result: HIGH LEVEL

Test	Result$_{(RU)}$	No Significant Level of Autoantibodies Detected	Moderate Level	High Level
CAGE autoantibody	<2.76	-X-	---	---
GBU4-5 autoantibody	1.06	-X-	---	---
NY-ESO-1 autoantibody	<1.01	-X-	---	---
p53 autoantibody	<3.09	-X-	---	---
SOX-2 autoantibody	7.02	---	---	-X-
MAGE A4 autoantibody	<3.91	-X-	---	---
HuD autoantibody	<3.99	-X-	---	---

* This test is not intended for patients who have previously had cancer (exception: basal cell carcinoma).

CLINICAL UTILITY:

The ACCP guidelines[a] recommend assessing the risk of malignancy of a pulmonary nodule, e.g., with the Swensen/Mayo nodule malignancy risk calculator[b], available at oncimmune.com/nodule-calculator. The calculated risk can be divided into three categories and the patient managed accordingly. *Early*CDT-Lung facilitates further risk characterization to assist with triaging difficult to assess nodules[c].

<10% risk of lung cancer*	Low Risk Group	High or Moderate *Early*CDT-Lung test result indicates risk raised to Intermediate risk.
10-65% risk of lung cancer*	Intermediate Risk Group	High *Early*CDT-Lung test result indicates risk raised to Intervention risk. Moderate *Early*CDT-Lung test result indicates >25% increase in risk, raising some patients to Intervention risk.
>65% risk of lung cancer*	Intervention Risk Group	Occasional use of *Early*CDT-Lung following biopsy or bronchoscopy where it is deemed further risk evaluation is of value.

* Risk categories according to the ACCP guidelines[a].

INTERPRETIVE COMMENTS:

A High Level result is reported when any one or more autoantibodies in the *Early*CDT-Lung panel are above the high cutoff value. For a patient with an intermediate risk (i.e., 10-65%) pulmonary nodule, a High Level *Early*CDT-Lung result will move the patient to intervention risk (i.e., >65%). Consider changing the patient's treatment pathway to that recommended by guidelines for a nodule with intervention risk of malignancy.

References:
a) Gould MK, et al. Chest 2013; 143(5):e93S-e120S.
b) Swensen SJ, et al. Arch Intern Med. 1997; 157:849-855.
c) Massion PP, et al. J Thorac Oncol. 2017; 12(3):578-584.
d) Chapman CJ, et al. Tumor Biol. 2012; 33(5):1319-1326.
e) Healey GF, et al. J Thorac Dis. 2013; 5(5):618-625.

Joseph P. McConnell, PhD, DABCC, FACB, Clinical Laboratory Director

*This test was developed and its performance characteristics were determined by
Oncimmune®™. It has not been cleared by the FDA. Oncimmune is a registered,
high complexity laboratory and is in compliance with all CLIA regulations.*

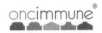

Leading early cancer detection

PDF version of the test results available through our results portal. Call 888-583-9030 to set up results portal.

DEFINITIONS

Test:	Indicates the autoantibody analyzed for testing.
Result:	Calculated reportable value of a given autoantibody in Relative Units (RU).
No Significant Level of Autoantibodies Detected:	Reportable result is below the low cutoff value.
Moderate Level:	Reportable result is between the low and the high cutoff value.
High Level:	Reportable result is above the high cutoff value.
Test Result:	Determined based upon the highest level of autoantibody measured relative to the cutoffs for each autoantibody.
Invalid:	Unable to determine result for this autoantibody. All other autoantibodies remain valid.
Cutoff:	Threshold value for each autoantibody assay above which the result is deemed to be abnormal, as established from results of clinical validation studies.[a,b]

CUTOFF VALUES FOR *Early* CDT-Lung

Autoantibody		Low Cutoff Value		High Cutoff Value
CAGE		4.25		4.52
GBU4-5		4.36		4.53
NY-ESO-1	No Significant Level	3.02	Moderate	3.39	High
p53	of Autoantibodies	5.79	Level	5.99	Level Result
SOX-2	Detected	5.48	Result	6.98	
MAGE A4		6.19		7.17
HuD		7.31		7.69

UNDERSTANDING YOUR RESULTS *(For Patient Use)*

*Early*CDT®-Lung test results are reported as High Level, Moderate Level, and No Significant Level of Autoantibodies Detected, depending on the level of autoantibodies in the blood compared to high and low cutoff values for each autoantibody. Answers to some frequently asked questions are given below. The patient should discuss the results with his/her physician for a clinical interpretation and recommendations for next steps.

What do I do if the result is "High Level"?

A "High Level" result means that one or more autoantibodies were detected above the high cutoff, which suggests that the likelihood of lung cancer is much greater than predicted by the patient's gender, age, smoking history, nodule characteristics and other clinical factors. This result does not definitively mean that lung cancer is present. A physician may recommend additional testing, including a PET scan, bronchoscopy, needle biopsy, or other testing. If lung cancer is not found, other age- and gender-specific screenings for other cancers (for example, breast and colon), as recommended by the American Cancer Society (www.cancer.org), should also be considered.

What do I do if the result is "Moderate Level"?

A "Moderate Level" result means that one or more autoantibodies were detected at an elevated level, which suggests that the likelihood of lung cancer is greater than predicted by the patient's gender, age, smoking history, nodule characteristics, and other clinical factors. This result does not definitively mean that lung cancer is present. A physician may recommend additional testing. If lung cancer is not found, other age- and gender-specific screenings for other cancers (for example, breast and colon), as recommended by the American Cancer Society (www.cancer.org), should also be considered.

What do I do if the result is "No Significant Level of Autoantibodies Detected"?

A "No Significant Level of Autoantibodies Detected" result suggests the patient's risk of having a lung cancer is unchanged. It does not rule out the possibility of the patient having lung cancer now or in the future. A physician may recommend that the patient continue a schedule of testing and examination based on the patient's personal history, nodule characteristics and/or clinical symptoms.

What do these autoantibody levels have to do with lung cancer?

In all types of lung cancer, some individuals have been found to have elevated levels of one or more of these autoantibodies[a-d]. Autoantibodies have been shown to be present in the blood up to four years prior to a tumor becoming visible on a CT scan[e-h]. Early detection of lung cancer has been shown to increase the potential for an improved outcome[i].

References:
a) Chapman CJ, et al. *Tumor Biology* 2012; 33(5):1319-1326.
b) Healey GF, et al. *J Thorac Dis* 2013; 5(5):618-625.
c) Massion PP, et al. *J Thorac Oncol.* 2017; 12(3):578-584.
d) Lam S, et al. *Cancer Prev Res* 2011; 4(7):1126-1134.
e) Chapman C, et al. *Chest* 2010; 138:s775A.
f) Trivers GE, et al. *Clinical Cancer Res* 1996; 2:1767-1775.
g) Li Y, et al. *Int J Cancer* 2005; 114:157-160.
h) Zhong L, et al. *J Thor Oncol* 2006; 1:513-519.
i) The National Lung Screening Trial Research Team. *N Engl J Med* 2011; 365:395-409.

Human Chorionic Gonadotropin (HCG) Test

Navarro Medical Clinic
Efren Navarro, MD
3553 Sining Street
Morningside Terrace
Santa Mesa, Manila 1016
Philippines
Evening phone calls after 6:00 p.m. CST at 847-359-3634
customer.service@navarromedicalclinic.com
www.navarromedicalclinic.com

THIS CHAPTER IS based on information obtained from www.navarromedicalclinic.com. Please refer to the Navarro website for more information and updates.

SUMMARY AND EXPLANATION

The HCG urine immunoassay detects the presence of cancer cells before the development of signs or symptoms. It was developed by renowned oncologist Dr. Manuel D. Navarro, who found that HCG was present in patients with all types of cancers. The HCG test is based on the theory that "cancer is related to a misplaced trophoblastic cell that becomes malignant."[1] This school of thought looks at how cancer is similar to pregnancy—from one cell come many others.

A fetus starts as one cell that divides repeatedly. Some cells become bones; others become organs, blood vessels, and so on. But after pregnancy that kind of frenzied division comes to an end, and strict order begins. Once a bone cell, always a bone cell. In much the same way cell division does not "play by the rules" during pregnancy, cancer cells do not play by the rules. Both cancerous cells and pregnant women secrete HCG. Therefore "a measurement of the amount of HCG found in the blood or urine is also a measure of the degree of malignancy. The higher the number, the greater the severity of cancer."[2]

Urine is the preferred specimen for the test because HCG is much harder to detect in the bloodstream. A 1980 study validated the use of urine specimens for the HCG immunoassay. The study showed that in 70 proven cancer cases, the immunoassay test produced 31 positive results (44.3 percent) using urine, while only 12 positive results (17.1 percent) were reported using blood.[3]

The Navarro Medical Clinic website reports "the test detects the presence of brain cancer as early as 29 months before symptoms appear; 27 months for fibrosarcoma of the abdomen; 24 months for skin cancer; 12 months for cancer of the bones (metastasis from the breast extirpated 2 years earlier)."[4]

INTERPRETATION

Results are sent directly to the patient's email address.

INTERPRETATION OF READINGS[5]			
Index	International Units	Readings	Interpretation
0	zero	(-)	Negative
1–3	1–49	(+/-)	Doubtful
4	50–400	(+)	Faintly Positive
5	401–999	(++)	Definitely Positive
6	1000–3000	(+++)	Moderately Positive
7	3001–5000	(++++)	Markedly Positive
8	5001–10,000	(+++++)	Very Markedly Positive
9	over 10,000	(++++++)	Excessively Positive

Levels can reach up to 10,000 international units (IU) or more in some cancers. However, most cancers have results anywhere from 50–90 IU. Repeated testing can be used to monitor progress and response to treatment.

When an index reading of 4 or more is given, it means the result is above 50 IU and is positive, meaning cancer may be present. If a reading of index 3 or lower is given, it means the result is below 50 IU and is essentially negative.

How to Obtain the Test

There are two options for preparing your sample. The first is to order a kit from www.joeballcompany.com. The cost is $64.99 for the US kit. Follow the instructions, and mail the completed test to the Navarro Medical Center.

The second is to make your own kit. You will need the following items to prepare a dry extract from your urine sample:

- 7 ounces of acetone (Nail polish remover is not an acceptable substitute.)
- 1 teaspoon of alcohol (ethyl, isopropyl, or rubbing)
- Coffee filter (white or brown)
- Plastic sandwich bag
- Glass container or jar
- Glass measuring cup
- Measuring spoon

Follow the simple test and mailing instructions on the clinic's website: www.navarromedicalclinic.com/preparation.php.

There cannot be any sexual contact for twelve days before collecting the sample for female patients. For male patients, there cannot be any sexual contact for forty-eight hours before collecting the sample. This test is not suitable for patients who are pregnant.

Accuracy

In research with seventy patients with documented cancer, the immuno-assay test gave thirty-one positive results using urine. Over 20 percent borderline false positive HCG elevations occurred in postmenopausal females.[6]

In serum HCG testing, blood is used. The Navarro Medical Clinic reports that results from a blood or serum sample are not as accurate because when HCG molecules pass through the liver, enzymes fragment them, so the reagent may not be able to identify them. With the Navarro test, whole HCG molecules are in the urine sample.

Cost

The test is $55 plus the cost of USPS first-class international mail. Payment instructions are online. The household items needed cost around $15.

PROCESS TIME

Allow three to four weeks for test results to be available when mailing from the United States, Canada, or Europe. Results are sent to the email address provided with the mailed test sample.

BENEFITS

+ This test is affordable.
+ It is a noninvasive screening test.
+ It's simple and can be done in the privacy of your home.
+ The test indicates the amount of cancer that may be present.

LIMITATIONS

See "Precautions" on the test website for activities and medications that should be temporarily stopped before a urine sample is collected. Substances such as thyroid hormones, steroidal compounds, female hormone supplements (estrogen, testosterone, progesterone), and vitamin D may interfere with results. If you are using these compounds, you must stop taking them for three days before collecting the urine sample. Always consult your physician before stopping any medications or supplements.

The test is not organ- or site-specific. The test cannot determine the stage of the cancer.

Note: A positive HCG test result can be caused by pregnancy, malignancy, and some pituitary gland issues due to an HCG-like substance (HCGLS) that may occur rarely in perimenopausal and postmenopausal women and some older men.

THOUGHTS

This test is affordable and can be done in the privacy of your home. It may seem silly to test for cancer with a coffee filter and a few household items, but I did it, and thousands of others have done it before me. This test is another useful tool in evaluating your cancer status. I like the numerical score that ranks the amount of HCG present as opposed to a simple positive or negative outcome. Increasing or decreasing levels can indicate the advancement or regression of disease. HCG is extremely sensitive; a tiny elevation in its level in women is highly indicative of cancer. In men, HCG is very good at diagnosing testicular cancer.

Note: The HCG hormone is what many pregnancy tests are based upon. After conception, the body dispatches HCG to maintain the lining of the womb and enable the production of progesterone hormone, which is essential in the first trimester of pregnancy. If a home pregnancy test kit reads positive, it is reacting to an increased level of HCG.

This same hormone is attractive as a weight-loss supplement because it can trigger the body's use of fat for fuel. Oncologists are not all of like mind on the issue of whether HCG used for weight loss has the potential to cause cancer. Some say because HCG is secreted by tumors, it is a marker and should not be confused as the cause of the tumor. Others say we do not yet know all there is to know about HCG and cancer and we should not put additional HCG in the body because hormones are very powerful. In an unrelated move, the United States prohibited the sale of over-the-counter and homeopathic HCG in 2011. The use of it now requires a prescription. See the notes for more information/additional references.[7]

SAMPLE TEST RESULTS

Dear Jenny,

Your HCG Test Result on 07/30/2013 is:

   Index + 4,(51.8 Int. Units)

This is within the POSITIVE range (0 I.U. - negative, 1 to 49 I.U. - doubtful [essentially negative], 50 I.U. and above - positive). A POSITIVE result indicates the presence of Human Chorionic Gonadotropin, a hormone found in the urine of pregnant women. Numerous medical reports show this to be present in the urine of cancer patients. However, the result must be correlated with the medical information (X-rays, CT scans, utrasounds, MRIs, etc.,). A biopsy procedure confirms the diagnosis of cancer. The elevated HCG is possibly coming from remnants (microscopic or otherwise) of the breast cancer. This serves as the baseline result.

Results can go up to 10,000 int. units or more especially in testicular cancer, some uterine cancers (H mole and choriocarcinoma) and germ cell tumor. However, most other cancers have results anywhere from 50 to 80 or 90 IU. The result must be correlated with the medical history together with other pertinent medical information (X-rays, CT scans, ultrasounds, MRIs, etc.). The test cannot determine the stage of the cancer but when it is done on a serial basis, say once a month, one can follow and monitor the progress of the disease.

Wishing you the best of health, I remain.

Sincerely Yours,

                    Efren F. Navarro, MD

Chapter 15

IvyGene®

IvyGene Diagnostics
1201 Cumberland Avenue, Suite B
West Lafayette, IN 47906
844-489-4363
www.IvyGeneLabs.com
info@ivygenelabs.com

THIS CHAPTER IS based on information provided by IvyGene Diagnostics. Please check the IvyGene website for updates.

SUMMARY AND EXPLANATION

"The IvyGene test is a blood test that uses advanced DNA sequencing methods to detect the DNA methylation pattern of circulating tumor DNA (ctDNA) in blood samples."[1] The test will confirm the presence of cancer. It can be used at all stages of disease, even before a tumor is detected. Unlike many genetic tests that analyze the ctDNA for cancer-related mutations, the IvyGene test identifies methylation patterns consistent with cancer's presence. The results include an IvyGene score that reflects the methylation status of target sites at the time of testing. If you want the technical verbiage, "the IvyGene test quantifies a DNA methylation marker within the promoter region of the MYO1G gene that has shown to be consistently elevated when cancer is present."[2]

INTERPRETATION

Results should be considered for each person individually. Increases or decreases in the IvyGene score are reflective of disease progression or regression. Healthy people may have an IvyGene score of less than 10. Scores over 10 or rising scores indicate the presence of cancer and should be investigated further.

HOW TO OBTAIN THE TEST

The test must be prescribed by a physician or clinician. Patients can have their personal physician order the test kit from www.IvyGenelabs.com.

ACCURACY

The IvyGene website reports that "the sensitivity is approximately 86% for patients who have clinically confirmed breast, colon, liver or lung cancer and are not currently undergoing cancer treatment. These numbers are subject to change as the use for the IvyGene test to confirm the presence of cancer for additional cancer types is investigated. The specificity is approximately 88%."[3] See the IvyGene website for additional information.

COST

The cost for the IvyGene test is approximately $400. This does not include the cost of the blood draw or the physician fee.

PROCESS TIME

This is approximately five business days from receipt of the blood sample at the IvyGene lab.

BENEFITS

+ Identifies the presence of cancer
+ Can be used to monitor disease progression or regression
+ Processed with a small blood sample; no biopsy required

LIMITATIONS

+ Does not indicate stage or type of cancer
+ Is not covered by most insurance companies at this time
+ Will not detect brain tumors due to limitations of the blood-brain barrier
+ Cannot identify the location of metastasis of the original cancer

THOUGHTS

This is amazing technology! Here is a blood test that has the ability to detect cancer at an early stage, and it's radiation-free. Research confirms that the methylation defect is a proven method to detect cancer. Be aware that IvyGene is formally validated for breast, colon, liver, and lung cancers. IvyGene is in preliminary testing and data collection for twenty other types of cancer. It plans to add those to the validated list soon. As usual, cancers originating in the brain will not be detected due to the blood-brain barrier. The IvyGene score will be a nice method to assess the success of therapies. Let's find it early and get those scores down with nontoxic integrative intervention. IvyGene rates high on my list! See "Overview of the Science" at www.IvyGenelabs.com for references.

SAMPLE TEST RESULTS

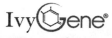

IvyGene®
LABORATORY REPORT

DOCTOR	SAMPLE	PATIENT
SAMPLE DOCTOR 123 Main Street Anytown, USA 12345 Customer Number: (0001)	**IvyGene® Number:** 1234 Unique ID: 5789-IVY Date Received: 1/8/2018 Date of Report: 1/10/2018	**SAMPLE PATIENT** DOB: 7/20/1060 AGE: 48 SEX: F

IvyGene® TEST RESULTS

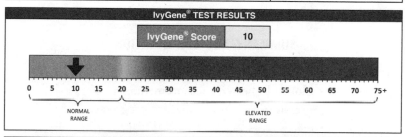

IvyGene® Score   **10**

0 5 10 15 20 25 30 35 40 45 50 55 60 65 70 75+

NORMAL RANGE   ELEVATED RANGE

TEST INFORMATION

The IvyGene® Test measures the methylation status of cell-free DNA extracted from blood samples at target sites within the MYO1G and the TNFAIP8L2 genes. These target sites have been demonstrated to be hypermethylated when certain cancers are present. Test results are reported as a quantitative IvyGene® Score, which indicates the methylation status of the target sites. The IvyGene® Score is calculated as a composite average of cell-free DNA that is methylated at the target sites as a fraction of the total cell-free DNA present.

IvyGene® Score
0-19 = normal range, **20-75+** = elevated range

The IvyGene® Test is an adjunct clinical test that is intended to be based on the independent medical judgement of the ordering physician in conjunction with the patient's complete medical history and the results of standard of care testing. The IvyGene® Test has been validated with four (4) cancer tissues of origin: breast, colon, liver and lung cancers. The presence of other cancer types may also result in an elevated IvyGene® Score. A large-scale clinical trial to demonstrate the efficacy of the IvyGene® Test as a cancer screening test has not been conducted. Cancer screening is not an approved utility of the IvyGene® Test.

The IvyGene® Test was evaluated and its performance characteristics determined by Mor-NuCo Enterprises Inc., a subsidiary of the Laboratory for Advanced Medicine (LAM). Mor-NuCo Enterprises Inc. is CLIA-registered and CAP-accredited to perform high complexity testing. The IvyGene® Test has not been cleared or approved by the FDA. Instead, the IvyGene® Test meets current U.S. Food and Drug Administration (FDA) requirements as a qualified laboratory developed test (LDT).

COMMENTS

This result has been reviewed and approved by Laboratory Director: David J. Taggart, PhD NRCC

Date of Review: 1/10/2018

Mor-NuCo Enterprises Inc. 1201 Cumberland Ave. Suite B, West Lafayette, IN 47906
P. 765-464-1583 Fax. 765-464-8769 Website: Ivygenelabs.com   Report Form v1.0

Chapter 16

Nagalase Test

Health Diagnostics and Research Institute (HDRI)
540 Bordentown Avenue, Suite 2300
South Amboy, NJ 08879
Phone: 732-721-1234
Fax: 732-525-3288
www.hdri-usa.com
info@hdri-usa.com

THIS CHAPTER IS based on information obtained from www.hdri-usa
.com and research done by the author. Please check the Health Diagnostics and Research Institute website for updates.

SUMMARY AND EXPLANATION

The test measures the activity of the enzyme a-N-acetylgalactosaminidase (nagalase) in the blood. Repeated measurements can be used to assess tumor burden, aggressiveness, clinical disease progression, and response to therapy.

Nagalase is a specific marker secreted only by cancer cells, certain pathogenic bacteria, and viruses (HIV, hepatitis B, hepatitis C, influenza, herpes, Epstein-Barr virus, and others). Nagalase is used by these invaders to ensure their survival by incapacitating the immune system. Nagalase is also secreted by the placenta during pregnancy to protect the fetus from being attacked as "non-self" by the mother's immune system. The more cancers grow, the more nagalase they secrete into the bloodstream. In response to effective treatment, nagalase levels go down as the cancer or infection is being effectively destroyed. Any treatment that lowers the number of cancer cells or viral particles will lower nagalase levels. For example, nagalase levels will drop after surgery when all, or a portion, of a tumor has been removed.

Chemotherapy and radiation also reduce nagalase levels. However, as you begin treatment, there may be an initial spike in the levels. As treatment continues, the levels should decrease. Studies show that nagalase decreased to near tumor-free control levels one day after surgical removal of primary tumors from cancer patients, suggesting the half-life of nagalase is approximately twenty-four hours. That short half-life makes nagalase an extremely valuable tumor marker to measure prognosis of the disease during various therapies.[1]

Patients with a wide variety of cancers, including prostate, breast, uterine, ovarian, colon, lung, esophageal, stomach, liver, pancreatic, kidney, bladder, and testicular cancer; mesothelioma; melanoma; fibrosarcoma; glioblastoma; neuroblastoma; and various leukemias, have been found to have increased nagalase activity in their blood. It is believed all cancers secrete nagalase; however, some types of tumors secrete more than others based upon the amount of biofilm coating present. It also "appears the secretory capacity of individual tumor tissue varies among tumor types, depending upon tumor size, staging, and the degree of malignancy or invasiveness."[2] Therefore it is important to know the tissue of origin to make the best use of this test as a predictive marker, as well as a test of therapeutic efficacy.

The test may be ordered before, during, and after therapies have begun. Obtaining a baseline value before therapy begins is best, followed by a series of tests to measure how an individual tumor is responding to treatment. A single test provides little actionable information for physicians.

"Studies correlating nagalase levels with tumor burden suggest that the measurement of this enzyme can diagnose the presence of cancerous lesions" sooner than other diagnostic means such as CT and PET scans.[3]

Cancer patients with high levels of nagalase have been treated with the administration of a naturally occurring protein called GcMAF—the short name for a vitamin D cofactor called "globulin component macrophage activating factor" or the technical name "group-specific component macrophage activating factor." GcMAF is the protein the body makes to activate anticancer activity in immune cells called macrophages (which means "big eaters"). However, cancer is clever. In its effort to survive and protect itself from being eaten by the macrophages, cancer cells ramp up their nagalase production in order to disable GcMAF, thus reducing the activation of the macrophages. Therefore, by giving the body more GcMAF, the immune system is better able to fight the cancer.[4]

Life Extension Foundation is studying the effects of GcMAF when used with dichloroacetate (DCA). "GcMAF has demonstrated some complete remissions on its own in patients who participated in three separate trials on breast, prostate, and colorectal cancer. The mechanism of action involves resupplying the Gc protein (also known as vitamin D binding protein), which cancer cells destroy by secreting an abundance of the enzyme nagalase. GcMAF restores the deficiency, which is a critical component in activating the macrophages, the immune system's cancer scavengers."[5] Vitamin

D has a powerful antitumor effect, which drives cancer cells to produce the enzyme nagalase in order to prevent vitamin D from binding to cancer cells. GcMAF disables the ability of cancer cells to shield against vitamin D attachment, thus improving its cancer-killing capabilities.

INTERPRETATION

Normal nagalase levels are considered to be less than 0.9 nmol/min/mg; however, out of an abundance of caution, many consider 0.65 nmol/min/mg a more appropriate upper limit of normal. Levels greater than 4 are regularly found in cancer patients as well as in patients with chronic fatigue syndrome or Lyme disease. Levels greater than 0.9 and less than 3 are commonly found in autistic children as well as in patients infected with various viruses.[6]

Regular nagalase testing can be useful as often as weekly in the early stages of treatment to measure the effectiveness of the therapy. Longer testing intervals can then be used to monitor progress once the most effective treatment is determined. Measuring serum nagalase levels is one way your doctor can help to answer your question "Is my treatment working?"

HOW TO OBTAIN THE TEST

The test must be ordered by a physician, who will need to contact HDRI Lab to order test kits at www.hdri-usa.com.

COST

The cost is $100 to the Lab. Additional physician fees may apply.

PROCESS TIME

Test results will be reported to your physician in approximately ten to fourteen days from the receipt of the sample.

BENEFITS

Nagalase activity is directly proportional to macrophage activation and is an excellent surrogate marker of immune response. Levels can be correlated to the degree of viable tumor burden when the tissue of origin is known.

Nagalase blood levels provide the basis for a sensitive test for monitoring the effectiveness of therapy in cancer. Your physician or oncologist can use the results to obtain a better understanding of the therapy's effectiveness and to fine-tune your treatment as it proceeds.

Because of the short half-life of nagalase, this test method is suitable

for monitoring various types of therapies and can be used by your doctor
to determine which therapy is working best for you. It can also be used
to determine when to switch or add new therapies to enhance effectiveness since cancers frequently become resistant to a particular treatment.[7]

If cancer is ruled out with other testing, the cause of a high nagalase
level can be further investigated with testing for viruses or pathogenic
bacteria.

LIMITATIONS

The test values may be affected by certain drugs used within the five
days preceding blood draw. Therefore the use of certain drugs, GcMAF,
vitamin D, and/or medical cannabis must be indicated on the question-
naire submitted with the requisition form.

This test does not identify the specific tissue of origin (organ) or the site
of the primary cancer or any metastases. Either pregnancy or an infection
can increase nagalase levels leading to a false positive. Autistic children
may have elevated levels of nagalase—it may not indicate the presence of
cancer.

THOUGHTS

After studying the benefits of this simple blood test, I have to say that it's
a good tool for assessing the amount of immune suppression while providing an indicator of therapy effectiveness. Testing every few months will
provide an overall view of your progress. See the notes for more informa-
tion/additional references.[8]

Chapter 17

OralID™

Forward Science
10401 Greenbough, Suite 100
Stafford, TX 77477
855-696-7254
https://forwardscience.com/oralid/

THIS CHAPTER IS based on information provided by Forward Science. Check the Forward Science website for updates.

SUMMARY AND EXPLANATION

Fluorescence technology is an optical light-based technology. Your dentist shines a blue light on your tongue, and on the oral mucosa inside your mouth to identify oral cancer, precancer, and other abnormal lesions that may not be apparent to the naked eye.[1]

If indicated, your dentist can collect a specimen for a cytology test and send it to a laboratory for further examination.

INTERPRETATION

During the fluorescence assessment the clinician is looking for dark lesions. If areas appear dark or abnormal, the area should be reassessed within two weeks. Any oral trauma sustained from extreme hot or cold foods or mechanical damage from chewing should have healed by that time.

If the lesion is still present after a two-week follow-up and continues to exhibit a loss of fluorescence, a gentle swab of the area is done to collect cells for a liquid-based Cytology Test (CytID). This is a simple test where the cells are sent to an oral pathologist to determine what is happening at the cellular level. Results take approximately one week. The results will be reported as negative (normal), atypical (suggestive of dysplasia), or malignancy. Additional notes on other conditions such as presence of fungus, bacteria, and leukoplakia are included. HPV testing is also available upon request.

HOW TO OBTAIN THE TEST

Simply ask your doctor or dentist if he or she offers oral-cancer screening with fluorescence technology.

ACCURACY

Forty-three percent of clinical lesions assessed by dentists with the naked eye are diagnosed incorrectly.[2] Fluorescence technology greatly improves this percentage.

COST

Some dental offices do not charge for the screening exam, and others may charge as much as $95. The cost is sometimes covered by dental insurance using code D0431. If a cytology test is required, the patient is billed $126.

PROCESS TIME

The initial screening exam is completed in about two minutes. If there is an area of suspicion, a few cells will be gently collected and sent to the lab for oral pathology analysis. These results take about one week.

BENEFITS

- The test is noninvasive, quick, and painless.
- It's an FDA-approved device.

LIMITATIONS

If you have burned your mouth with hot food or bitten your tongue while chewing, these areas will need to heal before you take the test, as they would appear suspicious.

THOUGHTS

I personally have several friends who have been diagnosed with oral cancer. Unfortunately their cancers were not caught early, and they dealt with multiple surgeries and radiation sessions. These treatments resulted in bone, tissue, and tooth loss—not to mention the loss of the function of their salivary glands. If your dentist does not offer this valuable screening service, I suggest you find one who does. Close to 70 percent of oral cancers are being found in the late stages (III and IV).[3] I have been told a cancer hospital in Houston diagnoses approximately ten cases of oral squamous cell HPV-related cancers per day. We can do better!

See the notes for more information and additional references.[4]

Chapter 18

Papanicolaou (Pap) and Human Papillomavirus (HPV)

THE NATIONAL CANCER Institute estimates 12,820 new cases of cervical/uterine cancer and 4,210 related deaths in 2017.[1] Many of these cases occur among women who are rarely or never screened for cancer. When cervical cancer is found early, it is highly treatable and survivable.

SUMMARY AND EXPLANATION

The Papanicolaou (Pap) test is used to detect cell changes on the cervix that might become cancerous if not treated, and to screen for existing cervical cancer. The Pap test can also screen for noncancerous conditions, such as infections and inflammation. Pap tests are the most effective method for early detection of abnormal cervical cell changes.[2]

Human papillomavirus (HPV) is a virus responsible for almost all cases of cervical cancer. There are about twelve identified types of high-risk HPV. HPV testing is used to look for the presence of viral DNA or RNA from high-risk HPV types in cervical cells. An infection from HPV is sexually transmitted and can also cause anal, vaginal, vulvar, penile, and oropharyngeal cancers.[3]

The Pap test and HPV test can be done at the same time. During a pelvic examination the doctor or nurse uses a small brush to collect a few cells from the cervix for testing. This takes only a few seconds. The collected cells are sent to a laboratory for analysis.

HPV infections are very common and are usually suppressed by the immune system within one to two years without causing cancer. The National Cancer Institute reports it can take ten to twenty years or more for a persistent infection with a high-risk HPV type to develop cancer.[4]

Current guidelines are as follows:

+ Women should have a Pap test every three years beginning at age twenty-one.

+ Women ages thirty to sixty-five should have Pap and HPV testing every five years or a Pap test alone every three years.

+ Women with risk factors may need more-frequent screening or continue screening beyond age sixty-five.

+ Women who have had the HPV vaccine still need regular screening.

+ Women who have had a hysterectomy may still need to be screened.[5]

If cellular changes are detected on the Pap test, often treatment can be done to prevent cervical cancer.

Information on the National Breast and Cervical Cancer Early Detection Program is available at www.cdc.gov/cancer/nbccedp.

INTERPRETATION

"Normal" or "negative" results of a Pap test mean there were no signs of cervical cancer, precancer, or significant abnormalities found. If your Pap test result is reported as anything other than normal or negative, it means some type of abnormality was found, such as abnormal tissue possibly related to an HPV infection or cervical cancer. An abnormality will not always indicate cervical cancer. However, the presence of abnormal cells can increase your risk of developing cervical cancer in the future. Many abnormalities will go away by themselves. Because of this some women will have a repeat Pap test in three to six months. You should talk with your physician about your results and what you should do next. Your physician may recommend further testing and/or treatment to reduce the chance of developing cervical cancer.[6]

The NCI uses the Bethesda system of classifying Pap tests. Lab specialists use the Bethesda system to report lab results to doctors. The report lets your doctor know if the cells were normal or abnormal or if there was an infection present. Abnormal results are put in categories, or typed, based on the severity of the problem:

+ "Cells that show minor changes but the cause is unknown may be typed as ASC-US or ASC-H. ASC-US stands for atypical squamous cells of undetermined significance. ASC-H stands for atypical squamous cells that cannot exclude high-grade squamous intraepithelial lesion.

+ Cells that show definite minor changes but aren't likely to become cancer may be typed as LSIL. It stands for low-grade squamous intraepithelial lesions.

+ Cell changes that are more severe and are more likely to become cancer may be typed as HSIL or AGC. HSIL stands for high-grade squamous intraepithelial lesions. AGC stands for atypical glandular cells."[7]

Follow-up screening options may include:

+ Repeat Pap tests

+ Colposcopy—Your physician will examine your cervix with a magnifying instrument.

+ Biopsy or endocervical curettage—a procedure in which a spoon-shaped instrument is used to scrape the mucous membrane of the passageway between the cervix and uterus, obtaining a small tissue sample, which is then sent to a pathology lab to be examined for abnormal cells[8]

If treatment is necessary, a surgical excision procedure, cryotherapy (freezing of the cells), or laser therapy may be done to remove or destroy the abnormal tissue and reduce the risk of cancer.[9] Most women with cervical cell changes or preinvasive cancer have no symptoms. Screening tests, therefore, are very important. The HPV test is reported as "negative" or "positive."

HOW TO OBTAIN THE TEST

Pap and HPV tests are available at doctors' offices, medical clinics, and local health departments.

Do not do the following for twenty-four hours before the test: douche, have intercourse, take a bath, or use tampons. Showers are fine. Avoid scheduling your Pap test during your period (menstruation). Blood may make the Pap smear results less accurate. Tell your doctor if you might be pregnant.

A Pap test can be part of a routine gynecologic exam. During the exam a sample of cells from the cervix are collected. To perform a Pap or HVP test, your doctor will use a swab or small brush "to collect samples of cervical cells from different areas of your cervix. These cells are sent to a laboratory where a technician examines them under a microscope for abnormalities. This procedure is sometimes referred to as a 'Pap smear' because the cells obtained are 'smeared' onto a glass slide to be examined under a microscope."[10]

ACCURACY

No test is 100 percent accurate. It is possible for the Pap test to miss the presence of cancer cells. However, if abnormal cells are missed on one test, they will likely be found during the next test. Generally about 10 percent of Pap tests have abnormal results; however, only about 0.1 percent of the women who have abnormal results actually have cancer. Most of the time abnormal cells are not likely to progress to cancer or are a result of benign conditions, such as natural post-menopausal cell changes.[11]

COST

There are two costs involved in having a Pap and/or HPV test: the consultation with the doctor or nurse, and the Pap/HPV lab fee. Pap and HPV costs can vary based on the doctor. The average rate can range from $50–$250 without insurance for the tests and exam. Independently the HPV test costs approximately $80–$100 compared with $20–$40 for the Pap test. Many insurance plans cover a Pap and HPV test with an annual exam. Check with your provider for coverage and deductibles.

Medicare Part B covers Pap tests and pelvic exams once every twenty-four months for all women. As part of the exam, women at high risk for cervical or vaginal cancer, or who are of childbearing age with an abnormal Pap test in the past thirty-six months, are eligible for screening tests once every twelve months. Most states also provide coverage for testing through their Medicaid programs for low-income women.

The National Breast and Cervical Cancer Early Detection Program (NBCCEDP) provides free or low-cost mammograms and Pap tests to low-income women with little or no health insurance. Contact them through www.cdc.gov/cancer/nbccedp.

PROCESS TIME

Test results are usually reported in two to three weeks.

BENEFITS

Pap tests done at regular intervals are very effective at detecting cervical cell changes before the changes become cancerous. Combining Pap and HPV testing improves detection rates.

LIMITATIONS

False positives can lead to overtreatment of cervical cell changes that would never become cancerous. Routine screening is necessary due to the possibility of false negatives.

THOUGHTS

The Pap smear has been in use since the 1940s to detect uterine and cervical cancer. Unlike mammograms and PSA screening tests, the Pap test has not been called into question as being plagued with a high rate of false results or leading to too much unnecessary intervention. It is also free of radiation, dyes, or invasive procedures—it is simple. It is still considered a gold standard for cancer screening.

Regular Pap and HPV tests are essential since they can spot abnormalities before they turn into cancer. Pap screening programs are credited with the decline in the incidence of cervical cancer over the past fifty years. To protect your health, follow your doctor's recommendations regarding how often you should get tested. Cervical changes caught early can be easily treated and prevent the pain and expense of a late-stage diagnosis. A Pap and/or HPV test can save your life.

See the notes for more information and additional references.[12]

Chapter 19

Prostate Health Index

Innovative Diagnostic Laboratory
8751 Park Central Drive, Suite 200
Richmond, VA 23227
855-420-7140
https://www.myinnovativelab.com/prostate-cancer
customerservice@myinnovativelab.com

THIS CHAPTER IS based on information provided by Innovative Diagnostic Laboratory and research done by the author. Check the Innovative Diagnostic Laboratory website for updates.

SUMMARY AND EXPLANATION

The Prostate Health Index offers an alternative to traditional PSA tests. History records that "over 1 million US men per year have prostate biopsies due to elevated PSA, but only around 25% actually have cancer."[1] Prostate-specific antigen (PSA) testing is the most common prostate cancer screening method. Innovative Diagnostic Laboratory's website notes:

> Prostate cancer causes changes to the prostate gland structure that can lead to increased "leakage" of PSA into the bloodstream. But increased PSA levels can also be caused by non-cancerous conditions such as enlargement of the prostate (known as benign prostatic hyperplasia, or BPH). This means that PSA testing often suggests that cancer is present when there is none. It also detects a high number of slow-growing tumors that otherwise may persist for many years with no ill effects.... As a result, PSA-based prostate cancer screening subjects many men to needless medical procedures.... Prostate biopsies can have complications such as fever, infection, bleeding, urinary problems, and pain.... Overtreatment due to prostate cancer misdiagnosis often causes lasting damage, including erectile dysfunction, urinary or bowel incontinence, and serious surgical complications.[2]

The Prostate Health Index measures three different types of PSA and provides a more accurate assessment of prostate cancer risk than standard

PSA tests. Prostate Health Index values are associated with increased probability of prostate cancer and more aggressive disease. They can also help differentiate prostate cancer from benign conditions, reducing the need for unnecessary biopsies.[3] The test includes the [-2]proPSA (p2PSA), which is a precursor of standard PSA.

INTERPRETATION

Results are reported on a predetermined scale. The physician will provide the interpretation.

HOW TO OBTAIN THE TEST

The test must be prescribed by a physician or clinician. Test kits can be obtained by contacting the lab.

ACCURACY

The Prostate Health Index (PHI) is three times more specific in detecting prostate cancer than PSA and free PSA alone.[4]

COST

Innovative Diagnostic Laboratory will verify possible insurance or Medicare coverage. The cash price is approximately $150. This does not include the cost of the blood draw or the physician fee.

PROCESS TIME

Results take about ten days from receipt of the test at the lab. Results will be sent directly to the ordering health care provider.

BENEFITS

+ Is processed with a blood sample
+ Is noninvasive
+ Provides early detection
+ May aid in ruling out the need for a biopsy
+ Provides more information than the standard PSA test

LIMITATIONS

+ Does not provide the stage of cancer

THOUGHTS

Prostate cancer is often asymptomatic in its early stages and progresses slowly. However, aggressive forms of prostate cancer can metastasize and be life-threatening. Early detection is important. Men are settling for standard PSA screenings. Help me spread the word about this test. Another company is also offering this test.[5] See www.myinnovativelab.com/scientific-papers/ for references.

SAMPLE TEST RESULTS

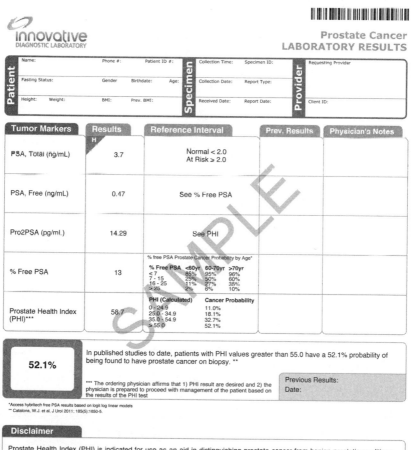

Chapter 20

Research Genetic Cancer Center Lab Tests

RGCC-USA LLC
3105 Main Street
Rowlett, TX 75088
214-299-9449
https://rgcc-group.com/
info@rgccusa.com

THIS CHAPTER IS based on information provided by Research Genetic Cancer Center (RGCC). Check the RGCC website for updates.

SUMMARY AND EXPLANATION

Research Genetic Cancer Center (RGCC) is a world-class laboratory specializing in cancer genetics and circulating tumor stem cell counts. The lab comprises advanced and innovative technologies focusing on molecular oncology. It offers several different tests used for:

+ The early detection and diagnosis of new cancers (years before most cancers would be detected)

+ Monitoring of existing cancers

+ Prognosis—providing information about the risk of recurrence of a current or previous cancer

+ Development of a personalized cancer treatment plan geared to achieve the best treatment outcome

+ Blending the very best of alternative and traditional therapies

The RGCC lab has a very sensitive test for isolating and counting circulating tumor cells (CTCs)—cancer cells that have broken away from the primary tumor and entered the bloodstream—in a blood sample.

Once malignant tumor stem cells are circulating freely in the body, they have the potential to generate metastatic disease. RGCC has proprietary technology to remove CTCs from a blood sample for further testing in the laboratory. This puts each individual's own isolated cancer cells in direct contact with the tested substances, not just a few cells from biopsied material. The lab also evaluates seventy-two tumor-related genetic markers on the tumor cells to predict outcomes of treatments and prognosis. RGCC can provide the following information:

+ A count of circulating tumor cells and cancer stem cells present in the blood, which may indicate tumor burden

+ Identification of the specific primary tumor site

+ Chemosensitivity testing—identification of chemotherapy drugs that are the most effective at attacking a person's individual cancer cells, as well as chemo resistance of a person's cancer cells

+ Assessment of natural substances for potency against the patient's CTCs and CSCs. Mechanisms of action and percentages of effectiveness are included.

+ Identification of immunity factors and metastatic risk

+ Blood tests for all cancers with CTCs. Brain and central nervous system cancers require a tissue sample.

+ Data on how an individual will react to specific chemotherapy agents. People's genetic makeup determines whether they are "accumulators" or "rapid metabolizers" of certain drugs. This can play a critical role in determining how effective a specific drug treatment is likely to be and how significant the side effects will be.

+ Testing of fifty-three chemotherapeutic agents and four resistance factors

+ Identification of specific markers on the tumor cells to assist the physician in forming a targeted approach.[1]

RGCC International was established in 2004 by Ioannis Papasotiriou, MD, PhD. Dr. Papasotiriou worked in the department of Experimental Physiology and Biochemistry in the Medical School of Thessaloniki in Greece. RGCC is a growing, innovative, and pioneering chemosensitivity/chemoresistance testing company. They have branches and representatives all over the world. The company's headquarters are in Switzerland; its lab is in Northern Greece. Branch offices are in locations such as the United States, the United Kingdom, Germany, and Cyprus.

The following tests are available:

aCGH (array comparative genomic hybridization)

The aCGH test "focuses on identification of chromosomal abnormalities, either deletions or amplifications." It aids in the identification of the primary origin of the cancer with 90 percent-plus accuracy. In 10–15 percent of cases no absolute primary site will be found. It is used when the type of cancer is unknown. For example, you can find out if the cells are coming from the colon, pancreas, lung, or other tissue. Results take longer than the other tests—approximately three to four weeks.[2]

Oncocount RGCC

This test "provides information on the presence and the concentration of circulating tumor cells (CTCs). It enumerates only the progenitor cells that are relevant to potent relapse and recurrence of the disease." (These are CD44 and CD133 for solid tumors, CD34 for blood-type cancers.)[3] It is used for follow-up and as a screening test.

Oncotrace RGCC

Oncotrace provides information about the presence of CTCs, their concentration, and their phenotype. It includes sixteen non-hematological markers and five hematological markers. It is used for patients with diagnosed cancer and for those in whom cancer is highly suspected.[4]

Oncotrail RGCC

Oncotrail tests for breast, colon, GI, lung, melanoma, prostate, and sarcoma cancers. It provides information about the presence of CTCs, their concentration, and their phenotype. "This test includes only markers relevant for a specific type of malignancy." It is used for follow-up and control.[5]

Onconomics RGCC

This test provides information about the efficacy of specific drugs on cancer cells. The test incorporates two procedures, the epigenetic analysis and viability assays.[6] Testing includes cytotoxic drugs and targeted therapies (MOAB and SMWM). New drugs are added periodically. Approximately fifty-three cytotoxic drugs are tested, as well as four resistance markers, sixty monoclonal antibodies/small molecules that inhibit specific targets, seventy-three tumor-related genes (analyzed for mutations), and seven markers. No natural substances are tested. As of 2018 the list is:

Cytotoxic drugs
Alkylating agents

- ACNU (nimustine)
- altretamine (Hexalen)
- BCNU (carmustine)
- bendamustine (Treanda)
- bleomycin (Blenoxane)
- carboplatin (Paraplatin)
- CCNU (lomustine)
- chlorambucil (Leukeran)
- cisplatin (Platinol)
- cyclophosphamide (Cytoxan)
- dacarbazine (DTIC)
- estramustine (Emcyt)
- hydroxyurea (Droxia, Hydrea)
- ifosfamide (Ifex)
- melphalan (Alkeran)
- mitomycin (mitomycin C)
- nedaplatin (Aqupla)
- oxaliplatin (Eloxatin)
- procarbazine (Matulane)
- temozolomide (Temodar)
- treosulfan
- trofosfamide (Ixoten)

Epothilones
- ixabepilone (Ixempra)

Inhibitors of topoisomerase I
- CPT11 (irinotecan, Camptosar)
- gimatecan
- topotecan (Hycamtin)

Inhibitors of topoisomerase II

- amrubicin hydrochloride (Calsed)
- dactinomycin (Cosmegen)
- daunorubicin (Cerubidine)
- doxorubicin (Adriamycin)
- epirubicin (Pharmorubicin)
- etoposide (VePesid)
- idarubicin (Idamycin)
- liposomal doxorubicin (Doxil)
- mitoxantrone (Novantrone)

Nucleus spindle stabilizer I

- Abraxane (nab-paclitaxel)
- cabazitaxel (Jevtana)
- docetaxel (Taxotere)
- eribulin (Halaven)
- paclitaxel (Taxol)

Nucleus spindle stabilizer II

+ vinblastine (Velban)
+ vincristine (Oncovin)
+ vinorelbine (Navelbine)

Nucleoside analogues

+ 5FU (5-fluorouracil, Adrucil)
+ capecitabine (Xeloda)
+ cytarabine (cytosine arabinoside, Cytosar-U)
+ fludarabine (Fludara)

+ FUDR (floxuridine)
+ gemcitabine (Gemzar)
+ MTX (methotrexate)
+ pemetrexed (Alimta)
+ raltitrexed (Tomudex)
+ UFT (uracil/tegafur)[7]

Resistance markers

+ MDR1
+ MRP
+ LRP
+ GST

Monoclonal antibodies

+ 5-azacytidine (Vidaza)
+ abiraterone (Zytiga)
+ afatinib (Gilotrif)
+ alemtuzumab (Campath)
+ anastrozole (Arimidex)
+ antiandrogen goserelin
+ atezolizumab (Tecentriq)
+ avelumab (Bavencio)
+ axitinib (Inlyta)
+ bevacizumab (Avastin)
+ bortezomib (Velcade)
+ brentuximab vedotin (Adcetris)
+ catumaxomab (Removab)

+ cetuximab (Erbitux)
+ crizotinib (Xalkori)
+ dabrafenib (Tafinlar)
+ dasatinib (Sprycel)
+ erlotinib (Tarceva)
+ everolimus/temsirolimus (Afinitor, Zortess/Torisel)
+ exemestane (Aromasin)
+ fulvestrant (Faslodex)
+ gefitinib (Iressa)
+ gemtuzumab (Mylotarg)
+ goserelin (Zoladex)
+ ibritumomab (Zevalin)
+ imatinib mesylate (Gleevec)

+ ipilimumab (Yervoy)
+ lapatinib (Tykerb)
+ leuprolide (Eligard, Lupron Depot)
+ nilotinib (Tasigna)
+ nintedanib (Ofev)
+ niraparib (Zejula)
+ nivolumab (Opdivo)
+ octreotide (Sandostatin)
+ ofatumumab (Arzerra)
+ olaparib (AZD-2281)
+ osimertinib (Tagrisso)
+ palbociclib (Ibrance)
+ panitumumab (Vectibix)
+ pazopanib (Votrient)
+ pembrolizumab (Keytruda)
+ pertuzumab (Perjeta)
+ ponatinib (Iclusig)

+ ramucirumab (Cyramza)
+ regorafenib (Stivarga)
+ rituximab (Rituxan)
+ ruxolitinib (Jakafi)
+ semaxanib (SU5416)
+ sorafenib (Nexavar)
+ sunitinib (Sutent)
+ tamoxifen (Nolvadex)
+ tositumomab (Bexxar)
+ trabectedin (Yondelis)
+ trametinib (Mekinist)
+ transtuzumab (Herceptin)
+ vandetanib (Caprelsa)
+ veliparib (ABT-888)
+ vemurafenib (Zelboraf)
+ vorinostat (Zolinza)
+ ziv-aflibercept (Zaltrap)

Tumor-related genes

Growth factors and proliferation stimuli

+ 5-LOX
+ ALK
+ BCR-ABL
+ CD117 (c-kit)
+ c-erb-B1
+ c-erb-B2
+ c-fos
+ c-jun
+ COX-2
+ EGF
+ EML4-ALK

+ estrogen receptor
+ IGF-1R
+ IGF-2R
+ IkB (a, b, c)
+ JAK1/2
+ mTOR
+ NFkB
+ NPM-ALK
+ NR3C4-B
+ p180
+ progesterone receptor

* NR3C4-A
* PTEN
* RAS/RAF/MEK/ERK

* RET
* SS-R

Self-repair resistance

* 06-methyl-DNA-tran.
* CXCL12
* CXCR4
* CXCR12
* DNA demethylase
* DNA methyltransferase 1
* gamma GC
* HAT

* HDAC
* histone deacetylase-dipeptide
* HSP27
* HSP72
* HSP90
* TGF-b

Angiogenesis

* ANG1
* ANG2
* FGF

* PDGF
* VEGF

Cell cycle regulation and immortalization/apoptosis

* BAX
* Bcl-2
* CD95 (FasR)
* CDC6
* E2F1

* hTERT
* p16
* p27
* p53

Angiogenesis-metastases

* 67LR
* c-MET
* KISS-1R

* MMP
* nm23

Drug metabolisms and targets

- CES1/2 (carboxylesterase)
- CYPB1
- DHFR
- DPD
- ERCC1
- GARFT
- NP

- ribonucleoside reductase
- RRM1
- SHMT
- TP
- TS
- UP

Markers

- CD20
- CD33
- CD52
- EpCAM

- PD-1
- PD-L1
- PD-L2[8]

Onconomics Extracts

This test "provides information about the efficacy of natural biological substances or extracts on cancer cells. The assessment is based on three methods: the direct cytotoxic effect, stimulation of the immune system and the inhibition of proliferative signals in the cancer cells."[9] New substances are added periodically. As of 2018 the fifty-three natural substances tested on every patient are:

- *Agaricus blazei* Murill
- alpha lipoic acid
- amygdalin (B17)
- Angiostop
- apigenin
- Aromat8-PN
- Artecin
- artesunate
- ascorbic acid
- Avemar pulvis

- Bio D Mulsion or NuMedica Micellized D3
- Boswellia serrata
- Breastin
- butyric acid
- C-Statin
- CoQ10
- Cordyceps sinensis
- curcumin (turmeric)
- DCA (dichloroacetate)
- DDG (2-deoxy d-glucose)

- doxycycline
- frankincense
- fucoidan
- GcMAF (Big Harmony)
- GcMAF (Big Harmony III)
- genistein
- indole-3-carbinol
- lycopene
- melatonin
- mistletoe
- Mito Booster
- Mito Booster II
- Mitochondrien Formular
- naltrexone
- OnKobel-Pro
- oxaloacetate (CRONaxal)
- pawpaw

- Poly-MVA
- Polyphenole CA
- Polyphenole CA III
- pure quercetin
- quercetin
- resveratrol
- Ribraxx
- salicinium
- salvestrol
- Super Artemisinin
- theaflavin
- Thymex
- Ukrain
- VascuStatin
- Virxcan
- Vitanox[10]

Results give the percentage of effectiveness for each substance. Substances are added yearly. See the website https://rgcc-group.com for the most recently tested agents.

Onconomics Plus RGCC

This test includes everything in the Onconomics and the Onconomics Extracts test. It is RGCC's most extensive test and is used to develop a personalized care plan.

Immune-Frame

This test "uses specific cellular markers and cytokine production to detect the type or types of cells responsible for the activation or repression of the immune system of a patient."[11] It provides a detailed report on the status of immune function.

Metastat

This test is a collection of specific markers. These markers on the CTCs point out the potential organ for relapse. This test evaluates cells of the primary tumor with ability to metastasize. The cells express specific genes and proteins according to the organ where a metastasis is most likely to occur. Genetic expression is evaluated.[12]

ChemoSNiP

This test uses pharmacogenomics, the science of examining "inherited variations in genes that dictate drug response." This test "explores the ways these variations can predict whether a patient will have a good response to a drug, a bad response to a drug, or no response at all."[13]

INTERPRETATION

Results are presented in a written report your doctor can use to guide your treatment options and choices. This test requires an experienced clinician to fully interpret the results. To make the results easier to understand, they are displayed in graph form.

If the submitted blood sample is negative for CTCs, no further testing can be done. The patient has a good prognosis, as no cancer cells were detected.

HOW TO OBTAIN THE TEST

+ Call the RGCC-USA branch office at 214-299-9449 to locate a registered physician in your area. Go to www.cancerteamusa.net, and select "Doctor Locator." (You will get a more complete list if you call, as all physicians may not be included in the directory.)

+ More information and sample tests can be located at https://rgcc-group.com. Email info@rgccusa.com with questions.

+ Payments can be made online. The company accepts credit cards, and payments are made in euros. The euro-to-dollar conversion rate is calculated at the time of payment.

+ RGCC recommends patients with active CTCs retest with an Oncocount every three to six months to monitor disease and effectiveness of treatment. Check with your ordering physician for specific recommendations.

SAMPLE TEST RESULTS

See https://rgcc-group.com for a complete display of all their test results.

Oncotrace RGCC®:

ONCOTRACE R.G.C.C. ®   1 / 1

R.G.C.C. - RESEARCH GENETIC CANCER CENTRE S.A.

Florina, __/__/____

Dear Colleague,

We send you the results from the analysis on a patient Mr.Ms._____ suffering from _____carcinoma stage ___. The sample that was sent to us for analysis was a sample of __ml of whole blood that contained EDTA-Ca as anti-coagulant, and packed with an ice pack.
In our laboratory we made the following:

- We isolated the malignant cells using Oncoquick with a membrane that isolates malignant cells from normal cells after centrifugation and positive and negative selection using multiple cell markers.

The results during the isolation procedure are presented below:

Table of markers:

CD45 positive cells (Hematologic origin cells)		CD45 negative cells (non Hematologic origin)	
CD15	NEGATIVE	CD34	NEGATIVE
CD30	NEGATIVE	CD99	NEGATIVE
BCR-ABL	NEGATIVE	EpCam	POSITIVE
CD34	NEGATIVE	VHL mut	Dim_POSITIVE
CD19	NEGATIVE	CD133	POSITIVE
		CD44	NEGATIVE
		Nanog	POSITIVE
		OKT-4	Dim_POSITIVE
		Sox-2	POSITIVE
		PSMA	NEGATIVE
		c-MET	POSITIVE
		CD31	NEGATIVE
		CD19	NEGATIVE
		MUC-1	NEGATIVE
		CD63	NEGATIVE
		panCK	Dim_POSITIVE

Index of marker: CD45: Hematologic origin cell marker, **BCR-ABL, CD30:** hematologic malignancy marker, **CD133, Sox-2, OKT-4, Nanog, CD44:** tumor stem cell marker, **CD15:** hematological malignancy marker, **CD19 (CD45 negative cells – Non Hematologic origin cells):** hematological malignancy, **CD19 (CD45 positive cells – Hematologic origin cells):** lung neuroendocrine malignancy, **CD31:** endothelial cell membrane antigen, **CD34:** hematological stem cell and blast cell marker, epithelioid sarcoma marker, **CD63:** melanoma cell marker, **CD99:** sarcoma marker, **EpCam:** epithelial origin marker, **MUC-I:** Breast cancer antigen, **PSMA:** prostate specific cancer stem cell membrane antigen, **VHL mut:** renal carcinoma marker, **c-MET:** membrane antigen that regulates the mesenchymal to epithelial transition, **panCK:** epithelial origin cell marker.

The final results after the isolation procedure are presented below: We notice that after isolation procedure there are remaining malignant cells. The concentration of these cells was isolated ___cells/ml, SD +/- 0.3cells.

Sincerely,

Ioannis Papasotiriou M.D., PhD
Head of molecular medicine dpt of
R.G.C.C.-RESEARCH GENETIC CANCER CENTRE S.A.

Index of circulating cells number: (If Over limit: Advanced or Progression of Disease, If Less than limit: Early disease or disease is responding to a treatment plan).
Breast cancer: < 5cells /7.5ml , Prostate cancer < 20cells/ml , Sarcoma: <15cell/6.5ml, Colon cancer: <5cells/ml, Lung cancer (Lc=0, r=0.99): <10cell/ml. All cancer types other than those listed above should be <5 cells/ml.

*This test will NOT DETECT cancers of the brain or other cancers that have been "encapsulated" by the body, not releasing circulating tumor or stem cells (CTC, CSC) into the blood stream or if any of these cells are dormant. We still recommend the use of biopsy, blood markers and/or various scans with this test when cancer is suspected or known to exist.No test is 100% accurate.

Mr./Ms.
Industrial Area of Florina, GR 53100 – Florina, Greece
Tel.: +30 23850 41950, 41951, 41960, 41961, Fax.: +30 23850 41931
Website: www.rgcc-group.com E-mail:papasotiriou.ioannis@rgcc-genlab.com   Day.__/__/____

Onconomics RGCC

The following are select pages of the sample test results. To see complete sample test results, go to www.rgcc-group.com/?page=test_onconomics-new.

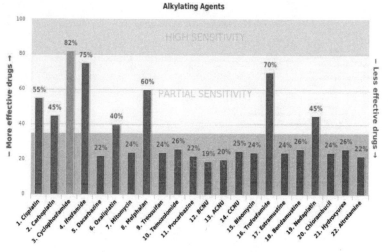

High Sensitivity: Cyclophosfamide
Partial Sensitivity: Cisplatin, Carboplatin, Ifosfamide, Oxaliplatin, Melphalan, Trofosfamide, Nedaplatin
No Sensitivity: Dacarbazine, Mitomycin, Treosulfan, Temozolomide, Procarbazine, BCNU, ACNU, CCNU, Bleomycin, Estramustine,
↳ Bendamustine, Chlorambucil, Hydroxyurea, Altretamine

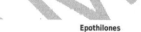

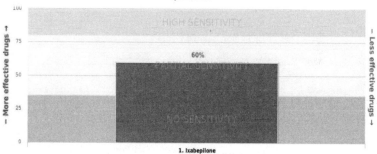

Partial Sensitivity: Ixabepilone

Mr./Ms. _____
Industrial Area of Florina, GR 53100 – Florina, Greece
Tel.: +30 23850 41950, 41951, 41960, 41961, Fax.: +30 23850 41931
Website: www.rgcc-group.com E-mail:papasotiriou.ioannis@rgcc-genlab.com

Day, ___/___/_____

SMW - Small Molecular Weight molecule

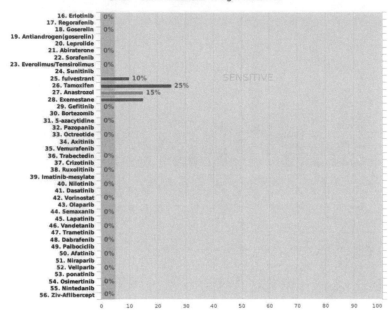

Tumor Related Genes

GROWTH FACTORS PROLIFERATION STIMULI

NAME	RELATED	RESULTS	OUTCOME	FUNCTION	CLINICAL RISK
p180	Tyrosin kinase growth f.	20%	HIGH RISK	Preprotein for Cellular stress	HIGH RISK
Bcr-abl	Resist phenotype	normal	LOW RISK	Fusion Protein	LOW RISK
PTEN	Tumor Suppressor Gene	30%	HIGH RISK	Repair Related Gene	HIGH RISK

COX2	Tumour Growth	25%	HIGH RISK	Eicosanoid related protein	HIGH RISK
5-LOX	Tumour Growth	normal	LOW RISK		

Mr./Ms. _____
Industrial Area of Florina, GR 53100 – Florina, Greece
Tel.: +30 23850 41950, 41951, 41960, 41961, Fax.: +30 23850 41931
Website: www.rgcc-group.com E-mail:papasotiriou.ioannis@rgcc-genlab.com

Day, ___/___/_____

PD 1		normal	LOW RISK	LOW RISK
PD-L2		normal	LOW RISK	LOW RISK

From the investigation above we concluded to the following:

1. From the whole neoplasmic population we have an expression of MDR1 in a percentage of 45% over control sample (positive in the check of resistance).
2. The activity of GST is stable in the low limits (no resistance to platinum compounds).
3. The activity of GammaGC is in normal range (no resistance to platinum compounds).
4. The activity of CES1 and CES2 is in low limits (no resistance to camptothecin compounds).
5. The concentration of p180 is in high range.
6. Increased activity of the Laminin and the MMP (increased invasive ability).
7. There is great sensitivity in taxanes (Docetaxel).
8. There is partial sensitivity in alkaloids of vinca.
9. There is no sensitivity in Eribulin.
10. Partial sensitivity noticed in MTX, in Gemcitabine, in Fudr, in UFT, in Raltitrexed, in Pemetrexed, no sensitivity noticed in Cytarabine, in Fludarabine but there is great sensitivity in (5FU, Capecitabine).
11. There is partial sensitivity in Epothilones.
12. Increased sensitivity in alkylating factors (Cyclophosfamide).
13. There is great overexpression of NFkB (10% over control), EGF (40% over control), TGF-b (55% over control) but there is normal expression of IkB(a, b, c).
14. It appears to have great sensitivity in the inhibitors of topoisomerase II (Epirubicin).
15. There is no sensitivity in the inhibitors of Topoisomerase I.
16. There is great over-expression of COX2 (25% over control), C-erb-B1 (40% over control), Estrogen-Receptor (20% over control), Progesterone-Receptor (10% over control) but there is normal expression of 5-LOX, SS-r, C-erb-B2.
17. We notice great neoangiogenetic ability (overexpression of VEGF-R 30% over control sample).
18. Finally, there is no sensitivity in Dacarbazine.
19. We notice that taurolidine cannot induce the apoptosis to the malignant cells (in IV route dosage).
20. We notice that taurolidine can induce the apoptosis to the malignant cells (in intraperitoneal route dosage).
21. We notice down-regulation of HSP27 (Heat Shock Protein) at 25% below control, HSP72 (Heat Shock Protein) at 15% below control and HSP90 (Heat Shock Protein) at 30% below control.
22. There is over-expression of ANG 1 at 10% over control, ANG 2 at 25% over control, IGF-r 2 at 10% over control, but we notice no down-regulation of ALK, EML-4-ALK, C-MET, NPM-ALK, CD 117 (c-kit), IGF-r 1, HDAC, HAT, NR3C4-A and NR3C4-B.

Conclusion:

- The specific tumor appears to have resisting populations because of the MDR1 overexpression that can be reversed by the use of inhibitors of ABCG2 pumps.
- The neoplasmatic cells have the greatest sensitivity in the alkylating agent (**Cyclophosfamide**), in the inhibitors of Topoisomerase II (**Epirubicin**), in the nucleous spindle stabilizer (**Docetaxel**) and in the antagonist (**5FU, Capecitabine**)
- Also can be used **Fulvestrant** as inhibitor of estrogen positive proliferative signal, **Tamoxifen** as inhibitor of estrogen positive feedback, **Anastrozol** as inhibitor of estrogen synthesis and **Exemestane** as inhibitor of aromatase enzyme.

Sincerely,

Ioannis Papasotiriou MD., PhD
Head of molecular medicine dpt. of
R.G.C.C.-RESEARCH GENETIC CANCER CENTRE S.A.

INDEX: M0: Abnormal p16, normal p53 and hTERT,
M1: Normal hTERT, abnormal p53, p16,
M2 crisis: over-expression of hTERT, p53, p16
Sample viability:<35% no sensitivity, 35%-80% partial sensitivity, >80% great sensitivity

*Be advised that any nutritional program suggested is not intended as a treatment for any disease. The intent of any nutritional recommendation is to support the physiological and biochemical processes of the human body, and not to diagnose, treat, cure, prevent any disease or condition. Always work with a qualified healthcare provider before making changes to your diet, prescription medication, lifestyle or exercise activities

Mr./Ms. _____
Industrial Area of Florina, GR 53100 – Florina, Greece
Tel.: +30 23850 41950, 41951, 41960, 41961, Fax.: +30 23850 41931
Website: www.rgcc-group.com E-mail:papasotiriou.ioannis@rgcc-genlab.com

Day, __/__/____

Onconomics Extracts

The following are select pages of the sample test results. To see complete sample test results, go to www.rgcc-group.com/?page=test _onconomics_extracts-new.

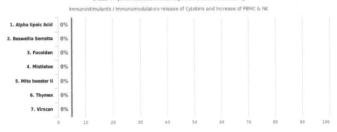

Class II (Immunostimulants/immunomodulators)

Immunostimulants / Immunomodulators release of Cytokines and Increase of PBMC & NK

1. Alpha lipoic Acid	0%
2. Boswellia Serratta	0%
3. Fucoidan	0%
4. Mistletoe	0%
5. Mito booster II	0%
6. Thymex	0%
7. Virxcan	0%

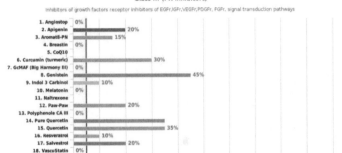

Class III (PK inhibitors)

Inhibitors of growth factors receptor inhibitors of EGFr,IGFr,VEGFr,PDGFr, FGFr, signal transduction pathways

1. Angiostop	0%
2. Apigenin	20%
3. Aromat8-PN	15%
4. Breastin	0%
5. CoQ10	
6. Curcumin (turmeric)	30%
7. GcMAF (Big Harmony III)	0%
8. Genistein	45%
9. Indol 3 Carbinol	10%
10. Melatonin	0%
11. Naltrexone	
12. Paw-Paw	20%
13. Polyphenole CA III	0%
14. Pure Quercetin	
15. Quercetin	35%
16. Resveratrol	10%
17. Salvestrol	20%
18. VascuStatin	0%

CONCLUSION: It seems that this specific population of malignant cell have greater sensitivity in Agaricus Blazei Murill, in Artecin, in Artesunate, in Ascorbic acid, in Bio D Mulsion NuMedica Micellized D3, in C-statin, in Lycopene, in Onkobel Pro, in Oxaloacetate (Cronaxal), in Salicinium, in Super Artemisinin, in Apigenin, in Aromat8-PN, in Curcumin (turmeric), in Genistein, in Indol 3 Carbinol, in Paw-Paw, in Pure Quercetin, in Quercetin, in Resveratrol, in Salvestrol and less in Amygdalin-(B17), in Avemar pulvis, in Butyric Acid, in Cordyceps Sinensis, in DCA (dichloroacetate), in DDG, in Doxycycline, in Frankincense, in GcMAF (Big Harmony), in Mito booster, in Mitochondrien formular, in Poly-MVA, in Polyphenole CA, in Ribraxx, in Theaflavin, in Ukrain, in Vitanox, in Alpha lipoic Acid, in Boswellia Serratta, in Fucoidan, in Mistletoe, in Mito booster II, in Thymex, in Virxcan, in Angiostop, in Breastin, in CoQ10, in GcMAF (Big Harmony III), in Melatonin, in Naltrexone, in Polyphenole CA III, in VascuStatin.

Sincerely,

Ioannis Papasotiriou MD., PhD
Head of molecular medicine dpt. of
R.G.C.C.-RESEARCH GENETIC CANCER CENTRE S.A.

DISCLAIMER

This study is known as an Ex-Vivo type study (testing the actual tumor stem cells of an individual outside their body). This test will tell us what natural substances will induce apoptosis via the cytochrome c (esp. caspase 3 & 9 pathways) after the tumor stem cells and a single product have been in contact, in a well plate for 48 hours. We have found this test to be very accurate over the past 10+ years and thousands of test. However, it cannot take into account the many combinations of natural substances or the physiological dynamics of each individual that are required for life. We are also aware that natural substances can have a wide variety of additional benefits that may assist healthy individuals, as well as those with cancer. Therefore, even if a product shows not to induce apoptosis in this test, it most likely will have many other benefits especially when used in combination with other therapies your health care provider may use. This is when you must rely on the skill, knowledge and training of your health care provider and their years of clinical experience (successes and failures) with the many various combinations which they have found to work in a clinical setting. The body is a wonderful, magnificent, dynamic organism and very complex.

Mr./Ms. _____
Industrial Area of Florina, GR 53100 – Florina, Greece
Tel.: +30 23850 41950, 41951, 41960, 41961, Fax.: +30 23850 41931
Website: www.rgcc-group.com E-mail: papasotiriou.ioannis@rgcc-genlab.com
Day, ____ /____ / _____

ACCURACY

In 2012 RGCC Ltd. received international validation from the Hellenic Accreditation System S. A. (Accreditation Certificate No. 860). The lab is accredited for the following:

- CTC/CSC isolation and immunophenotyping
- Cancer cell culture viability/cytotoxicity assays after exposure to substances
- Gene expression assays[14]

In early 2018 RGCC is planning to begin a new testing process that will be able to detect mutant cancer cells that were produced from the fusion of a macrophage (white blood cell) and a cancer stem cell. This process can occur in late-stage cancers. These mutant cells, along with anaplastic cells (cells with poor cellular differentiation), have been able to escape detection, resulting in a 10–12 percent false negative report.

COST

The following testing prices apply to the region of North America (United States, Canada, and North Central America). Prices will need to be converted to US dollars and are subject to change. Prices may vary from one region of the world to another and do not include the ordering office's charges or physician's fees. All prices are based on the euro.

- aCGH— €500
- Oncocount RGCC— €500
- Oncotrace RGCC— €700
- Oncotrail RGCC— €675
- Onconomics RGCC— €1695
- Onconomics Extracts—€1495
- Onconomics Plus RGCC— €1995
- Immune-Frame—€800
- Metastat—€800
- ChemoSNiP—€800

PROCESS TIME

Results take approximately two weeks and are emailed directly to the ordering practitioner.

BENEFITS

+ The test can identify the primary site or sites of cancer; in other words, it will tell you where the cancer is coming from.

+ CTCs can be detected long before cancer will be seen on a scan—this is early detection. Cancer cells often invade the bloodstream when the tumor size is only 1–2 mm or about 1/4 to 1/2 the size of a BB pellet.

+ The number of CTCs has shown to be directly related to disease progression/regression in most cases.

+ If CTCs are present, a personalized cancer treatment plan can be developed using the Onconomics Plus Test. This is the company's most inclusive test.

+ RGCC has a proprietary process that allows them to grow trillions of isolated cancer cells in a calf serum culture for sensitivity testing. This process keeps the identical genetic, epigenetic, and phenotype of the patient's cancer stem cells.

+ Drugs and natural substances are tested by direct contact with the patient's tumor cells, unlike predictive genomic tests where there is no contact between the cancer cells and tested substance.

+ All testing is done in triplicate, never single or double, as this assures unquestionable accuracy.

+ Gives percentages of effectiveness or resistance for each tested drug and nutrient.

+ RGCC can provide the patient with a list of the most effective chemo agents and natural substances for his or her particular cancer. Money and energy can be focused on the most effective substances. In the traditional setting, the patient would not be able to find out if a different chemotherapy drug would be more potent or effective at killing his or her cancer cells. (For example, a patient with breast cancer may be more effectively treated with a drug for prostate or even colon cancer.)

LIMITATIONS

- The test cannot identify brain or central nervous system cancers because of the blood-brain barrier. Actual tissue samples of a brain tumor must be provided to the lab for testing.

- The test cannot identify tumors that are completely encapsulated.

- The sensitivity tests for drugs and nutrients should be repeated every one to three years. This must be done to allow for changes due to genetic mutations cancer cells make during replication and growth. What tested well initially may no longer be effective.

- Not every practitioner is trained to interpret the results, but the number is growing. As of 2018 there are more than five hundred doctors using this test in the United States, Canada, and North Central America. Others are using this worldwide now.

- Most conventional oncologists in the United States are not familiar with this test and may dismiss its results and recommendations. In Europe this test is more widely used and accepted.

- Cost can be a limiting factor; this test is not currently covered by insurance.

A NOTE FROM RAY HAMMON, DC, NMD, DCBCN
MY PERSONAL EXPERIENCE WITH
RGCC CANCER TESTING

In April 2004 I began using the RGCC Ltd. cancer testing for all of our cancer patients and screening those who want to know if they have cancer. This was a powerful addition to my private clinical practice, which I started in January 2009. We have performed well over 1,000 RGCC tests during these years. During the past three years our branch, RGCC-USA (serving the US, Canada, and North Central America), has overseen many hundreds more tests administered by more than five hundred health care providers serving this region.

It never ceases to amaze me how different each test result is. Results

from the same types of cancers, even amongst family members, will yield
different results. I can accurately say the results of every test are at least
30%–60% different from every other. This is what really makes the RGCC
cancer test in a league of its own. I have yet to see any test that gives this
much diverse and useful information about every individual as this one,
and I have looked at many over these years.

This is the very reason our results for most of the patients we have worked
with have approximately a $\geq 35\%$ survival/stabilization rate. This is not just by
looking at the tumor shrinkage only, but the CTCs/ CSCs responsible for 95%+
of all metastases, which are responsible for 90%+ of all cancer-related deaths.
I feel it is crucial to target more than just the tumor. Circulating tumor and
stem cells must be addressed. The testing provided by RGCC allows the health
care provider to offer the cancer patient a true, unmatched Personalized Cancer Care. It has also allowed me to give my patients many options and design
a program just for them. My outlook on treating cancer has changed. I now feel
cancer can be managed much like other chronic diseases utilizing this vast
amount of accurate, scientific, and patient-specific information.

I am privileged to have been associated with RGCC Ltd. and Dr. Papasotiriou
for 11 years and to have been the first clinic on this continent to use this test.
For the past 4 years we have owned and operated RGCC USA. Our responsibili-
ties are many to the health care providers in the United States, Canada, and
North Central America. It is my pleasure to be a part in assisting patients and
their physicians to learn about the many benefits that RGCC Ltd. of Greece has
to offer. I truly believe RGCC has met the challenge and passed the test by providing the testing necessary to develop a Personalized Cancer Care Program.

I can assure everyone we have learned a great deal from Dr. Papasotiriou regarding his testing procedures, the accuracy, the technology, and
the clinical application of this test. It is a continued pleasure to share these
years of experience with those who want to learn a better way to care and
support cancer patients. I share in the opinion of many patients and colleagues around the world that RGCC is the very best world-class laboratory
in the field of oncology testing and development.

Dr. Papasotiriou is one of the very few true scientists I have known in my lifetime and the only one whom I have had the pleasure of working with. I can speak highly of his integrity, knowledge, humility, desire for accurate scientific methods, and complete dedication to his work.

> "Discovery consists of seeing what everyone has seen and thinking what nobody else has thought."
>
> —ALBERT SZENT-GYORGYI

Sincerely,

Ray Hammon, DC, NMD, DCBCN
Integrative and Functional Health Center
Rowlett, Texas USA

THOUGHTS

Most people are not aware that circulating tumor cells are present in the blood. Also, these cells are in the blood before a tumor is found and usually after cancer treatment is completed. We cannot be so focused on the tumor that we overlook the need to address CTCs. A positive test result can be alarming because it may be the first time you've been told you have cancer. Standard oncology methods of testing are not as sensitive. That's why this kind of early-detection test is so valuable—it allows you to intervene years before you might have otherwise.

If the Oncocount/CTC is 0, there is a low probability the patient has cancer. A 0 also can confirm whether prior cancer treatment has been effective. However, I recommend this test be used on an annual basis to monitor for a possible increase in CTCs and for early detection. Utilizing testing for natural substances is financially beneficial because you can use only the substances with the highest percentage of effectiveness. Likewise, the chemosensitivity testing will identify the most effective chemo drugs.

Please understand chemotherapy is a treatment, not a cure, and is toxic to both healthy and cancerous cells. Refer to the upcoming chapter about insulin potentiated therapy (IPT), a low-dose, less-toxic, yet effective method of giving a 10–20 percent dose of standard chemotherapy. Many practitioners using IPT are using the RGCC chemosensitivity panel to identify the most effective chemo drugs for IPT.

RGCC may find CTCs years before the primary tumor can be seen on a PET scan. This is true early detection. An integrative physician can then be consulted to help you implement therapies to reverse, halt, or slow the cancer growth. This test is money well spent.

In the summer of 2017 a group of physicians from around the world gathered for a conference at the RGCC lab in Greece, and I was privileged to receive an invitation. I immediately accepted and blocked my calendar for the trip. I never dreamed that I would get to tour the lab, the very lab whose work *I feel* saved my life. The lab was everything that I expected and more. I was able to suit up to tour the testing areas and sit in on lectures given by the cellular biologists who are doing this important work. They are brilliant! I soaked in every minute of my time there.

See www.rgcc-group.com for references.

Chapter 21

Thymidine Kinase Test

SUMMARY AND EXPLANATION

THE THYMIDINE KINASE (TK) test is a blood test for early cancer detection and monitoring of treatment. It is valuable for detecting cancer at its earliest stages, thereby increasing the chance of a better prognosis and effective treatment.

TK is an enzyme/functional protein common to all cells in your body that go through cell division. Most cancers have an increased rate of cellular division. TK levels increase when there is a rapid amount of cell division, thus providing a measurable indication of tumor growth. TK is responsible for DNA duplication during cell division and DNA repair.

Regularly monitoring TK levels in your blood can indicate when cancer is forming and provide an early detection tool. Changing TK levels can indicate whether your treatment is working.

For more than thirty years researchers from dozens of countries have documented the direct correlation of TK levels to more than eighteen different major categories of cancer. The research shows that rising TK levels show a clear correlation to the development and spread of cancer.[1] Studies show TK levels rise with cancer progression, decrease with effective treatment, and are at low levels for those who are normal or in remission. A healing injury, a viral infection, or pernicious anemia can also cause an elevated TK level.

The TK test cannot detect brain cancer due to presence of the blood-brain barrier or identify the specific type of cancer.

BENEFITS

+ The test is useful as a wellness profile.
+ It is a good early detection tool.
+ It is used to indicate progression or regression of disease.
+ The active form of TK that is measured has a short half-life, so the test can be repeated weekly to monitor cancer or rapid cell growth activity.
+ Remission can be confirmed and monitored.

LIMITATIONS

+ This test does not diagnose cancer. High TK levels indicate that cancer is a possibility and should be further investigated.

+ The test requires additional testing to confirm cancer.

+ Rare false positives can occur and be reported as higher scores. Reasons for this are injury healing, viral infection, or pernicious anemia.

+ The TK score in and of itself can't help with the identification of the origin site of any possible malignancy, except possibly for lymphoma or leukemia, which report extremely high scores.

HOW TO OBTAIN THE TEST

At the time of this printing, the test is not available in the United States.

THOUGHTS

The TK test is a simple blood test that has great merit. Even though it doesn't provide a definitive cancer diagnosis, it's a valuable monitoring tool to give you an indication of the presence of the rapid cell growth that's common with most cancers.

Monitoring your TK levels can prove valuable to uncovering a potential problem early. I might do an internet search to see if it has become available again.

Source for thymidine kinase testing: www.rndsystems.com (for research use only at this time).

Chapter 22

Videssa® Breast Test

Videssa® Breast
Provista Diagnostics
855-552-7439
www.provistadx.com/videssa-breast
ClientServices@ProvistaDx.com

THIS CHAPTER IS based on information provided by Provista Diagnostics and research done by the author. Check the Provista Diagnostics website for updates.

SUMMARY AND EXPLANATION

Videssa® Breast is the first protein-based blood test of its kind to assist in the accurate detection of breast cancer. The test fills a big void because mammogram results are not always black and white. It's well known that mammograms and other breast-imaging methods have limitations and that benign breast disease can mimic cancer. Often dense breast tissue and tiny lesions cause these unclear results. When this happens, the physician will either decide to order a tissue biopsy or repeat the imaging within a few months. This test offers a different approach that improves the accuracy and prevents delays of breast cancer detection. The test is recommended for women between the ages of twenty-five and seventy-five, and results are not affected by breast density. It's a simple blood test that looks for thirteen tumor-associated autoantibodies and eleven serum protein biomarkers. Solid science has validated the use of these blood markers. The test can bring clarity to an unclear mammogram report and, in many cases, rule out the need for a biopsy.[1]

INTERPRETATION

This test delivers real-time clinically actionable results to help guide a patient through the diagnostic process when clinical assessment is challenging. Test results are reported as either:

- Low-protein signature—likely indicating the absence of breast cancer

+ High-protein signature—may potentially indicate the presence of breast cancer

How to Obtain the Test

The test must be prescribed by a physician or clinician. If your physician is not currently using this test, the account registration form can be downloaded under the Healthcare Professionals tab at www.provistadx.com/videssa-breast. Once the account is set up, he or she can complete a test requisition form. It will include patient information and a copy of the patient's insurance card.

Accuracy

Studies done by Provista Diagnostics© report that combining Videssa® Breast and imaging detected 100 percent of breast cancers. Also, there is a negative predictive value (NPV) over 98 percent, which means a less than 2 percent probability of breast cancer in patients with a low-protein signature test result.[2]

Cost

Contact Provista for pricing information. For patients with health insurance, including Medicare, Provista will file a claim and appeals on your behalf.

Provista strives to make this test accessible and affordable to all patients who may benefit from testing. The company offers financial assistance to qualified patients who meet specific financial criteria based on household size and income.

Process Time

Patient test results will be reported in five to seven business days from the receipt of the sample.

Benefits

+ Processed with a small blood sample
+ Noninvasive
+ Reduces the need for biopsies and the rate of false positives
+ Improves cancer detection when combined with imaging

+ Accurately detects breast cancer irrespective of breast density

+ Accurately detects invasive breast cancer (IBC) and/or ductal carcinoma *in situ* (DCIS)

+ Usually eligible for insurance and Medicare coverage

+ Can be ordered independently; however, reported accuracy results are based on the patient having an unclear mammogram report.

LIMITATIONS

+ The test does not provide the stage of cancer.

+ The test should not be used as a stand-alone diagnostic tool but must be combined with imaging and patient history.

+ Data collected was limited to women between the ages of twenty-five and seventy-five with no history of breast cancer or biopsy within six months for one study and women between the ages of twenty-five and forty-nine with no history of breast cancer or biopsy for another study.

THOUGHTS

Thousands of women around the world have experienced the anxiety caused by an unclear or suspicious mammogram report. When this happens, there are usually two options. The first is the "watchful waiting" approach, which can delay diagnosis and intervention. The second is to perform a tissue biopsy. Studies report that 70–80 percent of breast biopsies are negative. That's a lot of needless medical procedures, not to mention the stress and the money involved. If you find yourself in this position, I would encourage you to insist on having this test run before any other intervention. If your doctor doesn't use the test, educate him or her. Show your doctor where he can order it. Stand strong and say no to the biopsy or watchful waiting until you get the results. The odds are that the results will *not* indicate the presence of cancer. See the "Resources" tab at www.provistadx.com/videssa-breast for publications and studies.

Chapter 23

Biofocus® Tests

Biofocus®
Biofocus GmbH
Berghäuser Str. 295
45659 Recklinghausen
Germany
Phone: +49 2361 3000 130
Please call from 7:00 a.m.–5:00 p.m. GMT
Fax: +49 2361 3000-162
www.Biofocus.de
prix@biofocus.de (Lothar Prix)

THIS CHAPTER IS based on information obtained from www.Biofocus .de and provided by the staff at Biofocus. Check the Biofocus website for updates. (The website has an option that can be utilized to view the content in English.)

SUMMARY AND EXPLANATION

Biofocus® is a laboratory located in Recklinghausen, Germany, that specializes in molecular detection and analysis of circulating tumor cells. It also offers chemotherapy and alternative-agent testing, as well as tests that examine related issues, including mutations, drug resistance, and immune function.

Biofocus uses a proprietary technique to isolate cancer cells. Results are based on measurements of gene expression. Tests are done with a blood sample.

Results are reported by email, in English, to the ordering practitioner and can be used as a guide for treatment option and choices.

The Biofocus test for circulating tumor cell (CTC) detection does not provide a numerical value of cancer cells present in the blood. It gives a yes-or-no answer as to whether CTCs are present, but if so, there is no measurement of how much. On average, Biofocus detection rates for CTCs in patients with a known carcinoma are 80 percent. For soft-tissue sarcomas (e.g., synovial sarcoma), detection rates are 40–50 percent. The test is not suitable for T-cell lymphomas.[1]

This test is preferably used for the monitoring of patients with known cancer. It is not necessarily an early-diagnostic test. It is useful in monitoring response to therapy and provides information about the risk of recurrence.

It's also used for the development of a targeted, patient-specific therapy by identifying chemotherapy drug agents that demonstrate the best response to an individual's cancer cell based on the predicted genetic expression of the cell.

Cost

Biofocus accepts Visa, MasterCard, and American Express. Payments are calculated in euros. Contact the lab for prices.

Process Time

Results take approximately two weeks.

Thoughts

I am a big fan of any test that uses a blood sample and allows patients to avoid a tissue biopsy.

This test does not include a numerical value for the number of CTCs in the tested blood sample. Lothar Prix at Biofocus told me:

> It is possible for us to correlate these figures with an absolute count of tumor cells. There may be fewer cells expressing the gene strongly, or more cells expressing weaker. So comparing between different individuals is not possible, but follow-up testing in the same individual may find indications for rise or fall of tumor-cell burden.

That said, my research does indicate obtaining a CTC count is valuable because increasing or decreasing counts can provide a tool for evaluating treatment and disease progression or regression. Results are based on predicted genetic expression and not the actual reaction of physically bringing the isolated CTCs in direct contact with the test drug or natural substance.

Biofocus is one of a handful of labs in the world that realize the efficacy of using natural substances to treat cancer, and I applaud the lab for its work in this area. It is one of the pioneers in this field, so check its website for updates. See www.Biofocus.de for references.

Chapter 24

CELLSEARCH®

CIRCULATING TUMOR CELL COUNT TEST

CELLSEARCH®
Menarini Silicon Biosystems Inc.
3401 Masons Mill Road, Suite 100
Huntington Valley, PA 19006
877-837-4339
www.cellsearchctc.com
us-support@siliconbiosystems.com

THIS CHAPTER IS based on information obtained from representatives of CELLSEARCH and from www.cellsearchctc.com. Check the CELL-SEARCH website for updates.

SUMMARY AND EXPLANATION

The CELLSEARCH® CTC Test is the first clinically validated, FDA-cleared blood test for counting circulating tumor cells (CTCs) in patients with metastatic breast, colorectal, or prostate cancer. The CELLSEARCH® CTC Test acts as a real-time liquid biopsy that predicts prognosis at any time during a patient's course of treatment.[1] The test requires a blood sample be sent to a registered CELLSEARCH lab for analysis.

The CELLSEARCH® test has not been identified as an early-detection test. The test is used in the conventional oncology setting as a supplemental test. It is used in the assessment of disease status in conjunction with laboratory analysis, imaging, biopsies, or other standard methods of monitoring known cancer. It is used to identify changes in disease status based on predictive prognosis at any time during cancer treatment. It increases the predictive accuracy of prognosis when other clinical parameters are conflicting.

INTERPRETATION

Abbreviations are as follows:

- mBC is metastatic breast cancer
- mPC is metastatic prostate cancer
- mCRC is metastatic colorectal cancer[2]

For breast and prostate cancers, a reduction of CTCs to less than 5 after initiation of therapy predicts a longer survival. An increase in CTCs to greater than or equal to 5 predicts a shorter survival. For colorectal cancer, a reduction of CTCs to less than 3 after initiation of therapy predicts a longer survival. An increase in CTCs to greater than or equal to 3 predicts a shorter survival.[3]

How to Obtain the Test

The test is available at several labs in the United States, including Quest Diagnostics, and must be ordered by a physician.

Accuracy

Clinical studies validate the predictive accuracy of the CELLSEARCH® CTC Test. Study results are available at www.cellsearchctc.com/clinical-applications/clinical-applications-overview.

Cost

The cost of the test may be covered by insurance. If insurance is not used, the cash price from Quest Diagnostics (as of March 2018) is approximately $770 for one of the tests—either breast, colon, or prostate.

Process Time

Patient test results will be reported in five to seven business days from the receipt of the sample.

Thoughts

I've included CELLSEARCH because it's an FDA-cleared CTC-count test. It's usually covered by insurance. This is the test you will likely receive if a recurrence of cancer is suspected in the conventional treatment setting.

CELLSEARCH does not promote this test as early detection because the test will only detect *metastatic* breast, colorectal, and prostate cancers. So beware, it is *not* early detection. With that said, using the test to monitor your CTC levels can help your physician in the clinical decision-making process.

Confusion begins when a patient is told his or her CTC from CELLSEARCH is zero. This can lead to a misunderstanding of the patient's condition. The patient may still have cancer, just not enough cancer for this particular test to be able to pick it up. I recommend you look into a more sensitive test, such as the Oncocount test provided by RGCC labs because it can detect cancer at its earliest stages and long before it has metastasized to other organs. Maintrac is another company that is offering a CTC count test.[4] See the "Clinical Applications" tab at www.cellsearchctc.com for reference information.

Chapter 25

Caris Molecular Intelligence®

Caris Life Sciences®
888-979-8669
www.CarisLifeSciences.com
www.MyCancer.com (patient education website)

THIS CHAPTER IS based on information provided by Caris Life Sciences and research done by the author. Check the Caris Life Sciences website for updates.

SUMMARY AND EXPLANATION

Caris Life Sciences offers genomic and proteomic tumor profiling known as Caris Molecular Intelligence®. The test requires that a sample of the tumor or malignant fluid be sent to the laboratory by your surgeon after collection. The lab will perform molecular testing on the DNA, RNA, and proteins to identify the biomarkers driving the cancer. This information may be a powerful tool to aid oncologists in personalizing your therapy.

INTERPRETATION

Reporting includes the identified genomic and proteomic alterations for the patient and provides information about immunotherapies, targeted therapies, chemotherapy, and clinical trials.

HOW TO OBTAIN THE TEST

The tests must be ordered by a physician. To order test kits, physicians need to go to www.CarisMolecularIntelligence.com to download the Profiling Requisition and complete and submit the requested information. A kit with specific instructions for the collection and shipping of specimens will be sent. Tumor tissue samples and malignant fluid samples must arrive at the lab within forty-eight hours from the time of collection. Sufficient sample volume must be sent to the lab for the analysis to be done. It requests at least a 5-mm-by-5-mm sample for tumor tissue.

If it is not possible to provide a current sample, the lab can also do an analysis of archived tissue; however, the lab requests that it be from the most recent tumor biopsy.

ACCURACY

Patients treated according to Caris Molecular Intelligence (CMI) results "experienced one year longer survival and received one fewer cancer drugs (avoiding potential toxicities and extra cost of therapy), vs patients not treated according to CMI recommendations."[1]

COST

Caris bills insurance companies directly as an independent service provider and works directly with them to process claims. Insurance companies usually take sixty to ninety days to respond to claims. Insurance companies may send out an explanation of benefits (EOB) during this time, but this is not a bill. Based on your health care plan, a bill for the deductible, coinsurance, or co-payment may be sent once the insurance company has processed the claim.

If insurance coverage is denied, Caris billing specialists will work with the insurance company to file appeals and pursue coverage on your behalf. If you have no insurance coverage, the cash price is $4,600. Please check with Caris for price changes.

Caris offers a Financial Assistance Program. It also has a Compassionate Care Program to help uninsured patients or patients who cannot afford associated out-of-pocket costs. Limits and conditions apply. Contact a Caris Patient Navigator at 888-979-8669 or visit www.CarisLifeSciences .com/order-now/billing-overview/faq for more information.[2]

PROCESS TIME

Reports will be available for your physician through a secure online portal approximately ten to fourteen days from the date of receipt of the specimen and required paperwork to begin testing.

BENEFITS

Caris Molecular Intelligence allows physicians to assess therapies for potential benefit; identify other therapies not previously considered; determine which drugs have a potential lack of benefit, thereby limiting unnecessary side effects and costs; and identify clinical trials that may benefit the patient.[3]

LIMITATIONS

The tests are not designed to predict recurrences of disease. Genomic testing only offers a predictive response to therapy. Patients need an identified tumor or mass for testing; it is not early detection.

THOUGHTS

If full-dose chemotherapy or one of the lower-dose approaches to chemotherapy is your choice, always insist on a personalized protocol. Our fingerprints are all different, and so are our cancers, which means that standard chemotherapy protocols may not be the most effective for you. Another way to say it is, treat the tumor's molecular profile and not the site of origin. Remember that genomic testing provides information on genomic alterations predicted to respond to specific drugs or targeted therapies. So carefully monitor your response to any therapy.

I describe several tests that provide genomic data in this book. Consider them all, then decide which is the best for you and discuss it with your doctor. Take an active part in your therapy decisions. Note that several of the labs don't require a tissue biopsy but rather use a blood sample, often referred to as a liquid biopsy. Maybe you can avoid an invasive procedure. References are available at www.carismolecularintelligence.com/publications/.

SAMPLE TEST RESULTS

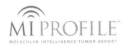

FINAL REPORT

PATIENT	SPECIMEN INFORMATION	ORDERED BY
Name: Patient, Test **Date of Birth:** XX-Mon-19XX **Sex:** Male **Case Number:** TN17-XXXXXX **Diagnosis:** Non-small cell carcinoma	**Primary Tumor Site:** Lung, NOS **Specimen Site:** Lung, NOS **Specimen ID:** ABC-1234-XX **Specimen Collected:** XX-Mon-2017 **Completion of Testing:** XX-Mon-2017	**Ordering Physician, MD** **Cancer Center** 123 Main Street Springfield, XY 12345 USA 1 (123) 456-7890

BIOMARKER HIGHLIGHTS (SEE PAGE 3 AND APPENDIX FOR MORE DETAILS)

Biomarker	Method	Result
Lineage Relevant Biomarkers		
ALK	IHC	Negative | 0, 100%
	RNA-Seq	Fusion Not Detected
	NGS	Mutation Not Detected
ROS1	RNA-Seq	Fusion Not Detected
PD-L1	IHC	Positive, High Expression, TPS: 100%
EGFR	NGS	Mutation Not Detected
KRAS	NGS	Mutated, Pathogenic
		Exon 2 | G12V
BRAF	NGS	Mutation Not Detected
PIK3CA	NGS	Mutation Not Detected
Her2/Neu (ERBB2)	NGS	Mutation Not Detected
cMET	NGS	Mutation Not Detected
	NGS	Amplification Not Detected

Biomarker	Method	Result
Lineage Relevant Biomarkers (cont)		
RET	RNA-Seq	Fusion Not Detected
Other Notable Biomarker Results		
Total Mutational Load		High | 36 Mutations/Mb
MSI	NGS	Stable
PBRM1	NGS	Mutated, Pathogenic
		Exon 5 | c.305-2A>C
TP53	NGS	Mutated, Pathogenic
		Exon 4 | c.375+1G>T
TS	IHC	Negative | 0, 100%
TUBB3	IHC	Negative | 1+, 10%
PTEN	IHC	Negative | 0, 100%
RRM1	IHC	Negative | 0, 100%

The therapies listed below are FDA-approved, on-NCCN Compendium® for the tested lineage or deemed relevant for this lineage by a panel of internal and external oncology experts. Complete therapy association information and Off-NCCN Compendium therapies are listed on pages (6-8).

THERAPIES WITH POTENTIAL BENEFIT	
atezolizumab, nivolumab, pembrolizumab★‡‡	**PD-L1**
docetaxel, nab-paclitaxel, paclitaxel	TUBB3
gemcitabine	RRM1
pemetrexed	TS

THERAPIES WITH POTENTIAL LACK OF BENEFIT	
afatinib	EGFR, Her2/Neu (ERBB2)
alectinib, brigatinib	ALK
ceritinib	ALK, ROS1
crizotinib	ALK, cMET, ROS1
dabrafenib, trametinib, vemurafenib	BRAF
erlotinib, gefitinib	EGFR, KRAS, PTEN

Results continued on the next page. >

Therapies associated with potential, uncertain, or lack of benefit, as indicated above, are based on biomarker results provided in this report and are based on published medical evidence. This evidence may have been obtained from studies performed in the cancer type present in the tested patient's sample or derived from another tumor type. The selection of any, all, or none of the matched therapies resides solely with the discretion of the treating physician. Decisions on patient care and treatment must be based on the independent medical judgment of the treating physician, taking into consideration all available information in addition to this report concerning the patient's condition in accordance with the applicable standard of care.

Chapter 26

FoundationOne®

COMPREHENSIVE GENOMIC PROFILE

Foundation Medicine Inc.
150 Second Street
Cambridge, MA 02141
Phone: 888-988-3639
Fax: 617-418-2290
www.foundationmedicine.com/

THIS CHAPTER IS based on information provided by Foundation Medicine and research done by the author. Check the Foundation Medicine website for updates.

SUMMARY AND EXPLANATION

This testing is only for patients with a confirmed diagnosis of cancer.

Foundation Medicine offers comprehensive genomic profiling tests to help physicians make informed, individualized treatment decisions for each patient. The process involves identifying specific genomic alterations implicated in cancer. These alterations are changes in the DNA and/or RNA sequences affecting the way a cell functions. Studies have shown tumors with specific genomic alterations respond better to certain treatments or targeted therapies.

There are three tests offered by Foundation Medicine:

+ FoundationOne®Heme—This is a test used for hematologic cancers (leukemia, lymphoma, and myeloma) and advanced sarcomas. It is validated to detect all classes of genomic alterations in more than four hundred cancer-related genes. In addition to DNA sequencing, FoundationOneHeme uses RNA sequencing across more than 250 genes "to capture a broad range of gene fusions, common drivers of hematological malignancies, and sarcomas." Testing is done from a tumor sample, blood, or bone marrow aspirate. Results are based on genomic factors.[1]

+ FoundationACT®—This is a blood-based circulating-tumor DNA (ctDNA) assay that provides new options,

183

often when a tissue biopsy is not possible. FoundationACT is validated to detect all classes of genomic alterations and to analyze more than sixty of the most commonly mutated genes in solid tumors. Testing is done with a blood sample.[2]

+ FoundationOne CDx™—This is a "single test that looks for all guideline-recommended genes in solid tumors." In the test 324 genes are evaluated. This test is FDA-approved, and results include companion diagnostics, biomarkers, and potential resistance. Testing is done from a tumor sample and is primarily used for non-small-cell lung, colorectal, melanoma, breast, and ovarian cancers. The test is FDA-approved for *all* solid tumors.[3]

Foundation Medicine reports its tests identify more potential treatment options than other available tests because they analyze all genes known to be relevant in human cancers. Additionally FoundationOneHeme, FoundationACT, and FoundationOne CDx measure important biomarkers of response, such as microsatellite instability (MSI) and tumor mutational burden (TMB), to predict which individuals are likely to respond to immunotherapies. These have been shown to be important independent biomarkers of response to many advanced cancers, including lung, breast, colorectal, and metastatic melanoma.

Foundation Medicine also offers FoundationInsights, which allows physicians to learn from other physicians treating patients with similar genomic profiles; they can assess information from experts in genomic alterations.

INTERPRETATION

The test report includes the identified genomic alteration for the patient and provides information about targeted therapies and clinical trials. Results may identify an approved therapy, an approved therapy for a different type of cancer, clinical trial options, or experimental treatments. The lab reports that 85 percent of tests identify a clinically relevant/potentially actionable mutation or biomarker.[4] These are related to targeted therapies, immunotherapies, or clinical trials. Approximately one in three patients with non-small-cell lung cancer, colorectal cancer, breast cancer, melanoma, and ovarian cancer will match with an FDA-approved therapy using FoundationOne CDx.[5]

How to Obtain the Test

All three tests must be ordered by a physician. Physicians need to contact Foundation Medicine to set up an account. To order test kits, they need to download the Test Requisition Form and complete the requested information. Requisition forms can be sent via fax or email.

Physicians receive a kit with specific instructions for the collection and shipping of solid tumor specimens, peripheral blood, or bone marrow aspirate. Pathology reports need to be included for the FoundationACT blood-based test.

Accuracy

All assays from Foundation Medicine report greater than or equal to 95 percent sensitivity and 99 percent specificity.

Cost

Foundation Medicine bills private insurance for the test on behalf of patients. If coverage is declined, Foundation Medicine will work to appeal and receive coverage. Applicable co-payments, coinsurance, and deductibles apply. Foundation Medicine will work with you regarding any costs not covered by insurance. Contact the FoundationAccess Program for payment options and assistance. Foundation Medicine's "FoundationAccess Program offers direct support and guidance during each step of the billing process." Contact Foundation Medicine's client services at 888-988-3639 or client.services@foundationmedicine.com for more information. The cost billed to your insurance company is as follows:

+ FoundationOneHeme—$7,200

+ FoundationACT—$5,800

+ FoundationOne CDx—$5,800

Process Time

Reports will be available for your physician through a secure online portal approximately two weeks from the date of receipt of the specimen at Foundation Medicine. Results can also be sent via fax to your physician.

Benefits

+ Detects genetic alterations on cancer cells' DNA and identifies associated pharmaceutical therapies

+ Informs you of clinical trials and experimental therapies that have been identified to target your tumor's DNA alterations

LIMITATIONS

Testing is only indicated for patients with previously diagnosed cancer. Tests are typically used for advanced or metastatic disease. The tests are not designed to predict recurrences of disease. Fifteen percent of patient samples will have alterations that are not mapped to FDA-approved agents or clinical trials.

THOUGHTS

For anyone considering chemotherapy, I feel it is very important that you ask for some sort of personalized testing. Standard chemotherapy protocols may not be the most effective for you. If genomic alterations are found, you and your doctor can consider them and tailor treatment for your individual cancer. As technology evolves, this tool is being used earlier in cancer care. This test can be particularly useful for people who have had chemotherapy that was not effective or have experienced a recurrence of cancer. As cancer grows back, it likely has gone through many different mutations during cellular replication. For example, a cancer can turn from being estrogen-positive to estrogen-negative. It pays to find out what your cancer looks like at the time you initiate therapy. It is important to understand that genomic testing only provides information on genomic alterations known to respond to specific drugs used as targeted therapies. So carefully monitor your response to any therapy.

The FoundationACT blood test falls in the category of what the industry calls a "liquid biopsy." Generally liquid biopsies use a blood sample to analyze circulating tumor cells and/or circulating tumor DNA (ctDNA) to evaluate a patient's cancer, prognosis, and treatment options. This new technology can be used in place of a tissue biopsy, especially if the tumor is difficult to access. It is definitely a less-invasive way to monitor patients during treatment, determine how mutations respond to chosen therapies, and help physicians decide which drugs will work best. Liquid biopsies are gaining traction as a viable alternative to more-invasive methods of screening. As of this writing, a number of companies are offering tests based upon some version of this technology.[6] Visit www .foundationmedicine.com for references.

SAMPLE TEST RESULTS

The following are select pages of the sample test results.

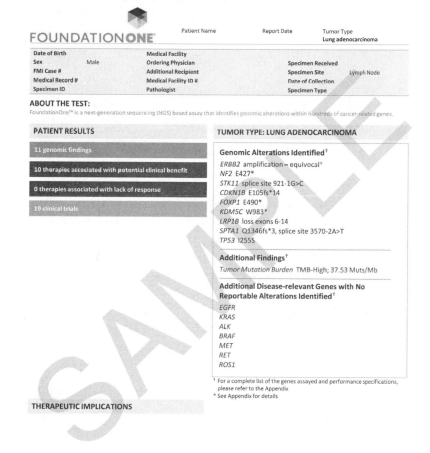

Electronically Signed by Jeffrey S. Ross, M.D. | Jeffrey S. Ross, M.D., Medical Director | CLIA Number: 22D2027531 | 10 August 2016
Foundation Medicine, Inc., 150 2nd Street, 1st Floor, Cambridge, MA 02141 | 1-888-988-3639

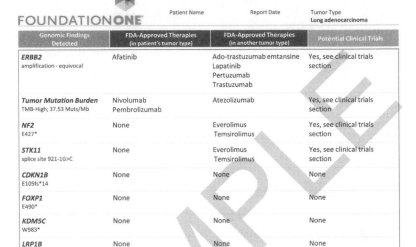

Genomic Findings Detected	FDA-Approved Therapies (in patient's tumor type)	FDA-Approved Therapies (in another tumor type)	Potential Clinical Trials
ERBB2 amplification - equivocal	Afatinib	Ado-trastuzumab emtansine Lapatinib Pertuzumab Trastuzumab	Yes, see clinical trials section
Tumor Mutation Burden TMB-High; 37.53 Muts/Mb	Nivolumab Pembrolizumab	Atezolizumab	Yes, see clinical trials section
NF2 E427*	None	Everolimus Temsirolimus	Yes, see clinical trials section
STK11 splice site 921-1G>C	None	Everolimus Temsirolimus	Yes, see clinical trials section
CDKN1B E105fs*14	None	None	None
FOXP1 E490*	None	None	None
KDM5C W983*	None	None	None
LRP1B loss exons 6-14	None	None	None
SPTA1 Q1346fs*3, splice site 3570-2A>T	None	None	None
TP53 I255S	None	None	None

Note: Genomic alterations detected may be associated with activity of certain FDA-approved drugs; however, the agents listed in this report may have little or no evidence in the patient's tumor type. Neither the therapeutic agents nor the trials identified are ranked in order of potential or predicted efficacy for this patient, nor are they ranked in order of level of evidence for this patient's tumor type.

For more comprehensive information please log on to the Interactive Cancer Explorer™
To set up your Interactive Cancer Explorer account, contact your sales representative or call 1-888-988-3639.

Electronically Signed by Jeffrey S. Ross, M.D. | Jeffrey S. Ross, M.D., Medical Director | CLIA Number: 2202027531 | 10 August 2016
Foundation Medicine, Inc., 150 2ⁿᵈ Street, 1ˢᵗ Floor, Cambridge, MA 02141 | 1-888-988-3639   page 2 of 33

Chapter 27

Nagourney Cancer Institute

FUNCTIONAL PROFILE CHEMOSENSITIVITY AND TARGETED AGENT TEST

Nagourney Cancer Institute
750 E. 29th Street
Long Beach, CA 90806
Phone: 562-989-6455; 800-542-4357
Fax: 562-989-8160
www.nagourneycancerinstitute.com
client.services@nagourneyci.com

THIS CHAPTER IS based on information provided by Nagourney Cancer Institute and research done by the author. Please check the Nagourney Cancer Institute website for updates.

SUMMARY AND EXPLANATION

Nagourney Cancer Institute offers personalized "functional profiling," which exposes an individual patient's living cancer cells to chemotherapy drugs, targeted agents, and combinations of drugs to determine their effectiveness. They use a real-time snapshot of how living human tumor cells behave in the laboratory. Some of the targeted agents tested are FDA-approved and commercially available; others may be available only at university medical centers or through the National Cancer Institute investigational drug trials. They are able to test most types of cancer, both solid and hematologic (blood).

The laboratory analysis determines which drugs kill cancer cells (the cells are "sensitive" to the drugs) and which ones do not (the cells are "resistant" to the drugs). Test results enable the patient's treating physician to prescribe the drugs with the best chance of improving the outcome and to avoid unnecessary or ineffective treatment.

This testing has a valuable place in the personalized treatment of cancer, as so many people don't receive a cancer diagnosis until a tumor is quite large. Tumor tissue can be collected and analyzed for development of a targeted treatment plan for the patient. Keep in mind, the tumor is not the whole problem when dealing with cancer. Circulating tumor cells, immune system depression, toxicities, and nutritional deficiencies need to be addressed as well.

Nagourney Cancer Institute tests "are disease-specific and based on your diagnosis and previous treatment history. [They] can customize the drugs tested based on your oncologist's request. A standard panel consists of 8–16 drugs/combinations."[1] Because this lab does not grow the tumor in the laboratory, the quantity of drugs analyzed is based on the quantity/ quality of the tumor tissue received; i.e., the more viable tumor it receives, the more drugs it can analyze.

Nagourney explains it this way:

> Currently, hundreds of drugs, drug combinations and targeted agents are used to treat cancer patients. With so many choices, how does your oncologist decide which ones are right for you? Generally, oncologists use established regimens developed through randomized clinical trials to prescribe chemotherapeutic agents. These regimens are average solutions for the "average" patient. Regrettably, average treatments provide average outcomes, with the majority of patients failing to show significant improvement from these protocols. Each cancer patient is unique and their response to therapy is very different from one person to the next. Drugs that work for one patient may not work for another, even if they carry exactly the same diagnosis....Functional profiling is a laboratory technique...that measures how cancer cells respond when they are exposed to drugs and drug combinations.[2]

Note: This test was formerly called Rational Therapeutics.

How to Obtain the Test

Call a patient relations representative at 800-542-4357 to get specifics regarding living tumor sample collection and transportation to the lab. If you wish, the lab will coordinate sample collection procedures with its sur- gical/hospital colleagues in California. Samples can be sent from all over the United States and internationally.

Specimen Criteria

Since the testing requires living tumor tissue, the specimen collection process is critical. The sample must be received at the laboratory within twenty-four to thirty-six hours of collection. If shipping on a Friday, please contact the laboratory for specific instructions. Contact the laboratory to order a specimen transportation kit, which includes the culture media tube, transport box, and return FedEx packaging.

To ensure the accuracy of the test results, the patient should be two to three weeks outside of any chemotherapy treatment when the specimen is collected.

* Solid tumor: A minimum of 1 gram of viable malignant tumor tissue is needed. Needle biopsies do not provide enough tissue for an accurate analysis.

* Malignant effusions: 500–1000 ml of heparinized, cytologically positive pleural or ascites fluid

* Blood (leukemia) specimen: 7–10 ml of peripheral blood in EDTA tube

* Bone marrow aspirate (leukemias and myelomas): 1–3 ml of heparinized bone marrow aspirate[3]

Clinical consultations with Robert Nagourney, MD, are available and include an overall assessment of the patient's condition, a physical examination, and a review of the patient's medical records and therapies. An interview is conducted to determine the patient's philosophy and treatment goals. Dr. Nagourney's opinion and recommendations will be provided in a written report. Phone and video consultations are also available. The fee for this is $395.

Cost

The fee for the functional profile is around $4,500–$7,500, depending upon the quantity and complexity of the agents tested. Payment is required at the time of service. The lab will file a claim with your insurance carrier to try to help you recover your out-of-pocket expense. Medicare/HMOs do not consider the functional profile test to be a covered service, but many private indemnity plans will cover part or all of the fee for the analysis. CPT codes are available to provide to your insurance carrier to determine level of reimbursement.

Financial assistance may be available from the Vanguard Cancer Foundation if you cannot afford the cost of the functional profile test. The foundation may be able to help cover part or all of the cost of the test. Assistance is based on financial need and must be approved before receipt of the sample by the laboratory. Contact Patient Relations at 800-542-4357 to request a Vanguard assistance application.[4]

Sample Processing Only

Occasionally the lab is unable to provide an adequate analysis because a specimen contained too few malignant cells for a reliable analysis. In these cases, there is a $500 sample processing fee to cover the cost of specimen transportation, laboratory personnel, reagents, and specimen processing.

If a specimen transportation kit sent out for use is not returned to the lab with a specimen for analysis, a $125 specimen kit fee will be charged to cover the costs associated with the kit. If a specimen is submitted, the cost of the kit is included in the test price.[5]

BENEFITS

The living tumor cells are kept in clusters (microspheroids) that mimic the body's environment. These microspheroids reflect the complex elements of the body's cellular environment, which has proved critical for the accurate prediction of clinical response. The test provides "real-time" analysis of how cancer cells actually respond when exposed to various treatment options.

Laboratory-validated data is provided to guide drug selection and treatment decisions. New options can be identified for patients who have failed therapy.

LIMITATIONS

The cancer must be advanced enough to be able to provide the required specimen. The testing kit must be on hand at the time of surgery.

PROCESS TIME

Once the sample is received at the laboratory, results are generally available within seven days.

THOUGHTS

There are a couple of misconceptions when it comes to the conventional treatment of cancer with pharmacological agents. First, people tend to accept the standard drug therapies as best. But that is the old-school, one-size-fits-all approach. We now know that a personalized selection of cytotoxic agents can greatly increase outcomes. Second, there is a misconception that chemosensitivity-resistance assays are only useful for patients in the relapsed state once they have failed conventional, standardized first-line therapy. It has been shown that standard protocols can induce drug resistance, diminishing the likelihood of a good outcome in subsequent therapy. I suggest you give it your best shot the first time.

If you were choosing chemotherapy, wouldn't it be best to start with the personalized approach? Chemo drugs are considerably toxic. Wouldn't it be best to use only those that will be most effective?

Chemosensitivity testing is not perfect; in fact, some would say it is still in its infancy. And experts in the field debate whether tissue or blood is better to use. But the bottom line is these tests are a significant step forward, and they provide guidance on which drugs may be most effective. Any clinically validated methodology that improves your chances for a better outcome is a tool to use. The results can also be utilized if you choose the low-dose chemotherapy option (discussed in chapter 32, "Low-Dose Approach to Chemotherapy").

I have to close this chapter by recommending you find cancer early. This book is full of tests to help you do exactly that. Remember, it can take years to grow a tumor large enough to obtain a large enough sample for this kind of testing. Early intervention can be lifesaving. References are available at www.nagourneycancerinstitute.com/the-science.

SAMPLE TEST RESULTS

EVA-PCD FUNCTIONAL PROFILE

NAGOURNEY
CANCER
INSTITUTE

Patient:	Assay Date:
Dx: Breast	Assay Quality: High Yield/Mod Viability
Prior Rx: Treated	Report Date:
Physician:	Specimen Number:

Drug	Ex Vivo Activity	EX Vivo Synergy	Ex Vivo Interpretation Response Expectation Compared with Database

SINGLE DRUG DOSE EFFECT ANALYSIS

Doxorubicin	Intermediate		Average
Taxol	Intermediate		Average
5-Fu	Resistant		Lower
Phenformin (Mitochondrial)	Resistant		Lower
Trimetrexate*	Resistant		Lower
Vinorelbine	Resistant		Lower

MULTIPLE DRUG DOSE EFFECT ANALYSIS

Vinorelbine & Lapatinib	*Sensitive*	*Synergy*	*Higher*
Vinorelbine & 5-Fu	*Sensitive*	Partial Synergy	*Higher*
Phenformin & Everolimus	*Sensitive*	Mixed Synergy	*Higher*
Vinorelbine & Lapatinib & Everolimus	*Sensitive*	Mixed Synergy	*Higher*
Cisplatin & Gemcitabine	*Sensitive*	N/A	*Higher*
Cytoxan & Doxorubicin	*Sensitive*	N/A	*Higher*
Cisplatin & Taxol & Lapatinib	Resistant	No Synergy	Lower
Cytoxan & Taxol & Lapatinib	Resistant	No Synergy	Lower
Taxol & 5-Fu	Resistant	No Synergy	Lower
Cisplatin & Taxol	Resistant	N/A	Lower
Cytoxan & Taxol	Resistant	N/A	Lower

DATA ANALYSIS:

Laboratory results represent only one part of the overall determination of therapy for patients and do not guarantee outcomes nor indicate the specific drugs that should be used in a particular patient.

* The following compounds serve as in vitro surrogates for their respective drug classes, e.g., Cytoxan: = Cyclophosphamide, Ifosfamide, Melphalan, Chlorambucil and related mustard alkylators; Cisplatin: = Carboplatin; Doxorubicin: = Daunorubicin and Idarubicin; Trimetrexate: = Methotrexate; 5Fu + Interferon: =Xeloda.

Ex Vivo best regimen (EVBR®) would be Cisplatin plus Gemcitabine $\cong$ AC $\geq$ VinoCAP.

Robert A. Nagourney, MD
Laboratory and Medical Director
Nagourney Cancer Institute

750 East 29th Street, Long Beach, CA 90806-1406 T 562.989.6455 F 562.989.8160 www.nagourneycancerinstitute.com

Chapter 28

Additional Labs Offering Chemosensitivity Testing From Live Tissue Samples

VIABLE (LIVING) TUMOR cells are required for this type of testing. The living cells must be handled and prepared for shipment to the lab using precise guidelines. Please call the lab a minimum of two days before surgery or other procedure to get the specimen requirements and the collection kit.

Here is a recap on this type of testing: You must have a malignant tumor or malignant fluid from which live cells can be collected. Each drug is tested with the cancer cells to see its effectiveness. Chemotherapy drugs that help one patient often don't help another patient with the same type of cancer. Testing *before* you receive chemo can identify exactly which drug or combination of drugs is the most effective for you and you alone. It can also detect differences in activity among different drugs within the same class of drugs, as well as identify drugs that don't work well.

Weisenthal Cancer Group

Personalized Cytometric Cancer Profiling (Chemosensitivity and Chemoresistance Testing)

> 16512 Burke Lane
> Huntington Beach, CA 92647
> Phone: 714-596-2100 or 866-364-0011
> Fax: 714-596-2110
> International: 011-714-596-2100
> www.weisenthalcancer.com
> mail@weisenthalcancer.com

Note: In addition to live cell chemosensitivity testing, it offers a test called the AngioRx™. It assesses the effectiveness of anti-vascular agents in mixed-cell micro-clusters. A genomic test can't do this. The new anti-angiogenesis drugs work for only a small percentage of patients and can cause serious side effects. In addition, they're extremely expensive—as much as $100,000 per year of treatment. If your physician is suggesting one of these drugs, this test is for you. Contact the Weisenthal Cancer group for more information.

AccuTheranostics™
ChemoFit™ (Chemosensitivity and Chemoresistance Test)

875 Ellicott Street
Suite 5080
Buffalo, NY 14203
Phone: 716-688-9600 or 877-402-2623
Fax: 716-688-9601
www.accutheranostics.com
info@accutheranostics.com

Note: ChemoFit™ is recommended for solid tumors, such as breast, cervical, colon, endometrial, lung, ovarian, prostate, and pancreatic cancers, and sarcomas. Use for leukemias and lymphomas is in the validation stages.

Part III

Additional Information to Consider

Chapter 29

Suggested Testing Uses

THE FOLLOWING IS a *suggested guideline* for the use of the tests in this book. It's important that you connect with an integrative physician who can support your path to being cancer-free using prevention, early-detection, nontoxic therapies as well as lifestyle interventions.

Refer to each chapter for additional information on each test. Just as we are all individuals, with our own set of DNA, your physician may have a very good reason for using specific testing. If he or she isn't aware of a test that you would like, share the test's website and be bold enough to explain why you're making the request. Many physicians are new to the integrative and prevention model and are happy to hear you out. Remember, it's your right to be able to choose a physician whose beliefs line up with yours. Most of the detection tests involve a simple blood draw and will not detect cancers originating in the brain due to limitations created by the blood-brain barrier.

Let the fear go! We've allowed cancer to become something big and scary by not stopping it early. Stop it while it's easily stoppable and before it's a big problem.

Detection—any site

(***Indicates my personal go-to tests for someone who has never been diagnosed with cancer)

+ Oncocount RGCC® (live cells/blood)***
+ IvyGene® (blood)***
+ CA Profile© (blood)
+ AMAS (blood)
+ Nagalase (blood)
+ Human chorionic gonado-tropin (HCG) (urine)
+ Thymidine kinase (blood)

Detection-specific sites

+ Videssa® Breast (blood)
+ EarlyCDT-Lung (blood)
+ OralID (oral mucosa using fluorescent light)

- Cologuard® (stool)
- Colon Health Home Test Kit (stool)
- Papanicolaou (Pap) and human papillomavirus (HPV) (cell scraping)

- Biocept (blood)—breast, prostate, colorectal, lung, and gastric
- BreastSentry™
- ColonSentry®
- Prostate Health Index

Progression or regression

- Oncocount RGCC® (blood)
- Oncotrail RGCC® (blood)
- Oncotrace RGCC® (blood)
- IvyGene® (blood)
- CA Profile© (blood)

- Nagalase (blood)
- Biocept (blood)—breast, prostate, colorectal, lung, and gastric—cell enumeration portion of the test

Chemosensitivity drug testing (assisting in the development of a personalized treatment plan)

- Onconomics RGCC® (live cells/blood)
- Onconomics Plus RGCC® (live cells/blood)—includes natural substances sensitivity
- Nagourney Cancer Institute (live cells/tissue or fluid)
- Weisenthal Cancer Group (live cells/tissue or fluid)
- AccuTheranostics™ ChemoFit™ (live cells/tissue)

Genomic drug testing (assisting in the development of a personalized treatment plan)

- Onconomics RGCC® (live cells/blood)—genomic and chemosensitivity
- Caris Molecular Intelligence (tumor tissue or malignant fluid)
- Biocept (blood)
- Foundation Medicine (blood, tumor tissue, or malignant fluid)
- Biofocus® (blood)

Natural-substance testing (assisting in the development of a personalized treatment plan)

+ Onconomics Extracts RGCC® (blood)—tests for approximately fifty natural substances shown effective against tumor stem cells

+ Biofocus® (blood)—tests for about fifteen natural substances

Immune-system testing

+ Immune-Frame RGCC® (blood)

+ Immune Cellular NK—BioFocus® (blood)

Metastasis potential

+ Metastat RGCC® (blood)

Response to cytotoxic drugs

· ChemoSNiP RGCC® (blood)

Chapter 30

Connecting With an
Integrative Physician

Assemble a Team if You Have Cancer

I F YOU FIND yourself with a diagnosis of stage I cancer or greater, I encourage you to assemble a team of experts. The organizations that follow have directories that can assist you in finding an integrative physician. Also, the free "Resources" download at www.cancerfreeexperts.com is a great tool. Interview doctors and ask lots of questions. Select a lead physician with whom you feel comfortable. Most doctors are willing to do a phone consult; however, they will charge a fee for their time. Don't hesitate to ask about real survival outcomes. Be willing to travel. Often once a personalized plan of care is developed, many physicians are willing to work with your local doctor.

If you only find indicators of an "ultra-early" cancer problem, you can seek out an integrative or functional medicine practitioner to help you establish a plan to stop and reverse the process, then monitor your progress with testing. I caution you against trying to doctor yourself! There is no need to reinvent the wheel. Connect with a doctor with a proven success record.

Consider a Cancer Consultant

There are a lot of qualified people treating cancer with great success, so put on your investigative "hat" and gather information. In my opinion, when dealing with a life-threatening disease, two heads are better than one. Having an advocate in your corner can be very valuable. I wish I'd found such a person at the time of my diagnosis. Remember, you don't get answers if you don't ask questions.

Here are a couple that I'm familiar with:

+ Dr. Janey Little (South Africa)—She offers Skype or telephone consults, and her approach is integrative.
+ Nasha Winters, ND, FABNO, L.Ac, Dipl.OM, of Optimal Terrain Consulting—She and her team of

physicians review your test results, lab work, pathology, and history, formulating a road map for you that includes both integrative and allopathic options. They'll work with your local physician. When you're dealing with a cancer diagnosis, calling in an expert is a good way to go.

+ Chris Wark (www.chrisbeatcancer.com)—Chris was diagnosed with stage IIIC colon cancer in December 2003. There was a golf ball–sized tumor in his large intestine, and the cancer had spread to his lymph nodes. He had the tumor surgically removed and declined chemotherapy, taking a natural approach to healing. Check out his cancer and health coaching program called "Square One" on his website.

ORGANIZATIONS WITH PHYSICIAN DIRECTORIES

Best Answer for Cancer Foundation
https://bestanswerforcancer.org
Search the "comprehensive Integrative Physician Directory" icon. Locate physicians by area, treatment, or disease.

Best Answer for Cancer Foundation is "a hybrid organization of doctors and patients working to shift the cancer paradigm from a one-size-fits-all disease-based approach to a patient-centered, integrative medical approach."[1] The organization offers education for member physicians as well as cancer patients.

Society for Integrative Oncology (SIO)
https://integrativeonc.org
Search under the "Directory" tab.

SIO is a professional organization for integrative oncology. It supports "communication, education, and research…by bringing together practitioners from multiple disciplines focused on the care of cancer patients and survivors."[2]

The American Association of Naturopathic Physicians
www.naturopathic.org
Search under the "Find a ND" tab.

"The American Association of Naturopathic Physicians (AANP) is the national professional society representing licensed naturopathic doctors.…Physician members are graduates of naturopathic medical schools accredited by the Council on Naturopathic Medical Education.... Members also include naturopathic medicine students, other health care professionals and corporate members who collectively strive to advance the profession of naturopathic medicine nationwide."[3]

Oncology Association of Naturopathic Physicians (OncANP)
https://oncanp.org
Search under the "Find an ND" tab.

Its vision is "to enhance survival and quality of life for people living with cancer through the integration of naturopathic medicine in cancer care."[4]

Academy of Comprehensive Integrative Medicine (ACIM)
www.acimconnect.com
Search under "Find a Health Practitioner."

The ACIM supports "the healthcare paradigm toward wellness by restoring hope, empowering people, training and supporting practitioners, conducting research, [and] implementing therapeutic innovations."[5]

Cancer Tutor
www.cancertutor.com
Click on the "Clinics" tab for the clinic directory, or search www .cancertutor.com/clinics.

Cancer Tutor is a leading voice in natural cancer treatments. It has a dedicated team that travels and evaluates clinics around the globe. The team members visit the clinics, interview the doctors, and follow up with past and current patients.

For your convenience, links to all these organizations are available on my website, www.CancerFreeExperts.com.

Chapter 31

Functional Testing Overview

CANCER IS MORE than a tumor and has many contributing factors. Think of a bucket with five holes in it, each hole representing burdens on your health and immune system. Cancer is the first hole. Even if you plug that first hole, you still have four other holes that haven't been plugged. Your bucket is still leaking. You're still at increased risk for disease. Those other holes represent things such as hidden dental infections, parasites, viruses, mercury toxicity, energy blockages, and stress. Once you've had cancer, you must pay careful attention to your health because you never want the disease to come back and metastasize. You may not be familiar with all the tests in this chapter, and some you most likely will have to seek a health care provider to access. But it's worth it—addressing these issues can produce big benefits long term.

What follows is a brief summary of each test. For more detail, go to www.cancerfreeexperts.com, and click on the "Free Downloads!" tab for a free download about functional tests.

BIOLOGICAL DENTAL EXAM

The relationship of the mouth to the rest of the body is often overlooked and may hold the key to finally being able to shake off chronic infections. Years of traditional dental work can leave you with a mouthful of toxic metals, unsuspected sites of infection deep in the bone, and interrupted flow of the body's natural energy pathways. The complex relationship of oral and systemic health within the whole person is inseparable. Exams should include an overall health history, testing for metal toxicities, special X-rays to identify silent infections, and energy pathway analysis, while being in a safe, mercury-free environment.

BIOLOGICAL IMPEDANCE ANALYSIS

This test measures the relationship of fat, muscle, bone, and water. It paints a different picture than the number on your bathroom scale. Its phase-angle measurement, for example, is an interesting way to chart the ongoing health of cell membranes and body mass.

BIOLOGICAL TERRAIN ASSESSMENT (BTA)

How well is oxygen getting around your body? What's the level of acidity in your tissues? What's your level of free-radical activity? Those answers and more can be had with a biological terrain assessment. Blood, saliva, and urine samples are analyzed by a computer, showing which biological systems are in good shape and which are weakened.

C-REACTIVE PROTEIN (CRP) TEST

This test gives a gauge of your level of internal inflammation by measuring a protein produced by the liver. Conditions such as cancer, arthritis, lupus, and inflammatory bowel disease can cause elevated CRP. So too can an infection. Chronically elevated inflammation causes damage to the body.

DARK FIELD MICROSCOPY

This is also called "Live Blood Cell Analysis." Dark field microscopy is the only way to observe *live* blood cells. A live blood analysis sees the blood in motion and is typically used to view the interaction of live blood cells with other factors such as fibrin, spirochetes, viruses, and elements of the immune system.

ELECTRODERMAL SCREENING

This combines time-honored Chinese medicine with the more modern technology of Dr. Reinhard Voll's electroacupuncture. It's a form of computerized information gathering that taps into the vast array of tiny electrical charges produced by every cell in the body. Use this test to identify energy blockages.

ESTROGEN PROFILE

Estrogen is a powerful hormone that can exhibit both protective and detrimental effects on estrogen-sensitive tissues. A twenty-four-hour urine sample captures the small "bursts" of hormone output throughout an entire day and measures many estrogen metabolites.

GALECTIN-3 TEST

Galectin-3 is usually found in small amounts in our blood; however, increased levels of galectin-3 are often found in patients with cancer proliferation and metastasis. This blood test can also reveal the process of fibrosis and potential for cancer progression.

Hemoglobin A1c Test

Sugar in the bloodstream is sticky, and it tends to stick to red blood cells. This blood test measures the amount of sugar/glucose bound to the hemoglobin in red blood cells. But unlike a finger prick, which gives only a momentary snapshot of your blood sugar level, a hemoglobin A1c test measures how thick the sugar coating has become on red blood cells over a three-month period—indicating recent *average* blood sugar levels.

Hormone Test

A comprehensive hormone test looks at levels of estrogen, progesterone, cortisol, melatonin, DHEA, and androgen. Hormones work in concert, and knowing where there are imbalances is important.

Lymphocytic Response Assay

Lymphocytes are your immune system's "soldiers." A lymphocytic response assay identifies how well those soldiers are dealing with substances such as foods, additives, environmental chemicals, molds, herbs, and dander. If you know what to avoid because your body does not react well to it, you can reduce the stress on your immune system.

Micronutrient Test

Are you running low on minerals, vitamins, key amino acids, or even CoQ10? These tests will tell you where you stand, whether you are absorbing your supplements, and how well nutrients are working in your body. Cancer has long been known as a disease of deficiency. It is important to identify deficiencies so you can "plug those holes" in your bucket.

Mycotoxin and Fungal DNA Testing

Mycotoxins—released by toxic mold species—are famous for their damaging effects on human cells. They're also associated with a wide variety of diseases, including cancer, kidney disease, immune suppression, neurotoxicity, depression, autism, and chronic fatigue syndrome. For example, aflatoxins, produced by a common household mold, are one of the most potent natural cancer-causing agents known to man. This testing can be done with a urine sample, nasal wash, sputum, or a tissue biopsy collected by a physician. An environmental test can be done using dust samples, as mycotoxins and fungi adhere to dust. Identifying a source of contamination can be very helpful.

PARASITE URINE AND STOOL TEST

A study published in *The Lancet Oncology Journal* in June 2012 reported that approximately one in six cancer cases started out as preventable or treatable infections caused by bacteria, viruses, or parasites. Each year these infections cause about two million cancer cases worldwide, resulting in 1.5 million deaths.[1] This test uses both stool and urine specimens to test for parasites.

PH ALKALINE/ACID TEST

pH is a measurement of how alkaline or how acidic something is. In a healthy person the pH of blood, spinal fluid, saliva, and urine should be in the middle of the scale, about 7.365. Cancer patients commonly have an acidic pH because tumors shed lactic acid, which makes the environment acidic. Measuring the pH of saliva or urine provides a snapshot of the body's extracellular pH.

SELF-ASSESSMENT OF THE HEART

A body under chronic stress is prone to developing disease. Chronic stress causes the adrenal glands to produce a lot of cortisol to help us handle that stress. If levels remain high, problems such as fatigue, insomnia, obesity, decreased insulin sensitivity, depression, and reduced immune function can develop. This test is not found in a lab. You must examine your own heart. See the "Functional Tests" download at www.cancerfreeexperts.com for a list of questions to ask yourself about emotional issues.

SPINAL ALIGNMENT ANALYSIS

The human body is part mechanical, part electrical energy. Pressure on nerves is known to block energy signals from reaching their destination. Imagine trying to steer your car when the steering wheel is not connected to the front tires. Get your spine checked for proper alignment.

THERMOGRAPHY EXAM

This one is for breast cancer. It is a better alternative to the routine, annual mammogram. Thermography was approved by the FDA in 1982 as an adjunct test for breast cancer risk assessment. This test is noninvasive, requires no compression, uses no radiation, and can provide earlier detection compared with a mammogram.

VIRAL SCREENING

Do you have an infection dragging down your immune system? Viral screenings most often use a blood sample and can look for viruses commonly implicated in cancer, such as human papillomavirus (HPV), Epstein-Barr virus (EBV), cytomegalovirus, hepatitis B, hepatitis C, human immunodeficiency virus (HIV), human herpesvirus 8 (HHV-8), and the human T-lymphotropic virus type 1 (HTLV-1).

GLYPHOSATE TEST

Glyphosate is the world's most widely produced herbicide and is the primary chemical in Roundup™ as well as in many other herbicides. It's a broad-spectrum herbicide that is used in more than seven hundred different products, from agriculture and forestry to home use. Usage of glyphosate has increased since the introduction of genetically modified glyphosate-resistant crops that can grow well in the presence of this chemical. It's damaging to the gut flora of humans and animals. Check out the research of Zach Bush, MD, online and on YouTube. Eating organic is not enough. A urine test can check for levels of this chemical in your system. I suggest testing your water as well. The Great Plains Laboratory offers both (www.greatplainslaboratory.com).

DIRECT-TO-CONSUMER LAB AND IMAGING TESTING

If you don't have insurance or don't want to deal with the co-pays, or if you want a test your doctor has not ordered, you can use a direct-to-consumer company. Sometimes those companies' cost is less than your insurance co-pay because they negotiate pricing based on large volumes. You can order the test yourself, usually online, pay for it, and get the results sent to you. Also, many imaging centers are offering discounted cash pricing on MRIs and PET and CT scans.

Many people tell me they can't afford to get basic testing because they have no insurance or a huge deductible. Today you have options with low-cost testing. And if a problem is noted, the lab report alerts you to see a doctor. The earlier a problem is detected, the easier it is to be treated and the more likely it is to be treatable.

We have direct access to clinical laboratory testing throughout the United States for those important blood chemistry and wellness tests, such as a complete blood count, a urinalysis, a liver function panel, allergy testing, a C-reactive protein test, hormone tests, HIV testing, vitamin D levels, and more.

As always, if you find a problem, seek professional advice.

Go to www.cancerfreeexperts.com to read more detail on each of these functional tests.

Chapter 32

Low-Dose Approach to Chemotherapy

OR DECADES WE'VE known cancer has one big weakness: it needs sugar to survive. We've also known we can use sugar to target a very low dose of chemotherapy to cancer cells and spare patients the toxicity of larger doses. This method, insulin potentiation therapy (IPT), is championed by the Best Answer for Cancer Foundation, which provides education and certification for medical doctors practicing IPT.

Information was provided by the Best Answer for Cancer Foundation, a 501(c)3 based in Austin, Texas.

INSULIN POTENTIATION TARGETED LOW-DOSE (IPTLD) THERAPY

Insulin potentiation therapy (IPT) is a time-proven and powerful method of treating cancer. It has been in use since 1946. It is often called "a kinder, gentler approach."

IPT, also called insulin potentiation targeted low-dose (IPTLD) therapy, uses traditional chemotherapy drugs but is very different from conventional chemotherapy.

IPTLD is able to selectively target chemo drugs directly to cancer cells, largely bypassing healthy cells. Because of this, patients undergoing IPTLD experience far fewer side effects; their quality of life is higher. Whereas most people undergoing conventional chemotherapy can be instantly recognized by their bald heads, for example, most IPTLD patients do not lose their hair.

IPTLD uses about one-tenth the chemotherapy drug dosages used in conventional oncology.

IPTLD is also different because most physicians who make use of IPTLD realize chemotherapy, even at reduced dosages, is not the only tool available. They make use of complementary therapies to eliminate cancer and rebuild the immune system.

IPTLD physicians also typically make use of chemosensitivity tests to determine which drugs and complementary therapies would be most effective and which would not be. This process of selection and elimination spares patients unnecessary exposure to the effects and costs of a regime that would have little opportunity for a good outcome.

THE INSULIN ADVANTAGE

Each of our cells has a membrane, an outer layer, to protect it from toxins. Conventional chemotherapy needs to flood the body with drugs to force penetration through that membrane.

IPTLD, on the other hand, recognizes the membrane of cancer cells is built differently than healthy cells. Cancer cells use sugar as their primary fuel; healthy cells use fat as their primary fuel. The membrane of a cancer cell is built to give it plenty of access to glucose moving through the bloodstream.

Cancer cells love glucose. The faster they get glucose, the faster they can grow and spread. PET scans find cancer by looking at the cellular uptake of sugar. A radioactive tracer is mixed with glucose (sugar water) and injected into a vein. The cancer cells take in the radioactive agent as they take in the sugar. The resulting three-dimensional images of tracer concentration within the body are then constructed by computer analysis to reveal a mass, the tumor.

This need for glucose—sugar—also creates a vulnerability, however, and IPTLD uses that vulnerability to full advantage.

Insulin is the same natural hormone we hear about in diabetes, and it is what actually "escorts" glucose into cells. Cancer cells are equipped with more insulin receptors, upwards of sixteen times more, than healthy cells. Insulin cannot pump glucose into a cell without an insulin receptor, and cancer cells have a lot of them. Glucose is so important to cancer cells that they have the ability to secrete their own insulin to ensure their supply of fuel.

What if we pair a small dose of chemo drugs with insulin and glucose, in much the same way a PET scan pairs sugar with a tracer? The cancer cells take in the chemotherapy drugs in their effort to get at the sugar. Think of it as a Trojan horse effect.

To administer IPTLD, a physician first carefully lowers the patient's blood sugar level with insulin. As the blood sugar drops, the patient's healthy cells rely on fat metabolism, but the patient's cancer cells become seriously compromised. Cancer cells sense the threat to their survival, and their insulin receptors open wide to get at whatever sugar is left in the bloodstream. When the blood sugar level has dropped sufficiently—what is called the "therapeutic moment"—the physician administers a low dose of chemotherapy followed by glucose to bring the patient's blood sugar back to a normal level.

Potentiation means to make more effective. Because insulin and glucose target the delivery of the drugs, IPTLD uses only about 10 percent of the chemotherapy used in conventional treatment, meaning patients can maintain their lifestyle without many of the side effects normally caused by chemotherapy.

Insulin also has another benefit. Chemotherapy is most effective when it targets cancer cells when they are dividing because that is when they are most vulnerable. Insulin prompts cancer cells to divide, further enabling the chemo to effectively target the cancer cells.

Without the use of insulin, the conventional large dose of chemotherapy forces itself through the membrane of any cells that happen to be dividing. The cells that divide the most are those in the intestine, bone marrow, mouth, and hair follicles. That is why the side effects of conventional chemotherapy can often include hair loss, nausea, lower red and white blood cell counts, mouth and stomach ulcers, and even organ failure. By using insulin to target the drugs to the cancer cells, the healthy cells are largely spared.

Conventional use of chemotherapy comes down to whether we can kill the cancer without killing the patient. To summarize the process that takes place with IPTLD:

+ Insulin enables the differentiation of cancer cells and normal cells.

+ Insulin targets the drugs to the cancer cells, largely bypassing healthy cells.

+ Cancer cells take up more of the chemotherapy drugs than they would without the use of insulin.

+ Insulin prompts cancer cells to divide, making them more sensitive to the toxic effects of the drugs. The result is a level of cancer cell death and growth control comparable to, or even better than, standard chemotherapy.

+ The lower dose means there are far fewer side effects. Patients do not experience severe side effects that lead to the debilitating loss of hope and lowered quality of life.

+ The lower dose does not affect the immune system's ability to protect against other infections the way traditional chemotherapy protocols do.

+ Because of the lower dose being used, IPTLD treatments can continue as long as necessary without long-term toxicity to healthy cells and tissues.

+ IPTLD enables the aggressive pursuit of simultaneous
  immune therapy and chemotherapy, a combined treatment
  not usually possible with standard chemotherapy protocols.

IPTLD has been reported to work especially well for breast, colon, lung, prostate, and stomach cancers, as well as lymphoma and melanoma. IPTLD has also been reported to bring responses and remissions to patients with pancreatic, ovarian, renal cell, blood, bone, cervical, esophageal, lip, mouth, neck, small intestine, testicular, throat, thyroid, uterine, and vaginal cancers.[1]

CHEMOSENSITIVITY TESTING BEFORE IPTLD

Today chemosensitivity testing provides real-time information about specific drugs and more natural therapies that will be effective for you, even at different times during therapy, and the tests correlate with treatment success.[2] Chemosensitivity testing is an essential component in the use of IPTLD. Most physicians who utilize IPTLD will not do so without having first identified the best drugs for you. They typically use chemosensitivity testing or genomic testing to do this.

WHAT IT IS LIKE TO RECEIVE IPTLD

The patient is seated in the physician's office, usually in a comfortable lounge chair. Medical staff will insert an IV into a vein or port. The patient will be given a dose of insulin based on his or her body weight to reduce the blood glucose level. The patient will start to feel light-headed, or even weak, hungry, and flushed. The insulin dose will keep the patient in this state for several minutes, giving the cancer cells time to open their insulin receptors.

Think of lowering your blood sugar as you might think of holding your breath. You know you can do it for maybe three minutes, but much longer, and you would die. If it were possible to completely deprive cancer cells of glucose, they would die within a matter of minutes. Unfortunately to keep you alive, we cannot do that. However, IPTLD can lower the amount of glucose by about 70 percent, enough to make cancer cells more vulnerable to chemotherapy drugs.

At the therapeutic moment, the chemotherapy drugs are delivered, followed immediately by an intravenous infusion of glucose. Anti-inflammatory, antifungal, antibacterial, antiviral, and liver support substances are also often administered at this time.

Clinical experience with the IPTLD protocol has demonstrated the therapeutic moment comes approximately twenty-five to thirty minutes after insulin is given. A session of IPTLD lasts about two hours.

On days when IPTLD is not administered, patients may undergo a number of complementary therapies—from intravenous vitamin C or a Myers' cocktail to chelation or ozone therapy.

Each person is treated on a case-by-case basis, but generally doctors advise between fourteen and twenty-five IPTLD sessions combined with complementary therapies and lifestyle changes.

TECHNICALLY SPEAKING

Insulin plays an important role in the mechanisms of malignancy. Fractionated low-dose chemotherapy "utilizes insulin as a biologic response modifier to target just the cancer cells and not the immune system or vital body organs."[3] IPTLD manipulates the way cancer cells function to therapeutic advantage by employing insulin to enhance anti-cancer drug cytotoxicity and safety.

It is well known that "cell-cycle phase-specific anticancer drugs work best on cells in S-phase of the growth cycle.... Because of the much richer distribution of insulin and IGF-1 receptors on cancer cell membranes versus normal somatic cells, these drug potentiating effects will predominate in the cancer cells with a relative sparing of normal tissues."[4]

Insulin has been found to increase the cell-killing effects of methotrexate (a chemotherapy drug) in breast cancer cells in tissue culture by a factor of up to 10,000.[5] In a study of three cases where IPTLD was used in the treatment of metastatic tumors following failure of standard chemotherapy, the findings were:

> We achieved remission for 15, 21 and 8 months, respectively. The first patient was lost to follow up after June 2008 and the other two are in remission until now, receiving maintenance treatment. Their quality of life improved rapidly after the first 2–3 courses and gave the patients the opportunity to restore their normal work activity after 2–3 months from the beginning of treatment. The third patient was additionally treated with LHRH agonist.
>
> Treatment was very well tolerated, the only complaints being weakness and sleepiness during the first day. Lab examinations showed no significant toxicity. In our 3 patients we observed insignificant increase of liver function tests in the first 6 weeks, while these normalized without any additional measures during treatment.[6]

In another study of 196 patients diagnosed with a variety of neoplastic diseases:

> Laboratory tests demonstrated that the dose related toxicity of chemotherapeutics could be largely mitigated when applied in conjunction with insulin, at a fractionated dose in accordance with a dose dense regimen. Upon follow-up, eighty-five of 106 patients (80%) with advanced metastatic disease reported a subjectively significant improvement in their quality of life....Only two of the 148 patients with initially low Hb level needed blood transfusion while in active treatment....Patients easily tolerated IPTLD.[7]

Good scientific evidence exists to affirm the formulation of IPTLD. The way IPTLD functions makes it an excellent candidate for treating cancer because it is consistent with the natural biology of cancer cells.

Since most diseased cells have an excess of insulin receptors, IPT can be used to treat conditions as diverse as arthritis, herpes, hepatitis C, and AIDS, as well as cardiovascular, respiratory (including pneumonia), neurological, and intestinal disorders.

IPT is an off-label use of both chemotherapy and insulin; however, off-label use of drugs is common practice.

WHY DON'T MORE ONCOLOGISTS USE IPTLD?

IPTLD uses significantly less of the pharmaceutical drugs used in conventional chemotherapy. For understandable reasons, the pharmaceutical industry does not want to encourage doctors to use less of their products. Medical associations and schools dependent upon pharmaceutical funding have not been motivated to embrace it.

Insulin potentiation therapy was developed by a family of physicians in Mexico. Dr. Donato Perez Garcia and his son and grandson have collaborated with other doctors to provide scientific evidence for the validity of the therapy and to get clinical studies published in the scientific/medical journals. Their goal is to get IPTLD properly studied in the United States so more physicians and patients will use it.[8] The Best Answer for Cancer Foundation offers physician training and is spearheading the collection of data.

The side effect of insulin is hypoglycemia, or low blood sugar. Patients undergoing IPT are closely monitored by professionals and given glucose intravenously to offset the insulin. Patients will feel hungry and may experience other mild and temporary symptoms, including fatigue, headache, or sweating. Note that diabetic patients administer and manage their own insulin without the daily oversight of professionals.

Since chemotherapy drugs have considerable toxicity associated with their use, there is always a risk. But because IPTLD uses much lower doses than conventional chemotherapy, the risk is significantly reduced. Patients may experience some constipation and nausea after the first two IPTLD treatments. Anemia and decreased white blood cell and platelet counts are unusual; rarely are decreases so severe as to require transfusions.

Most conventional cancer treatment focuses on only controlling cancer growth. While that is obviously essential, the rest of the body must be included in the process. The cancer must be eliminated or brought under control, and the patient's compromised immune system function must be optimized. A wide array of complementary therapies can be used to:

- "Provide more effective and targeted cancer treatments that leave surrounding healthy tissue unharmed"
- "Utilize other cancer-killing agents and thereby decrease dependency upon chemo drugs"
- "Help the body detoxify"
- "Provide nutrition to a depleted body"
- "Nurture and strengthen the immune system"[9]

Cancer is a case of immunological tolerance—the immune system tolerates it; it does not see the cancer cells as something to be sought after and killed. Some complementary therapies work to break that tolerance. Others work to strengthen the immune system, to give the body healing nutrients and restore good health long term. Some of these therapies do double duty as preventive therapies. There is a detailed discussion of them in chapter 34, "The Toolbox."

SHIFTING THE CANCER PARADIGM

Best Answer for Cancer Foundation is at the forefront of the emerging shift from the traditional one-size-fits-all approach to an enlightened integrative cancer treatment approach, one more personalized and more patient centered with an emphasis on better outcomes. It is the foundation's mission "to improve the quality of life and treatment of cancer patients with a holistic platform, targeted cancer therapies, and a patient-centered approach."[10]

IPTLD allows patients to devote their full attention to achieving wellness, increasing their chances of recovery and improving both the quality and length of their lives.

Two books the foundation recommends about IPTLD:

+ *The Kinder, Gentler Cancer Treatment: Insulin Potentiation Targeted LowDose^{TM} Therapy* by Best Answer for Cancer Foundation, 2009

+ *Treating Cancer With Insulin Potentiation Therapy* by Ross A. Hauser, MD, and Marion A. Hauser, MS, RD; 2002

For more about the Best Answer for Cancer Foundation and the International Organization of Integrative Cancer Physicians, see www .bestanswerforcancer.org and https://bestanswerforcancer.org/physicians/.

As an added note, many integrative physicians are using the principles of IPTLD for natural therapies such as IV vitamin C.

Chapter 33

Cancer—Beat It, Don't Feed It

W E'LL KNOW AMERICA is serious about reducing the incidence of cancer when we see organizations such as the American Cancer Society wage a "war" on sugar.

I saw an invitation from a major hospital in the Houston area to attend "A Survivor's Celebration of Life." The program included culinary creations from local bakeries and a cake-decorating contest. Since we know many of these survivors will have a recurrence, and we know cancer cells use sugar for their metabolism, it is simply wrong for people entrusted with the care of these survivors to feed them something that fuels their disease. I was speechless.

I attended another event for survivors, a luncheon. As each woman left, she was handed a beautifully wrapped iced cake pop—pink, of course. You can safely assume I declined the parting gift.

I have photos of a large basket of candy in the surgical waiting area of one of Houston's well-known cancer treatment centers as well as the sugary items offered in the hospital cafeteria, such as the pastry and beverage counters. To be fair, I did find a small basket of red and green apples near the register in the cafeteria.

How can the medical establishment say it is waging a war on cancer while passing out candy? Simply, it can't. The establishment has not taken what is arguably the first step in fighting cancer, which is to wage war on sugar.

On February 4, 2014, front-page newspaper headlines read "Too Much Sugar Tied to Heart Problems."[1] The accompanying articles explained a major CDC study—the biggest of its kind—had concluded consuming added sugar clearly increases the risk of death from heart disease. People who consumed the highest amounts of added sugars were more than twice as likely to die from cardiovascular disease.[2]

Wow. That is straight to the point. Finally we are turning the corner and coming to a more enlightened approach to heart disease. We have been blaming heart disease on cholesterol, something the body makes because it needs it to survive and thrive.

The next day news headlines proclaimed "Cancer to Skyrocket

Worldwide, Study Says: WHO Report Faults Smoking, Obesity, Rise in Population."[3]

The American Cancer Society posted an essay for World Cancer Day 2014 and said,

> Avoiding tobacco, maintaining a healthy body weight, eating right and getting enough exercise, and getting appropriate cancer screening tests can all make a significant difference.[4]

No wow there. As usual, smoking leads the list. I agree quitting smoking is a great preventive thing in terms of avoiding cancer, but since only 15.5 percent of Americans smoke anymore, that advice does not apply to more than four out of five people. Eating added sugar applies to many, many more people. Are the powers that be afraid to take on the sugar lobby and put sugar front and center in the war on cancer?

ARE WE SERIOUS ABOUT BEATING CANCER?

Lifestyle choices are an overwhelming factor in cancer development. If we removed artificial sweeteners, high-fructose corn syrup, added sugars, inflammatory vegetable oils, excess refined salt, genetically modified foods, antibiotics, hormones, pesticides, and so on from the standard American diet, I predict cancer rates would drop substantially.

Unfortunately eating in today's world has become more about convenience and pleasure than about eating for nourishment. I have to admit, given the bounty of easily accessible processed foods with their attractive packaging, it's challenging to give your body what it needs in terms of quality fats, proteins, and carbohydrates on a daily basis. It can seem like a treasure hunt to find nourishing foods while avoiding toxic, empty-calorie foods.

Merriam-Webster defines *food* as simply "something that nourishes."[5] Check out your local vending machine, and see if you think the items in it meet the definition of *food*. (Hint: they don't.)

Headlines were generated by the Susan G. Komen organization when it took money from chocolate-candy makers (sugar), a fried-chicken restaurant chain (fried foods are linked to cancer), and a number of companies that make processed foods. No organization serious about winning a war on cancer would pick these kinds of sponsors.

SUGAR ACTS AS FERTILIZER FOR CANCER

Sugar is a major enemy of your body's immune system. And cancer is the ultimate immune system disorder. We've known this for decades. A 1973 study showed simple sugars (including fructose, glucose, sucrose, honey, and even orange juice) can decrease the white blood cells' ability to fight infection for up to five hours after ingestion.[6] This study used high dosages of sugar, but the evidence strongly suggests chronic consumption of sugar suppresses immunity. We all need a robust immune system to recognize and kill cancer cells.

In 1800 the average American consumed about 18 pounds of sugar per year. Today it's 75–170 pounds a year, depending upon who produces the statistic.[7] Sugar needs to be removed from the pantry and diet of anyone who wants to be cancer-free.

On a personal note, I encourage anyone who is not worried about risking cancer with sugary foods to be sensitive to those who do have cancer. For us cancer patients, the fight is tough enough without watching people around us drink sodas and eat candy bars, cookies, and chips.

I cannot emphasize enough how important diet is, whether you are in treatment, recovering, or trying to prevent cancer. Starchy carbohydrates and processed sugar have become toxic, addictive staples of our diets.

I understand these foods are comforting to the patients. I understand doctors don't take time to address diet because they are busy with test results, chemo, surgery, and so on. But this practice of turning a blind eye must end if we're going to reduce the incidence of cancer. So it is up to you. You must take charge of all aspects of your health, even those not addressed by your doctor or covered by insurance.

Don't forget that starchy carbs are a sugar. A seemingly harmless slice of whole-wheat toast will raise your blood sugar at least as much as eating a small candy bar. Many people incorrectly believe processed grains such as bread or pasta are good for us, but the body rapidly breaks down refined grains into sugar.

PROCESSED FOODS—A POOR NUTRITIONAL CHOICE

Processed foods are easy to recognize—they are nearly always in a package to make them more convenient. There is little or no nutritional content in most of what you find in a bag or box. The contents have usually been heated, milled, or irradiated, and contain artificial additives. Foods are usually processed to extend their shelf life. This is important for food that travels long distances or sits in supermarkets for long periods. For example, natural fats go rancid much more quickly than refined trans fats and interesterified fats that can extend shelf life by months. But the changed molecular structure of refined fats is not body-friendly; these creations have been linked to heart disease and cancer. For decades the American Heart Association advised people to eat trans fats to prevent heart disease. The FDA belatedly revoked its "generally recognized as safe" (GRAS) status for "partially hydrogenated" trans fats in 2015.[8] Refined bread is "enriched" with synthetic vitamins, for example, because so many natural vitamins are removed in processing. Much has been written warning of the synthetic, fractionated vitamins used to "fortify" flour and milk. (Hint: pasteurized/homogenized milk and commercial bread are not "whole" foods.)

Artificial sugars, flavorings, corn syrup, and refined salt are often added to improve flavor and disguise the taste of low-fat and low-quality, inexpensive ingredients. Use only natural sweeteners such as stevia or raw honey in limited quantities.

Most processed food is made with genetically modified organisms (GMOs), which, I believe, time will prove are not safe to eat.

Check the label for the presence of sugar, salt, fat, monosodium glutamate, and gluten. These five elements are often added to processed food because they have an addictive quality. Dr. David Kessler, former head of the FDA, said food companies have literally captured our brains to keep us coming back for more processed food products. Remember that marketing jingle for potato chips? You cannot eat only one. Right. Dr. Kessler told us food companies scientifically experiment with how foods taste, smell, and look, adjusting the sugar, fat, and salt content as needed, to come as close as possible to eating's "bliss point—the point at which we get the greatest pleasure from sugar, fat, or salt."[9]

At some point you have to just say *no*.

Recently several Latin American countries essentially said no in an attempt to lessen the obesity epidemic. In 2014 Brazil released dietary guidelines warning against processed foods: "Limit the use of processed foods, consuming them in small amounts as ingredients in culinary preparations or as part of meals based on natural or minimally processed foods.... When eating out...avoid places where unlimited food is offered for a set price.... Eat in places that serve fresh meals at good prices. Avoid fast food chains."[10] The city of Buenos Aires installed vending machines with fruit. And Mexico, which is high on the list of most populated countries in obesity statistics, passed a groundbreaking soda tax expected to prevent up to 630,000 cases of diabetes by 2030.[11] Billboards across Mexico City ran photographs of a man with amputated feet—a consequence of diabetes. Billboards warned that a roughly twenty-ounce bottle of soda contained twelve teaspoons of sugar and asked, "Would you eat 12 spoonfuls of sugar? Why do you drink soda?"[12] Remember that the next time someone offers you a soda.

REDUCING SUGAR—KETOGENIC DIET AS A THERAPY

The Paleo and the ketogenic diets are becoming popular ways to remove sugar from the diet. Both involve eliminating refined carbohydrates and focusing on healthy, beneficial fats and organic/grass-fed sources of protein. The ketogenic diet is stricter; it is about 70–80 percent fats, 10–20 percent protein, and 5–10 percent carbohydrates (veggies, not starches). Since cancer cells need glucose (sugar) to thrive, and starchy carbohydrates turn into glucose in your body, cutting out processed carbs literally starves cancer cells by taking away their primary fuel source.

When doctors prescribe a ketogenic diet, it is because they want you to burn fat, not sugar. Cancer cells cannot adapt to a fat- (or ketone-) burning mode, while healthy cells can. In fact, most people were fat burners until recent times, when sugar became such a large part of the diet. Good fats include olive oil, coconut oil, butter, avocados, egg yolks, grass-fed meats, and raw nuts. Protein recommendations are usually about fifty to seventy grams per day. Always consult a holistic nutritionist or doctor when considering a diet change.

In my research into a nutrition plan that would deprive cancer cells of the sugar they need to survive, I met Ellen Davis and read her book *Fight Cancer With a Ketogenic Diet*. It's well researched and referenced. Her insights will help you make dietary changes.

Ms. Davis told me the following:

> Making the statement that "cancer feeds on sugar" sounds like a fringe chant from some alternative health guru on television, but I can assure you, that statement is backed up with real scientific evidence from as far back as the early 1920s.

In her book Ms. Davis wrote:

> In 1928, Dr. Otto Warburg, a Nobel Prize-winning physician and biochemist...proposed the hypothesis that cancer is a metabolic disease. Dr. Warburg showed in his studies that cancer cells exhibited a preference for the utilization of sugar (glucose) as a fuel, even when the oxygen that normal cells use for energy creation is available. He commented:

Cancer, above all other diseases, has countless secondary causes. But, even for cancer, there is only one prime cause. Summarized in a few words, the prime cause of cancer is the replacement of the respiration of oxygen in normal body cells by a fermentation of sugar.

Until recently, Dr. Warburg's hypothesis…has been marginalized by the persistent belief in the oncology world that cancer is a genetic disease.[13]

Ms. Davis went on to comment that Thomas Seyfried's *Cancer as a Metabolic Disease: On the Origin, Management, and Prevention of Cancer* began to shed light on the hypothesis that cancer is instead a metabolically based disease and that the genetic markers that the cancer research community has focused on for so long are really just downstream effects of the cancer cell's broken metabolism.

Metabolic diseases are conditions in which metabolism, or how the body makes energy from the food we consume, is in some way messed up or abnormal. Normal cells create energy by using food and oxygen (cellular respiration). Most energy production occurs in the mitochondria, the energy factories of the cell. There are two main types of food-based fuels cells use for energy production:

1. Glucose (blood sugar or blood glucose)—Glucose is a product of carbohydrates. It is converted into energy through a process known as glycolysis. In normal cells "glycolysis is a source of other molecules that flow into the mitochondria to complete normal oxygen dependent cellular respiration."

2. Fatty acids—There are several kinds of fatty acids. They come from fats in the food we eat or from stored fat in our cells. When blood glucose is low, these fats are used to make up the fuel deficit. They are then broken down by the liver into ketone bodies, a process called ketosis.[14]

Normal cells will use ketone bodies for fuel when glucose levels drop. Even highly glucose-dependent brain and nerve cells can utilize ketone bodies for fuel if there are a sufficient number of them in the bloodstream. The ability of most normal cells to use ketones indicates that the cell's mitochondria are healthy and functioning properly. Cancer cells, on the other hand, cannot use ketones for energy.

Normal cells are "metabolically flexible"—they can use either glucose or ketones. This metabolic flexibility, or lack thereof in the case of cancer cells, is exactly why a ketogenic diet can force cancer cells to literally run out of fuel.[15]

The ketogenic diet is a powerful tool for fighting cancer. But for all its metabolic power, it has very few side effects, and instead of being toxic to normal cells, it actually strengthens the body. People who adhere to the ketogenic diet have reported less physiological stress when undergoing mainstream chemotherapy and radiation treatments.

A ketogenic diet is an effective tool for just about any disease system involving metabolic derangement. See Ellen Davis' website, www .ketogenic-diet-resource.com, for more information on this diet. I want you to have all the options. Another great option is Dr. Joseph Mercola's book *Fat for Fuel*. He also offers an online course. Or check out Amazon.com for a nice list of books with Keto recipes.

WHEN CANCER WAS RARE AND FOOD WAS NATURAL

In the 1930s Weston A. Price, DDS, embarked on a novel expedition to investigate the causes of physical degeneration in people. It was a unique window in time. The world was still small enough that he could readily find isolated populations who had had little or no contact with the foods of "modern" civilization, yet technological advances allowed him to document his findings with photographs and films that spoke volumes. He traveled to hundreds of places within multiple countries, from Switzerland to Alaska, from Africa to the South Seas Islands. He found overall excellent health in people eating their indigenous foods. However, where traders established trading posts, they had brought sacks of sugar and white flour, canned goods, pasteurized milk, and refined vegetable oils. Soon after, signs of degeneration became evident. Dr. Price found that dental cavities, arthritis, and low immunity to tuberculosis became rampant after the "modern foods of commerce" were introduced. Dr. Price found good health could be restored when modernized foods were removed from the diet.

As he surveyed the world, he saw people eating different diets, depending upon what was available. The Eskimo, for example, ate a lot of animal protein and fat but rarely vegetables. In some parts of Africa protein came primarily from bugs, not animals. But all healthy populations had diets containing at least four times the minerals of the American diet of his day and ten times the amount of fat-soluble vitamins (A, D, E, and K).[16]

Today Americans have not been taught how to eat well. I find most people actually don't know they are eating poorly. They make decisions with their taste buds, not with nutritional intelligence. And the food is addictive. Nutrition advice from the government and some associations is grossly colored by corporate lobbyists. Most doctors have precious little education in nutrition. It is up to you to educate yourself.

> Why spend money on what is not bread, and your labor on what does not satisfy? Listen, listen to me, and eat what is good, and you will delight in the richest of fare.
>
> —ISAIAH 55:2, NIV

Chapter 34

The Toolbox

Cancer is a complex, systemic disease. To achieve better outcomes, treatment must go beyond just addressing the tumor. The conditions leading up to cancer's presence in the body also must be addressed. Too often conventional treatment focuses only on the cancer, ignoring the toxicities, poor cellular respiration, and compromised immune system function that allowed cancer to develop in the first place. In this section you'll learn that there is a lot you can do to promote good cellular function, encourage good gene expression, assist the body with detoxification, and discourage cancer.

I'm a big believer in the body's ability to heal, but it needs the necessary building blocks. Every day is a new day, and you can birth new, healthy cells. Estimates are that an adult human will produce fifty to seventy billion new cells each day. Those healthy cells will come from the necessary fats, minerals, vitamins, enzymes, and proteins needed to function properly.

An estimated 5–10 percent of cancers are genetically driven, meaning caused by the genes over which we have no control, leaving the vast majority of cancers as *epigenetically driven*, meaning caused by diet and environmental factors we can control. We can prompt our genes to express in healthy ways.

When the Human Genome Project concluded in 2003, we finally had a map of the human genes. Experts were surprised to find humans have around twenty thousand genes, not the hundred thousand expected. This pretty much put an end to the idea that one gene gone wrong was the cause of any one disease. Something else and more complex was at work. Scientists began to focus on the epigenome—a network of internal chemical switches—influenced by diet and environment, constantly tweaking how our genes express.

We inherit one copy of a gene from our mother and one from our father. We may inherit one bad gene, but we likely inherit at least one good gene. That's enough for most people to live with one good gene expressing. But if we stress the good gene, then it may no longer express in healthy ways.

The BRCA1 and BRCA2 mutation makes a person more susceptible to breast cancer, but not everyone with this mutation will have breast cancer. Why? Epigenetics. Our network of chemical messengers is affected positively by a nutrient-dense diet and affected negatively by exposure to toxins such as pesticides and radiation or by the stress of a divorce or job loss, for example. A study in *The Lancet* in February 2018 titled "Germline BRCA Mutation and Outcome in Young-Onset Breast Cancer (POSH): A Prospective Cohort Study" found that there is "no significant difference in overall survival or distant disease-free survival between patients carrying the BRCA1 or BRCA2 mutation and patients without these mutations after a diagnosis of breast cancer."[1] This report is another confirmation that we are more than our genes. We can learn how to encourage our bodies to produce a healthy outcome.

How do you start? I'll share a few things I learned along the way—things I wish I had known at the start.

Don't eat within four hours of bedtime.

You can have a one hundred–calorie snack before bed but not a whole meal. This may seem hard, so let me explain why this is important. When we go to bed with a full stomach, digestion gets priority. Nutrients and energy will be spent processing what's in the stomach instead of doing the usual nighttime jobs of detoxing and healing.

Hydrate.

Drink lots of "clean" water. Proper hydration will open up the body's detoxification pathways and assist with alkalinity. Start the day with a cup of warm lemon tea. I squeeze the juice of a fresh lemon in warm water for an alkalizing drink. I try to drink one ounce of water for every two pounds of body weight. I often add a tablespoon of organic pure hydrolyzed collagen. I use a whole-house catalytic carbon filter system. It does a great job of removing toxins from my drinking and bath water.

Be aware of chemical pesticides.

Get friendly with nontoxic fertilizers for your backyard. If you have a gardener, talk to him about the products he uses. In the produce aisle buy organic to reduce ingesting pesticides used on fruits and vegetables. The Environmental Working Group puts out lists called the "Clean 15" and the "Dirty Dozen"; see www.ewg.org. Pesticides can be carcinogenic and disrupt hormonal activity. Wheat, corn, and soy are major sources of pesticides. Approximately 90 percent of corn and soy are GMOs, meaning they are not organic.

Avoid fluoride.

Use non-fluoride toothpaste because fluoride has been implicated as a carcinogen, and this chemical also affects how our bodies use iodine. Even the small amounts in typical toothpaste brands you get at the grocery store have been shown to displace iodine in the body.[2] By displacing the iodine, fluoride interferes with the working of the thyroid gland—the master controller of our metabolism. Fluoride is often added to municipal drinking water. Better filtration systems can get rid of most of the fluoride and chlorine.

Avoid BPA, BPS, phthalates, atrazine, and other xenoestrogens.

These are endocrine disruptors that have estrogen-like effects. They build up in our fat cells and are linked to many conditions, including breast, prostate, and testicular cancer, and obesity.[3] They're found in plastics, cosmetics, children's toys, cash register receipts, nonstick cookware— pretty much everywhere around us today. Opt to store food in glass containers and drink out of glass bottles.

A great source of information about environmental toxins can be found in a free PDF download titled *State of the Evidence* at www.bcpp.org/resource/state-evidence-2017/. It is produced by Breast Cancer Prevention Partners, one of the few organizations on a mission to prevent cancer. The document was written for the breast cancer audience, but the information applies pretty much to anyone with any type of cancer.

Beware of synthetic hormone replacement.

With the increase in hormonally driven cancers, it pays to limit our exposure to synthetic hormones. Birth control pills are comprised of synthetic hormones and have been linked to cervical and breast cancers. Bioidentical hormone replacement was thought to be safer, but I wonder if we know all there is to know yet. Do women really need more estrogen of any kind? Or do women just need natural progesterone to balance the excess environmental estrogens? Check out the book *Breast Cancer Boot Camp: Dr. Hobbins's Breast Thermography Revolution* by Dr. William Hobbins and Wendy Sellens.

Understand man-made electromagnetic fields.

When we use a cell phone, for example, we are exposing ourselves to microwave radiation. Modern technology surrounds us 24/7 with an invisible web of man-made electromagnetic fields (EMFs). There is a possible link between cancers of the brain, breast, and blood and prolonged

EMF exposure, and it is wise to limit exposure, especially at night, when the body is detoxing.

For more information on the hazards of electromagnetic fields, check out the book *Overpowered* by Martin Blank, PhD, or the writings of Magda Havas and Camilla Rees for a well-rounded take on everything from cell phones and smart meters to dirty electricity and silver clothing.

I enjoy walking barefoot on the grass; it is a great way of transferring electrons and grounding yourself! Pick up a copy of Clint Ober's book *Earthing: The Most Important Health Discovery Ever?* He says when a person's bare skin touches the ground, the contact provides a neutralizing charge to the body and naturally protects the nervous system from extraneous electrical interference. Electrons from the ground enter the body and work like antioxidants, disarming free radicals that set the stage for illness. Consider earthing products such as a computer pad to ground yourself while working.

Discourage parasites and yeast.

It's difficult to avoid all the damaging environmental assaults aimed at our gut flora—herbicides, GMOs, antibiotic residues, and so on. Plus, dietary sugar feeds undesirable "beasties and yeasties" in the gut. Parasites and yeast are implicated in cancer. Cut out the sugar and carbs to stop feeding them, and take steps to heal a leaky gut. Check out the book by Robert Scott Bell and Ty Bollinger, *Unlock the Power to Heal*, or Martie Whittekin's Digestive Health Education Series, available at www. HBNShowUniversity.com.

Maintain a healthy body weight.

Obesity has been linked to cancer. Excess body fat produces estrogen that fuels hormone-driven cancers. Excess sugar also can fuel the growth of cancer.

Exercise.

Movement increases oxygen, detoxifies, and reduces insulin and blood sugar levels. All these benefits discourage the growth and spread of cancer cells. Exercise often because it also increases the release of endorphins in the brain, creating a sense of well-being and elevating your mood.

Not into exercise, you say? Most people can walk for twenty minutes, and it doesn't cost a dime. Advance to the point where you walk thirty minutes a day. Include short bursts of aerobic activity to get your heart rate up, followed by walking. Start out slow, and build up strength and endurance. Exercise is potent medicine for chronic disease because it optimizes your insulin and leptin receptor sensitivity.

Enjoy the sunlight—optimize vitamin D levels.

Spend at least twenty minutes daily in the midday sun with at least 40 percent of your skin exposed. This increases your vitamin D and elevates your mood. Vitamin D was meant to be made by the skin, but most of us are still deficient even with sun exposure, so we need to supplement with the pill form. Vitamin D is one of the best anticancer tools. A big mistake in American health happened in the 1980s when we were sold on the idea that it was not safe to go outside without slathering on sunscreen. It turns out sunscreens had toxic chemicals in them, and vitamin D levels plummeted because people blocked their ability to create it naturally. Mounting research suggests the rise in skin cancers in the last thirty years has its roots in omega-3 deficiencies, not prudent sun exposure.[4] The hormonally active form of vitamin D, calcitriol, or 1,25-dihydroxyvitamin D3, is being widely used for cancer prevention and treatment. D3 has been proved to inhibit the growth of many kinds of cancers.[5] It promotes apoptosis, inhibits the invasion of other tissues, inhibits metastasis, and is antiangiogenic. Vitamin D also has anti-inflammatory properties.[6] New genes are frequently discovered that vitamin D either up-regulates or down-regulates in the body's attempt to keep us healthy.

Maintain your vitamin D levels over 50 ng/ml. I try to keep mine around 75. There is a free one-hour presentation on the subject at www .Mercola.com; find the search box, and type in "vitamin D lecture." You can also look at the navy's table; it gives you exact calculations of the sun's height in the sky on any day of the year and at any location. Use it to see whether the midday exposure where you are located is likely to generate vitamin D: http://aa.usno.navy.mil/data/docs/AltAz.php. If the altitude number is above 35, it is believed the sun is high enough to enable us to make vitamin D. Also, check out the phone app "dminder."

Sweat every day for detox.

This can be accomplished during exercise. I also use a far-infrared sauna to raise my core body temperature and trigger deep sweating. My dear friend Shirley Williams, who was diagnosed with terminal stage IV breast cancer, used a sauna daily to restore her health; check out her book at www.shirleymwilliams.com.

Make sure you *go* every day.

The processed-food diet and the chemical assault on our gut biome are huge factors in bathroom issues such as constipation. Normal bowel "transit time" is twelve hours, meaning the remains of what you eat should make their exit about twelve hours later. Enzyme supplementation with meals and probiotics can be helpful, but the best remedy is less processed food and more whole and raw food.

Get a good night's rest.

Sleep boosts the immune system, lowers cortisol levels, and helps with the production of important hormones. Melatonin, the anticancer hormone, is best produced when you sleep in a dark room. Nighttime is when our bodies do a lot of detoxification and repair work. Get to bed at a reasonable hour, and consider wearing an eye mask to block out all light.

Relax, smile, and laugh.

Find time each day to de-stress. If someone or some situation is causing chronic stress, take steps to remove the source. Stress is strongly implicated in cancer. Check out a book by Brenda Stockdale, *You Can Beat the Odds: Surprising Factors Behind Chronic Illness and Cancer*. She is a pioneer in psychoneuroimmunology. Her stress-reducing techniques have been implemented in hospitals, cancer centers, and primary-care settings around the United States.

Health education

Get on the email list at www.Mercola.com, www.thetruth aboutcancer.com, and www.GreenMedinfo.com. You will get daily insights on groundbreaking health news and information that will empower you. For expert information on cancer therapies, detection, and prevention, enroll in Cancer Free University at www.CancerFreeUniversity .com and use coupon code CANCER 50 for 50 percent off.

Cold caps

This is a bit different from what I've talked about so far, but I definitely wish I'd known about cold caps. I could have kept most of my hair while undergoing chemotherapy. A cold cap is like a thick swimming cap you wear on your head before, during, and after a chemo session. It chills your scalp, constricting the blood vessels. This appears to reduce the amount of chemo reaching hair follicles and prevents hair from falling out. My research says that most people keep around 75 percent of their hair. There are several companies offering the caps. Do an internet search for them.

GOOD NUTRITION IS CRITICAL

Many of your food preferences were established when you were a young child, and they continue to be influenced by your current environment—an environment where almost one out of two people get cancer. When choosing what to eat, employ your brain, not just your taste buds. Instead of thinking how delicious a piece of thick chocolate cake would taste, take a minute to consider the fats, sugar, artificial chemicals, and empty calories that will permeate your body if you eat it. Tell yourself your body deserves better. The standard American diet is making us fat and sick. We need to go back to basics. If the label has a lot of ingredients, and ones you cannot pronounce, move on to something more natural and healthy. Love yourself enough to feed your body according to its needs. This may require a change in thought process. Instead of living to eat, you eat to live. I am personally doing this, and I invite you to join me.

I look at labels with the word "natural" with a raised eyebrow because the term does not have any legal meaning and food producers love to slap it on everything. Americans are often eating hamburger from cattle given hormones (including estrogen because it puts on weight) and fed an unnatural diet of genetically modified corn and soy, plus steroids and antibiotics. The meat counter may have a sign saying "all natural," but God would say otherwise. Grass-fed beef is truly natural; grain-finished is not.

Get friendly with farmers' markets and vegetable co-ops. If you play golf or tennis, bring your own unsweetened ice tea in a thermos; don't buy the sugared teas and sports drinks in bottles and cans. When you go out to eat, bring your own salad dressing; simple olive oil and balsamic vinegar in a glass container works. Tell the server you don't want the bread basket. Ask for the gluten-free or Paleo menu options. Ask the chef to use butter, not oil.

It's my opinion that cancer treatments will produce marginal benefits if nutrition is not addressed. You eat at least three times a day. It matters what you eat. Feed yourself as if you want to live to see your grandchildren grow up—or whatever in life is fulfilling for you.

It's important to define what I mean by the term *food*. Basically food will rot, spoil, and decay. It has life in it and can give life to us when we eat it. Digestion of highly processed, dead food will deplete the body's reserves of vitamins, minerals, and enzymes.

Living food

Eat about half of your food in its natural or fermented state, which means before cooking. The living enzymes in raw and fermented food are great for the immune system. Check out the book *Wild Fermentation* by Sandor Ellix Katz. Be sure to check the labels in the grocery store. Fermented foods don't contain vinegar and are found in the refrigerator section.

Fresh juice

Many cancer patients have an increased nutrient requirement, and fresh juices are a great way to provide it. Juices allow the body to absorb nutrients without expending a lot of energy on digestion. If a cancer patient is very nauseated or unable to eat, a rectal implant of a small amount of fresh juice can be lifesaving. It's important that juices are primarily made from vegetables. Fruits are too high in sugar. An organic Granny Smith apple will do. If you can't make your daily batch from scratch, substitute with an organic dehydrated green food supplement. A great resource is Cherie Calbom, www.juiceladycherie.com.

Spices

Processed foods tend to rely on salt for flavor instead of herbs and spices, which provide both flavor and medicinal properties. Purchase fresh herbs at your local grocery store or farmers' market. You can also grow many of them on your patio in pots. Garlic, ginger, curcumin, mint, sage, parsley, oregano, thyme, basil, black pepper, and onions are all powerful sources for anticancer phytonutrients.[7]

High-quality protein

Cancer patients need adequate amounts of protein to prevent muscle wasting. But it's a balancing act. You need enough protein to build, repair, and maintain the body, but not so much you inadvertently feed the growth of cancer cells. Excess protein is believed to stimulate the mammalian target of rapamycin (mTOR) pathways, which facilitate the building of muscles. However, this can be detrimental when treating cancer, as the mTOR pathway increases cellular proliferation as it increases growth hormone and IGF-1. Interestingly the pharmaceutical drug metformin, which has anticancer activity, also inhibits the mTOR pathway.

I calculate my daily protein consumption by dividing my weight in pounds by 2.2 to convert it to kilograms, and then multiplying by 0.8. This gives me my total daily amount of protein in grams. If math is not your strong point, just aim for fifty to seventy grams of protein a day. An egg is roughly six grams of protein, and four ounces of meat, chicken, or fish is approximately thirty grams of protein.

Protein sources should be nutrient-dense and high-quality—eggs and chicken from pastured farms, grass-fed beef, and wild-caught fish (not farm-raised). Meat from animals slaughtered in large feedlots has residual hormones and antibiotics in it.

Fats and oils

Many nutrition experts are saying the biggest dietary mistake of the last sixty years was to turn our backs on butter and other natural fats that nourished mankind for centuries. Instead, we were erroneously told to embrace refined vegetable oils. It did sound healthy, didn't it? But mankind never ate these oils before. Processed oils made from corn, soy, and cottonseed are high in omega-6 fatty acids, which throw off our anti-inflammatory balance. They are refined with heat, bleached, and deodorized to give them longer shelf life. The process changes their molecular structure into something that is not body friendly. Canola oil initially has omega-3s, but they turn into trans fats when the oil is heated and processed. And most of the canola, corn, soy, and cottonseed crops are genetically modified.

Good sources of anti-inflammatory omega-3 fats are fatty fish such as wild-caught salmon (not farmed), krill oil, walnuts, and pastured eggs. Omega-3 deficiencies are a common underlying factor in cancer. Evening primrose oil can have a balancing effect on hormones, which contributes to healthy breast tissue, and it can lessen menstrual cramps and PMS symptoms. Stay with natural fats such as butter and other animal fats, coconut and palm oil, extra-virgin olive oil, and avocado oil. Some 50 percent of our cell membranes are made up of fat—make it the best quality possible.

GMOs

Almost all corn, soy, cotton, canola, and sugar beets are genetically modified organisms (GMOs). They have altered DNA and are risky—avoid them. GMO corn and cottonseed oil have been genetically altered to produce their own systemic insecticide. The same insecticide enters your gut when you eat those foods. These genetically modified crops are not the same ones our Creator intended for us to eat. Studies are clearly linking GMOs and their associated chemicals to negative changes in our gut biome and our ability to detoxify. Corn chips were the hardest for me to give up. Being from Texas, I love chips and salsa. I often substitute the corn chips for plantain chips, or eat my guacamole with a fork.

Gluten

Wheat—the staff of life, it was called. But no more. In the last sixty years much crossbreeding and gene splicing have taken place to produce greater yields. The result is "dwarf wheat," a mutant plant with a genetic code that never existed in nature before, and an inflammatory gluten content upwards of fifty times greater than wheat of biblical times. Additionally, wheat is often sprayed with the herbicide glyphosate, which the WHO declared to be "probably carcinogenic to humans."[8] Dr. William Davis, in his book *Wheat Belly*, says modern wheat is a high-glycemic-index carb that produces documented effects of exaggerated blood sugar swings, exposure to brain-active exorphins, glycation processes that underlie aging, and altered immune responses.[9] Few foods have as high a glycemic index as wheat. Two slices of wheat toast will raise your blood sugar more than two tablespoons of sugar. Whole wheat is worse. Go gluten-free or grain-free; it's much more than a fad.

Soy and flax

The topic of soy is very controversial. Soy products are high in plant estrogens (also known as phytoestrogens and isoflavones). And flax is even *higher* in phytoestrogens yet commonly recommended as being a good source of plant-based omega-3s. However, according to William Hobbins, MD, and Wendy Sellens, DAOM, phytoestrogens should be avoided by the 80 percent of women who have estrogen-positive breast cancers.[10]

Phytoestrogens, or other similar compounds, attach to the estrogen receptors in breasts and may increase risk for breast cancer by stimulating those receptors. These include bioidentical estrogens, flax, soy, black cohosh, and red clover. Flax is nineteen times more potent than soy.[11]

Our culture bombards us with estrogenic substances in food (soy is in many processed foods, for example) and the environment (think BPA). Avoidance is good advice.

Since a picture is worth a thousand words, check out the thermographic images from Wendy Sellens in *Breast Cancer Boot Camp* to see the difference in breast vascularity with and without flax in the diet.[12]

On the opposite end of the spectrum, fermented soy has shown to have strong anticancer properties—specifically the component genistein. Check out the product Haelan 951. Give them a call at 866-360-2193. They will be happy to send you lots of helpful information. Be prepared, the taste and smell are less than appetizing, and the product is a bit costly.

Restrict dairy products.

The Weston A. Price Foundation, Dr. Ron Schmid, and others have pointed out the many problems with modern pasteurized and homogenized milk "products." Many people have a difficult time breaking down the casein protein due to allergies, which can be a sign of a leaky gut membrane and immune dysfunction. I attempt to limit my dairy consumption to organic butter. On the other hand, *raw* milk, butter, and cheeses are used by many people as part of a healthy diet. The proteins in raw dairy are intact and not damaged by the heat used in the processing of standard grocery store dairy products. Raw dairy products can often be purchased directly from a farm.

Avoid fructose and sugar.

You absolutely *must* avoid all forms of sugar if you are in treatment, and most of the rest of us eat far too much of it. There is a strong relationship between sugar, insulin, and insulin-like growth factor. All provide fuel for, and signal the growth of, cancer cells. When consuming fruit, stick to those lower in sugar, such as green apples, berries, and cherries. Dr. Hammon tells me for every serving of fruit you consume, you should have two servings of a vegetable. Also, remember, carbohydrates such as bread, potatoes, corn, pasta, chips, tortillas, and rice break down into sugar, so consume them sparingly.

Avoid artificial sweeteners and MSG.

Don't be fooled by the zero-calorie marketing. Artificial sweeteners are not beneficial for our health. Also, studies repeatedly have shown that diet beverages make you gain weight faster than non-diet, in part because they keep you craving sweets and starchy snacks.

Avoid all glutamate additives, such as monosodium glutamate (MSG), yeast extract, hydrolyzed vegetable protein, and hydrolyzed plant protein, because these additives are thought to stimulate tumor growth and invasion.

Avoid alcohol.

Besides the sugar and yeast in alcohol, which are fuels for cancer, alcohol breaks down to acetaldehyde, which is a carcinogen. If it sounds hard to give up the evening cocktail, try the KeVita® brand of fermented "sparkling probiotic" beverage.

Anticancer Natural Substances

Integrative oncologists have been using whole foods and natural substances to treat cancer for many decades.

Dr. William Li, president and medical director of the Angiogenesis Foundation, has done a tremendous amount of research on the health benefits of natural foods. For example, cancer cells support themselves by creating new blood vessels, a process called angiogenesis. Dr. Li found that some foods discourage that process by producing angiogenesis inhibitors.

Healthy cells have a natural system of checks and balances to regulate the growth of blood vessels—angiogenesis stimulators and inhibitors. However, we know cancer cells make errors in DNA replication, and this appears to allow cancer cells to hijack the body's system of checks and balances. It's been reported that a tiny, microscopic tumor, given a steady supply of blood, can grow to up to sixteen thousand times its original size in as little as a few weeks.[13] This process helps us understand how a CTC can escape a tumor—travel to another location in the body—and start the process of growing blood vessels to support a metastasis.

Angiogenesis-inhibiting foods include turmeric, cinnamon, parsley, garlic, berries, apples, green tea, olive oil, bok choy, and kale. Apoptosis agents—meaning they promote cancer cell death—include marine oils, omega-3s, onions, radishes, resveratrol, and berberine.

Artemisinin

This supplement is made from a Chinese herb; it is also called wormwood extract. It has been used for thousands of years in treating malaria, and more recently, cancer. Artemisinin becomes cytotoxic (cell killing) in the presence of ferrous iron. Once inside the cell, artemisinin reacts with iron inside the cell, spawning highly reactive chemicals called free radicals. The free radicals attack other molecules and the cell membrane, breaking it apart and killing the cells. The process selectively targets cancer cells, leaving healthy cells alone.[14] Dr. Robert Rowen says artemisinin is a close cousin to oxygen therapy because it delivers a knockout oxidative stress to cancer cells.[15]

Ashwagandha

Ashwagandha leaf extract from the ginseng plant has been used in traditional Indian medicine for decades. This powerful extract has demonstrated the ability to kill cancer cells.[16]

Astragalus

This herb is revered for its ability to boost the immune system. In Asia, and even in some North American hospitals, astragalus is used to protect patients from a common side effect of chemotherapy, the depletion of red and white blood cell counts. This depletion makes cancer patients more susceptible to infection and serious illness. In laboratory studies, astragalus extracts enable the body to produce more immune system macrophages and natural killer cells. Research also suggests that astragalus can be useful in managing cancer-related fatigue. The dried root is used in tea, encapsulated as a supplement, or added to a smoothie as a powder.

Berberine

Berberine is a natural alkaloid found in a variety of traditional herbs, such as barberry, goldenseal, and Oregon grape. It is a very handy supplement because it positively affects so many things—glucose metabolism, lipid levels, insulin sensitivity, cardiac issues, weight management, immunity, and gastrointestinal health.[17] Berberine has antibacterial, anti-inflammatory, and immune-enhancing properties. Berberine targets 5' adenosine monophosphate-activated protein kinase (AMPK), which regulates metabolism. Berberine increases the activity of AMPK, sometimes called the "metabolic master switch." It's one of my favorite supplements because it can lower blood sugar about as well as the prescription drug metformin.[18] It's a natural solution to help with insulin resistance and diabetes.

Beta-carotene

Beta-carotene is a carotenoid compound responsible for giving fruits and vegetables their orange pigment. It's a powerful antioxidant that's been found to help protect against cancer and target cancer stem cells. Good sources are carrots and dark green leafy vegetables such as spinach, kale, mustard greens, collard greens, and Swiss chard.

Beta-glucan

This supplement is made of natural extract from baker's yeast, shiitake mushrooms, and cereal grains such as barley, oats, rye, and wheat. It has shown antitumor activity in many cancers. Studies show this extract enhances the production of immune cells in the bone marrow. Also, white blood cells called phagocytes, or "eating cells," have been shown to engulf more invaders and digest them faster with beta-glucan bound to their receptor cites.[19] Beta-glucan is often described as the substance that puts microscopic glasses on your immune cells. Studies suggest the product Transfer Point is best for this.

Bone broth

Nutrient-dense food is making a comeback, and bone broth is part of that. Note: We're talking homemade broth made from pasture-raised animals fed naturally without antibiotics or hormones. We are not talking about bouillon cubes or powders that are mostly salt, MSG, corn maltodextrin, wheat gluten, caramel color, and preservatives. Real bone broth contains gelatin that protects and heals the mucosal lining of the digestive tract (leaky gut) and helps aid in the digestion of nutrients. Bone broth also contains amino acids, especially glycine and proline, which are the key building blocks the body needs to manufacture collagen.

Colostrum

Colostrum is often called "the perfect first food." Newborn mammals receive colostrum from the mother's breast immediately after birth. Initially, colostrum's big molecules readily pass through a permeable gut wall and gain entry to the bloodstream. Colostrum carries the "software programming" to lay down the foundation of the immune system. About twenty-four hours later colostrum begins the second part of its mission—sealing the intestinal wall nice and tight so the gut can act as a barrier against things that shouldn't get to the bloodstream. But as we grow up, years of antibiotics, painkillers, and an inflammatory diet open up the gut wall and make it permeable again. This is called "leaky gut," and it is estimated that up to 80 percent of American adults have a leaky gut. Inflammation in the gut damages the immune system's ability to produce IgA, without which pathogens can escape into the bloodstream and infect any part of the body.

Supplemental colostrum is said to be able to heal a leaky gut and help the immune system make its army of macrophages, T-cells, and natural killer cells—better equipping the body to defend against cancer. As you first begin to use colostrum, you may experience a Herxheimer reaction, an uncomfortable detoxification effect. If your abdomen hurts, this is usually a sign you need to go more slowly so your body can keep pace with the destruction of pathogens and continue to heal.

Beware of brands air dried with a high-heat method that destroys virtually everything in the colostrum but a few immunoglobulins—what's left is little more than powdered milk. I like Sovereign Laboratories' colostrum because it is flash pasteurized, which protects the active ingredients. Its cows are pasture-fed US grade-A dairy cows certified to be free of BST, hormones, antibiotics, and mad cow disease. Perhaps most of all, I like its use of a liposomal delivery system. Douglas Wyatt, the founder of Sovereign Laboratories, said "Raw fresh colostrum has a liposomal surrounding of the active, sensitive molecules and so, we know that this is critical for processed supplements."[20] You can order it at https://colostrumld.com/CancerFree.

C-Statin

This is a food-based supplement isolated from a common garden weed called bindweed. C-Statin acts as an antiangiogenesis factor, meaning it stops new blood vessels from growing. Cancers build a network of small blood vessels to get nourishment. If angiogenesis is inhibited, cancer cells will have a hard time growing.

Curcumin

Curcumin, a root, is the subject of some five thousand peer-reviewed studies that find it does an amazing job of fighting cancer and other chronic illnesses. Curcumin is the active ingredient in the bright yellow Indian spice turmeric, and studies of this herb reveal immense therapeutic potential in preventing breast cancer metastasis. It has been shown to inhibit "proliferation of cancer cells by arresting them at various phases of the cell cycle."[21] Curcumin supplements are available in oral liposomal form. It is also being administered intravenously as an integrative therapy.

Enzymes

As we age, our natural enzyme levels drop, and supplementation can be beneficial. There are two different types of enzymes. The first is digestive enzymes. I recommend that you take digestive enzymes about fifteen minutes before meals to help with the complete breakdown of food and better absorption of nutrients.

The second is systemic proteolytic (protein eating) enzymes. They work differently. For cancer patients, these enzymes are typically used to weaken biofilm around cancer cells, yeast, and other pathogens. As the biofilm is weakened, the immune cells can go to work. Another function of proteolytic enzymes is that they eat away at fibrin. Cancer cells contain a fibrin meshwork perhaps fifteen times thicker than that of normal cells. Fibrin is believed to be a key component of cancer cells' ability to defeat attacks by the immune system. Fibrin impedes the ability of lymphocytes, phagocytes, and cytokines to make contact with cancer cells and destroy them.[22] Proteolytic enzymes can also reduce inflammation; help kill off bacteria, viruses, molds, and fungi; clean the blood of debris and fibrin; and work on incompletely digested proteins that make their way into the bloodstream, where they can trigger food allergies and autoimmune disease. Systemic enzymes should be taken away from meals and on an empty stomach or in the middle of the night. Dr. Nicholas Gonzalez documented the success of enzymes in creating cases of exceptional survival and tumor reduction.[23] Integrative cancer care almost always includes aggressive enzyme supplementation.

Epigallocatechin-3-gallate (EGCG)

EGCG is an active compound in green tea. Studies have shown that it disrupts cancer stem cell metabolism, diminishes cell proliferation, and reduces cell invasiveness.[24] It can be bought in supplement form or enjoyed by the cup.

Essential oils

These are naturally occurring, volatile aromatic compounds found in plants and extracted through steam distillation or cold pressing. They are a highly concentrated essence of the plants from which they were derived. Some can improve quality of life for cancer patients by sending chemical messages to the brain that affect mood and emotion. Some are anticarcinogenic. Various species of frankincense (Boswellia) are used for breast and skin cancer. Clove essential oil, for example, has been found to kill cancer cells known as MCF-7.[25] Essential oils from cinnamon, thyme, chamomile, and jasmine have been found to be significantly potent against breast cancer cells lines.[26]

Ginger (6-shogaol and 6-gingerol)

Ginger is a root plant and a cousin to curcumin. Studies repeatedly demonstrate it is an anti-cancer powerhouse. It's effective not only against cancer cells but against the resistant cancer stem cells. It has even outperformed chemotherapy.[27]

Haelan 951

Many naturopaths and integrative oncologists make use of this unique liquid dietary supplement, usually as an adjunct to an existing cancer treatment protocol. It is made from non-genetically modified *fermented* soy. It's used to boost the immune system and suppress cancer cell progression. The company reports the product reduces the amount of estrogen circulating in the body by favoring the beta receptors.[28] To learn more, go to https://haelan951.com. The taste is definitely disagreeable, and it is pricey, but there is a lot of research supporting it, and many people have favorable reports about its effectiveness.

Honokiol

Honokiol is a polyphenol found in the bark and seed cones of the magnolia tree. Polyphenols are antioxidants and give plants their color and flavor.[29] Honokiol is considered a unique compound that can exert many powerful actions against cancer and chronic illnesses. Research indicates it works on the cellular level to halt cancer growth and disable the metastatic process.[30] It also works against inflammation and infection. As an antioxidant, it is one thousand times more potent than vitamin E. Preclinical research suggests honokiol is helpful with various cancers—bladder, breast, colon, esophageal, lung, myeloma, ovarian, prostate, and sarcoma. Unlike most polyphenols, this one can cross the blood-brain barrier.[31] This holds promise for its ability to treat brain tumors. Honokiol also shows potential in preventative health by reducing inflammation and oxidative stress.[32] There is currently no clinical data on the use of honokiol in humans. It's available in 98 percent pure extract in capsule form as a supplement.

HCL supplementation

According to Dr. Jonathan Wright, most of us don't make enough stomach acid.[33] This is called hydrochloric acid, or HCL, and we need it to break down foods completely. Many people take antacids to relieve what they think is too much stomach acid. But actually when you have *too little* acid, food doesn't digest quickly enough, it begins to ferment, and gases travel up into the esophagus (i.e., heartburn). The stomach was meant to be a very acidic environment to break down food, especially proteins. Proper digestion is key to health and immune function.

Inositol hexaphosphate (IP6)

This is a powerful antioxidant. It enhances the immune system and boosts natural killer cells. IP6 is a derivative of the B vitamin inositol. It is found in beans, brown rice, corn, sesame seeds, wheat bran, and other high-fiber foods. It has been called a "natural cancer fighter," and studies suggest it induces apoptosis in various forms of cancer, including colon and prostate cancers.[34] Dr. AbulKalam Shamsuddin, a pathologist at the University of Maryland School of Medicine, pioneered the studies of IP6. He discovered it can control the rate of abnormal cell division and help fight bacterial and fungal infections.

Iodine

You'll find iodine in almost every organ and tissue of the body. It's an essential trace element, yet many, if not most, of us are deficient. We may not get enough in our food, and our body's ability to use iodine is compromised by environmental toxins such as fluoride and perchlorate.

Iodine-deficient breast tissue shows alterations in DNA and estrogen receptor proteins.[35] Breast cancer cells readily "absorb iodine, which in turn suppresses tumor growth and causes cancer cell death."[36] Iodine also is critical for thyroid function and metabolism. Seaweed, scallops, and cod fish are natural food sources; Lugol's iodine is a useful supplement. It's a good idea to have your iodine levels checked.

Lycopene

Lycopene is a carotenoid, a pigment made by plants. Lycopene is found in many fruits and vegetables, including tomatoes, carrots, apricots, and watermelons. Studies have shown supplementing with lycopene can reduce PSA levels in men; prostate cancer cells treated with lycopene had changes in their cell division cycle, leading to less cancer cell growth.[37]

Modified citrus pectin

The naturally occurring soluble fiber that joins the cells of fruit together is called citrus pectin. Modified citrus pectin (MCP) is a supplement made from purified pectin obtained from the inner pith of citrus peel. Natural pectin is indigestible and passes through the intestinal tract. A great deal of research has been done on the benefits of MCP. It has been shown to prevent abnormal cellular growth, modulate immune function, remove heavy metals and toxins from the body, and block the creation of fibrotic scar tissue. MCP has also been shown to inhibit galectin-3 activity in the extracellular matrix and bloodstream. Galectin-3 is a protein, and cancer patients typically have elevated levels of it, which can increase the probability of metastasis. Refer to the chapter "Functional Testing Overview" for information on a test for galectin-3 levels. There are many forms of MCP, and I caution you not to buy blindly. The molecular weight and structure of the pectin molecules must be extremely small so they can enter the bloodstream and be effective at the cellular level. I had the opportunity to visit with Isaac Eliaz, MD, of Santa Rosa, California; virtually all the clinical trials in the last two decades have used his formulation, PectaSol-C by ecoNugenics.

Mushroom extracts

These have been traditionally used to activate natural killer cells, thus reducing tumor growth. Some extracts have antiviral, antibacterial, and antifungal properties.

Parthenolide (feverfew)

Feverfew is a perennial herb, a member of the daisy family that grows along roadsides and wild in fields. It contains an active ingredient, parthenolide, which is effective against cancer stem cells.[38]

Pawpaw

This is an edible bean-shaped fruit native to North America also called *Asimina triloba*. In vitro (outside-the-body) studies demonstrated pawpaw extract is cytotoxic to cancer cells, including those resistant to

Adriamycin (a chemo drug), and has antiangiogenic properties. Another reported mechanism of action is a drop in the ATP, or energy, of the cell, thus promoting apoptosis/cell death.[39]

Poly-MVA

I was introduced to Poly-MVA® in 2009. It's a one-of-a-kind, powerful liquid nutritional supplement. It can be taken orally or intravenously. I am impressed by the case studies and positive reports shared by patients and doctors.

Poly-MVA is a bit expensive but worth it, especially if you're dealing with or have had cancer or a degenerative disease. Note: Cancer rates are on the rise in pets, and Poly-MVA is available for them also.

I want to share a bit of information on Poly-MVA because of its usefulness in cancer and many other chronic medical conditions.

The following information is provided with permission from AMARC Enterprises Inc. Statements have not been evaluated by the Food and Drug Administration, and the product is not intended to diagnose, treat, cure, or prevent any disease.

> Poly-MVA is a powerful, patented dietary supplement that is the first in a remarkable new category of supplements known as Lipoic Acid Mineral Complexes. Poly-MVA is a unique, patented proprietary blend of palladium, alpha-lipoic acid, vitamins B1, B2 and B12, the amino acids formyl-methionine and acetyl cystiene, and trace amounts of molybdenum, rhodium, and ruthenium.[40]

MVA stands for minerals, vitamins, and amino acids. Poly-MVA "is designed to provide energy for compromised body systems by changing the electrical potential of human cells and facilitating aerobic metabolism within the cell."[41] In other words, it shuttles energy for proper metabolism. As a nutritional supplement, Poly-MVA works at the cellular level in the electron transport chain in mitochondria while protecting the cell and its DNA/RNA.[42]

Poly-MVA travels easily throughout the body and can cross the blood-brain barrier. Poly-MVA is showing "great promise in cases where other means of supplementing cell nutrition are ineffective" and in combination with many other protocols.[43]

In more scientific terms, the proper transfer and movement of energy/electrons are how cells process all their various functions, communicate, and survive. Normal cells use oxygen and energy/electron transfer one way, and abnormal cells, a different way. Poly-MVA targets this cellular pathway and therefore can support *all* normal cell functions. This electron dysfunction in abnormal/anaerobic cells is how many chemotherapeutics and radiation therapies try to target abnormal cells, and the effort requires the presence of electrons. A lipoic acid palladium complex can generate and shuttle energy/electrons; it therefore can be used in some cases as adjunctive support to potentiate—make stronger—various therapies. This polymer/complex both protects the cell and donates energy to the normal cell's electron transport chain via the mitochondria, which then provides energy to the cell by supporting the ATP cycle, helping to stabilize cell metabolism.

The benefits of the lipoic acid palladium complex in Poly-MVA may:

+ Discourage abnormal cell growth
+ Improve metabolic function
+ Slow the aging process from cellular breakdown
+ Support cellular function and raise energy levels
+ Support appetite
+ Protect cellular DNA
+ Convert free radicals into an energy source
+ Have many mineral, vitamin, and antioxidant functions[44]
+ Support oxygenation of cells and tissue
+ Support the liver in removing harmful substances from the body
+ Support nerve and neurotransmitter function[45]

Poly-MVA has undergone numerous cell line studies, safety, animal, and human tests, since 1992, when it was formulated. Among those:

+ Board-certified oncologist Dr. James W. Forsythe, MD, HMD, of Nevada conducted an outcome study on over five hundred adults with various stage IV adult cancers over a seven-year period. He observed a 70 percent overall positive response rate. He concluded Poly-MVA is an essential component of his patients' protocols for improved results, health, and overall outcomes:

    In stage IV adult cancers of any origin, improvement in quality of life issues is directly proportional to improvement to overall response rate. Even stable disease can be tolerated and changed into a chronic livable condition.[46]

+ Ongoing research and studies by independent laboratories have confirmed Poly-MVA's effectiveness in a variety of cancer types, including brain, breast, liver, lung, prostate, and skin.[47]

+ Ischemia studies demonstrated that administration of Poly-MVA limits damage and protects cellular function.[48]

+ "Phase One human safety trials have been conducted in the PUNCH Study (Poly-MVA Utilized as Neuroprotection against Chronic Hypertension)," paving the way for a glioblastoma study and multiple myeloma and MS studies.[49]

+ "A 1000-patient animal study with a veterinary oncologist resulted in an 86 percent improved quality of life response in the animals' health."[50]

Poly-MVA has been approved by the FDA's review process for further investigation in human clinical use for efficacy in cancer and degenerative disease care.

I encourage you to see the "Poly-MVA/Information Packet," "Testimonials," and "Scientific Research" tabs at www.polyMVA.com and www.polymvasurvivors.com. Numerous articles, studies, and in-depth data are available on its website.

Probiotics/prebiotics

Supplement your diet with a good multi-strain probiotic. When choosing a probiotic, remember, it's not about the number of microbes but about finding a brand that has more than just two or three strains. Look for at least eight different strains. And once you take your probiotics, don't forget to feed them with a prebiotic such as acacia senegal. Or enjoy a fresh slice of jicama or asparagus—natural prebiotic options to taking another pill. The immune system is based in the gut; feed the "good bacteria" for good function. An added benefit is good bowel function, which is also important.

Quercetin

This is a type of plant-based phytochemical known as a flavonoid. Findings suggest quercetin displays antitumor activity by triggering apoptosis (cell self-destruction).[51] It has been shown to downregulate the expression of an anti-apoptosis protein and upregulate the expression of pro-apoptosis proteins. It also promotes activation of a mitochondrial pathway to induce apoptosis. Good sources include grapefruit, apples, onions, red wine, and black tea.

Restore™

Our modern lifestyle can be very hard on our gut. Most of us have been liberally dosed over the years with prescription antibiotics that kill off the good gut flora. In addition, the standard American diet is full of chemicals, GMOs, gluten, and environmental toxins such as herbicides and animal antibiotics—none of which is friendly to the gut. The net result is a loss of friendly bacteria and bacterial diversity in the gut, combined with injury to the tight junctions in our intestinal lining. Think of those tight junctions as our "firewall" protecting us against these very toxins. Intestinal permeability, or "leaky gut," means the junctions aren't so tight anymore. The natural barrier has been compromised, and toxins and undigested food can find their way into our bloodstream. The immune system then sees foreign objects in the bloodstream and attacks them. Leaky gut distracts the immune system from its priorities of handling legitimate pathogens and cleaning out errant cancer cells.

Remember, at least 70 percent of our immune system resides in the gut, and 90 percent of our neurotransmitters are made in the gut. I know people who have healed leaky gut with a liquid supplement developed by Dr. Zach Bush called Restore™. It strengthens and supports the integrity of the gut lining, creates an environment for the diversification of good gut bacteria, and promotes balanced immune function. Restore utilizes a lignite extract that is stabilized and made bioavailable through a proprietary process, yielding the functional compound Terrahydrite™, shown in cell culture studies to be uniquely effective in strengthening the tight junctions.

Resveratrol

The skin of red grapes and other fruits gives us resveratrol that acts to induce apoptosis. Resveratrol is also a powerful antioxidant; it can neutralize free radicals. Free radicals feed the cancer process by causing mutations in a cell's DNA or by promoting inflammation.

Salvestrols

Salvestrols are a class of natural chemicals recently identified in plants. They are reported to have the ability to recognize and enter cancer cells. Once inside the cancer cell, they go through a process of molecular activation by a special enzyme, CYP1B1, and cause the cells to cease growing or die.[52] CYP1B1 is pronounced "sip one bee one" and is an intrinsic component of cancer cells.[53] Salvestrols are available in fruits, vegetables, and herbs such as strawberries, blueberries, broccoli, bell peppers, basil, parsley, and mint. The attention salvestrols receive confirms why a plant-rich diet has traditionally been considered to offer protection against cancer.[54]

Silymarin (milk thistle)

Silymarin is the active ingredient in the plant, milk thistle. The National Cancer Institute reports that "laboratory studies demonstrate that silymarin stabilizes cellular membranes, stimulates detoxification pathways, stimulates regeneration of liver tissue, inhibits the growth of certain cancer cell lines, exerts direct cytotoxic activity toward certain cancer cell lines, and possibly increases the efficacy of certain chemotherapy agents."[55]

Spirulina

Edible freshwater algae produce spirulina. The blue-green color comes from phycocyanin, a pigment-protein complex that absorbs light and then transfers that energy to chlorophyll. People like to describe spirulina as an Aztec superfood, claiming that gram for gram, it is about the most nutritious food on the planet. It has more beta-carotene than carrots, is high in bioavailable copper and iron, contains the trace minerals selenium and manganese, is high in protein, has all the essential amino acids, has vitamins B_1 and B_2, plus a balance of both omega-3s and omega-6s. It is easy to digest. NASA chose to use it as a food for astronauts. Animal and test tube research suggests spirulina can reduce cancer occurrence and tumor size, improve white blood cell count, and stimulate antibodies.[56] In 2014 Czech researchers found it helpful with pancreatic cancer.[57] Note that spirulina absorbs nutrients from water. Spirulina from water that is polluted or contains heavy metals will have concentrations of the pollutants, so quality counts. Generally spirulina from the United States (especially Hawaii) and Europe tends to be cleaner than spirulina from China. Spirulina supplements come in powders, flakes, and tablets.

Transfer Factor Multi-Immune™

This supplement is made by Researched Nutritionals and is available through licensed practitioners. It is typically dispensed to cancer patients for immune system support. It contains a blend of colostrum, IP6, shiitake and maitake mushrooms, beta-glucan, astragalus, green tea and pomegranate extracts, 5-methyltetrahydrofolic acid, methylcobalamin (vitamin B_{12}), zinc, and selenium. It's all in one product.

Vitamin C—oral

Did you know the orange is a relative lightweight when it comes to vitamin C content compared to papaya, red bell pepper, broccoli, strawberries, and even pineapple? Vitamin C is a potent antioxidant with the power to boost immune function. Typically at oral supplement doses above 1,000 mg a day, we absorb about 50 percent of the dose. The other 50 percent is broken down in the gut and sent out via the urine.[58] A method of increasing absorption is to take a liposomal form of vitamin C. Liposomal means the nutrient is encapsulated in a phospholipid (a fatty membrane) so the nutrient can bypass destructive digestive juices in the stomach and move fairly intact through the gut lining and into the bloodstream.

INTEGRATIVE THERAPIES

In the toolbox there are also a number of integrative therapies. Some of these tools are supportive in nature; some are used specifically for treatment of patients with cancer. Some are administered by a physician in an office setting. Some can be used at home under a physician's direction. Poly-MVA, for example, can be taken orally at home or can be administered by physicians intravenously in the clinic for greater therapeutic effect. Many people are searching for options to conventional cancer therapies (such as cytotoxic chemotherapy), which have limited success rates and potential life-altering side effects. Patients are increasingly educating themselves about the risks and benefits of conventional therapies, and many are choosing evidence-based alternative therapies that are more humane and have fewer side effects.

It is important to understand that no treatment should be undertaken without the supervision of a trained clinician. You need to work with a professional who has experience with these therapies. Just as chemotherapy doesn't work for everyone, all integrative therapies don't work for everyone. By monitoring your therapy with appropriate testing, you can tell if your therapy is working. And if not, you can switch to a different intervention.

Intravenous vitamin C

This may be one of the best documented natural cancer treatments. Vitamin C—ascorbic acid—has the documented ability to kill cancer cells.[59] However, oral doses don't pack enough punch to kill cancer; for that job, high doses of ascorbic acid must be delivered intravenously. The molecular shape of ascorbic acid is very similar to glucose, so cancer cells rapidly absorb it. As it begins to accumulate, it interacts with intracellular copper and iron and generates hydrogen peroxide (H_2O_2). Cancer cells don't have the enzyme to break down H_2O_2 into water and oxygen, so it builds up in the cells. Eventually the hydrogen peroxide breaks apart cell membranes and effectively kills the tumor from the inside out. Clinics are using this therapy alone and also in conjunction with other therapies, including chemotherapy.

Before using high-dose IV vitamin C, a G6PD lab test must be done to ensure the patient can tolerate higher doses—it is a simple blood test. If you have a deficiency of the G6PD enzyme, you are not a candidate for high-dose vitamin C.

Today many integrative cancer clinics are having patients fast before IV vitamin infusions, causing the cancer cells to be hungry for glucose. The vitamin C will be attracted to the insulin receptors on the cancer cells, adding in quick absorption. They are sometimes using a small dose of insulin to lower blood sugar levels before starting the vitamin C infusion. Both methods are used to make the therapy more powerful.

Vaccines

Tumor cells make defensive molecules that repel or destroy T cells and B cells, the white blood cells that help the body fight diseases. Much research is being done on developing vaccines to prompt dendritic cells to stimulate other immune cells to act against specific cancers. Dendritic cells are also part of the immune system; they interact with T cells to initiate and direct an immune response. Personalized dendritic vaccines are created by isolating the patient's cancer cells to identify the most frequently expressed protein (epitope) on the surface of the cancer cells. This cancer protein is then imprinted on to the dendritic cells. The dendritic cell population is then augmented (increased in number) in the vaccine. The goal of the vaccine is to educate T and B cells (immune cells) to identify the body's own cancer cells to mark them for destruction. If a vaccine "takes," it will give long-term immunity to the patient's cancer cells.

Immune-stimulating vaccines are in use in many other countries but have not been widely accepted in the United States. Cost estimates are around $10,000–$25,000.

Immunotherapies

These are the "new kids on the block," new pharmaceutical drugs trying to assist the immune system in its job of seeking out and destroying abnormal cells. These drugs often come with substantial side effects because when man-made substances interact with the immune system, there can be devastating consequences. But as time provides for more experience, results should improve, and immunotherapies could be a game changer in cancer treatment.

Oral and IV chelation

Heavy metals compromise our immune system's ability to ward off all pathogens—viral, fungal, and bacterial. The level of lead in our bones is five hundred to one thousand times higher than people who lived in the preindustrial age.[60] Lead's toxicity interferes with production of energy in our cellular mitochondria. Today we also have higher levels of other heavy metals, including mercury, aluminum, barium, and cadmium. Oral and intravenous chelating agents can pull heavy metals out of the body. EDTA, for example, is a semisynthetic amino acid commonly used to lower lead levels. DMSA and DMPS may be preferred to target mercury.

EDTA is a powerful antioxidant, so it dramatically reduces the level of damaging free radicals. That action then conserves our glutathione, permitting it to function more effectively as our own natural, powerful detoxifier. EDTA also thins the blood by increasing prothrombin levels. Thinner blood leads to increased blood flow, which means oxygen levels are increased. A small Swiss study published in 1989 found that cancer was reduced 90 percent during an eighteen-year follow-up of patients treated with calcium-EDTA compared with people not treated at all.[61]

Myers' cocktail

The Myers' cocktail is an intravenous vitamin and mineral protocol developed by Dr. John Myers at Johns Hopkins University. Dr. Myers used intravenous vitamins and minerals in the treatment of a wide variety of medical conditions, including cancer. Doctors often customize the "cocktail" for each patient; the formula typically includes vitamin C, the B vitamins, magnesium, calcium, and glutathione. A Myers' cocktail is used to help nutrients go directly into the cells through the bloodstream, bypassing the digestive system, which can be beneficial for cancer patients who have compromised digestive systems and are nutrient deficient.

Photodynamic therapy

Photodynamic therapy (PDT) "is a treatment that uses special drugs, called *photosensitizing agents*, along with light to kill cancer cells. The drugs only work after they have been activated or 'turned on' by certain kinds of light. PDT may also be called *photoradiation therapy, phototherapy,* or *photochemotherapy.*"[62]

The photosensitizing agent can be given either intravenously to reach the bloodstream or be applied topically on skin, depending on the location of the cancer. Cancer cells absorb the agent, "then light is applied to the area to be treated. The light causes the drug to react with oxygen, which forms a chemical that kills cancer cells. PDT might also help by destroying blood vessels feeding cancer cells and by alerting the immune system to attack the cancer."[63] Read more about it at www.cancer.org/treatment/treatments-and-side-effects/treatment-types/photodynamic-therapy.html.

Ultraviolet (UV) light blood irradiation therapy

Ultraviolet therapy is a time-honored medical procedure used to treat disease since the early 1900s. Some of a patient's blood is withdrawn, exposed to ultraviolet light, and then reintroduced into the patient's bloodstream. The treated blood shares its photonic energy with the rest of the blood, creating an oxygen-rich environment and stimulating immune cells. Some effects are:

+ Improved circulation
+ Improved oxygenation of tissues
+ Deactivation of pathogens such as bacteria, viruses, and fungi
+ Stimulation of the immune system
+ Increased tolerance of chemotherapy and radiation
+ Cardiovascular protection
+ Anti-inflammatory and anti-infection protection

This therapy is often used in conjunction with ozone. A couple of good books on the use of UV light in the treatment of cancer and other microbial diseases are:

+ *Into the Light—Tomorrow's Medicine Today* by Dr. William Douglass, MD
+ *Light—Medicine of the Future* by Jacob Liberman, OD, PhD

Hyperbaric oxygen therapy (HBOT)

Hyperbaric oxygen therapy involves the use of a hyperbaric chamber. "Pure oxygen is delivered under pressure, which has the effect of dissolving oxygen into the plasma—delivering as much as 10 times more oxygen" than the bloodstream normally delivers and better reaching body tissues. The increase of oxygen provides fuel for healing. Cancer cells prefer an oxygen-poor environment, so oxygen is cancer's enemy.[64]

Ozone therapy

The regular oxygen we breathe is made up of two oxygen atoms; ozone is made up of three. That third oxygen atom makes ozone a "super-charged" form of oxygen and gives it effective, nontoxic medicinal properties. Remember, cancer cells prefer an oxygen-poor environment. With more oxygen, tumors behave less aggressively and demonstrate a reduced ability to metastasize. Ozone increases the delivery of oxygen to tissues and cells, kills bacteria and viruses, and increases cellular energy production because it stimulates the mitochondria. Ozone therapy both heals and detoxifies. Ozone is usually administered intravenously or through vaginal and rectal routes.

Oncothermia and hyperthermia

Heat has been used as a means of therapy for centuries. The human body uses heat in the form of a fever to kill pathogens. Heat can cause significant damage to cells, and the body can only survive for a short period of time in temperatures over 42 degrees Celsius (107.6 degrees Fahrenheit). However, heat can be used to treat cancer when its damaging capabilities are applied with skill. In fact, "malignant tumors can be controlled or even recede as a result of targeted oncothermia."[65] This therapy can be challenging to find in the United States. Check out these clinics in Santa Monica, California: www.i2med.com and www.ThermalOncology.com.

DMSO

Dimethyl sulfoxide, or DMSO for short, is "an organic, sulfur-rich substance found in the woody part of trees."[66] DMSO is a transporter—it is absorbed into the human body with incredible ease. It has long been a favorite therapy of holistic and integrative physicians because it has been shown to calm inflammation, scavenge free radicals, block radiation damage, and improve the effect of cancer therapies such as high-dose vitamin C, laetrile, colloidal silver, chlorine dioxide, and chemotherapy. DMSO can be taken orally, applied topically, or given intravenously. It targets cancer cells and is used to open ports on the cells' surface to allow the therapy to get inside. One downside of DMSO's use is that it creates a body odor similar to sulfur. Two good books on the subject:

+ *The DMSO Handbook for Doctors* by Archie H. Scott
+ *DMSO: Nature's Healer* by Dr. Morton Walker

GcMAF

Two substances in the body, nagalase and GcMAF, are in relationship with each other as cancer ramps up. Nagalase is an enzyme/protein secreted by cancer cells for their survival, and GcMAF (globulin component macrophage activating factor) is the body's weapon to defeat nagalase. When Gc protein combines with vitamin D in the body, it is used by the immune system's macrophages to kill cancer cells. But when Gc protein cannot be converted to GcMAF, the immune system is compromised. Cancer cells are smart, and they create nagalase, which blocks the Gc protein from attaching itself to vitamin D. When patients are given GcMAF, some have substantial recoveries. In other cases, it is thought the immune system is just not strong enough to use it. GcMAF comes in a vial, and you inject it much like diabetics inject insulin with a small needle under the skin. If nagalase levels are high, the dosage of GcMAF should be increased. Beware of knock-off, substandard products.

MSM (methylsulfonylmethane)

MSM is a sulfur-containing natural compound we often see as a supplement for joint health. A recent study shows it also inhibits breast cancer growth—including the dreaded triple-negative breast cancer   and without any toxicity.[67] MSM promotes healthy circulation, connective tissue, and digestive tract detoxification. It purifies the blood, supports liver function, supports healthy bone and muscles, and is used to produce glutathione. This is an oral protocol and should be used under a clinician's guidance. Garlic and onions are the best food sources of sulfur. Others are raw milk (not pasteurized), meat, fish, fruits, vegetables, and grains. Unfortunately processed food greatly reduces the amount of this nutrient in our diet. MSM therapy is often used in combination with cesium chloride. To learn more about its clinical uses, visit www.msm-info.com.

Colloidal silver and mild silver protein

Silver has been used for many centuries as an antimicrobial/antibiotic substance. It can be taken orally, applied topically, or given through IV. It has demonstrated antitumor activity with human breast cancer cells.[68] Researchers say it works by disrupting the oxygen metabolism process of viruses, fungi, and single-cell bacteria—it basically suffocates the organism. Silver has been shown to selectively target pathogens and leave healthy cells alone. It also has immune-enhancing effects. Check out a product called Argentyn 23 (the professional line) or Sovereign Silver (the company's consumer line).

Medical cannabis

A great deal of research has been done on chemical compounds secreted by the oils of cannabis flowers. THC is most well-known of its compounds, or cannabinoids, as they are called, because it produces the "marijuana high." But that is just one of at least eighty-five compounds in this plant. Another compound, CBD, is the primary focus of medical cannabis. Studies have shown some cannabinoids have antitumor effects, including induction of cell death; inhibition of cell growth; and inhibition of tumor angiogenesis, invasion, and metastasis.[69] Cannabinoids work by binding to receptors throughout the body. Therefore, it is critical to aim the right cannabinoids at the right receptors. I strongly encourage anyone considering medical cannabis to not buy blindly. With cancer and other conditions, it is critical the correct ratio of cannabinoids be utilized; there are different ratios for different cancers and conditions. United Patients Group (UPG), based out of California (415-524-8099, www .UnitedPatientsGroup.com), is a leader in information and education for cannabinoid therapeutics, including CME courses for physicians. UPG provides essential guidance needed to make critical decisions about your treatment. A phone consultation with its oncology nurse or nurse practitioner is approximately $200. The group will review your records, labs, and scans, and discuss your options. To learn more about medical cannabis, search for the online series "The Sacred Plant."

Cesium chloride

Cesium chloride is a concentrated ionic liquid mineral supplement, an alkaline mineral salt. Inside the cell, alkalinity pulls potassium from the blood and blocks the cell's intake of glucose, stopping fermentation and starving the cell. It also works to neutralize the cancer cell's lactic acid production. Lactic acid is the main component of the deadly cachexia cycle (wasting syndrome), which develops in about half of all cancer patients. Cesium chloride is often used in combination with MSM. In using it, there can be issues about a person's levels of potassium and uric acid, and swelling caused by die-off and detoxification overload. More information is available at www.essense-of-life.com/healthtopics/A-203/ cesium-chloride.html.

3-bromopyruvate (3BP)

Energy production fuels all cells, including cancer cells. 3BP is a small molecule drug, a glycolytic inhibitor, which targets cancer cells by shutting down their ability to make energy. 3BP works on all PET scan–positive cancer cells.

3BP acts as a kind of "Trojan horse." It tricks cancer cells into thinking they are receiving a useful nutrient when, in fact, they are getting a powerful cancer-killing molecule. Unlike healthy cells, tumor cells have elevated levels of monocarboxylic acid transporters, and the small 3PB molecule uses those transporters to get inside, where it quickly destroys the ability of tumor cells to generate energy (glycolysis and OxPhos). Tumor cells very quickly die; normal cells are left unaffected.

3BP is an inexpensive, common chemical that cannot be patented. It looks promising but has not yet gone through human trials. In July 2013 the FDA accepted an investigational new drug (IND) application for the use of bromopyruvate for a phase I clinical trial in liver cancer. Dayspring Cancer Clinic in Scottsdale, Arizona, is one of only a few cancer clinics in the United States currently making 3BP available to patients with all types of cancer through the use of an Institutional Review Board (IRB) study.

Mistletoe

This is a semiparasitic plant that grows on some types of trees. Mistletoe extract is called Iscador. Extracts of mistletoe have been shown to kill cancer cells in the laboratory and to boost the immune system.[70] The Germans have used mistletoe for cancer since the 1920s. In some European countries extracts made from European mistletoe are among the most prescribed therapies for cancer patients, but not in the United States, where the FDA has not approved the use of mistletoe as a treatment for cancer.[71] However, there is a clinical trial going on at Johns Hopkins with mistletoe. Mistletoe must be ordered by a physician and can be given intravenously or via subcutaneous injections.

Laetrile (also called amygdalin or B17)

I mention laetrile because it's a therapy that I'm asked about quite often. I've spoken to people who claim that it was a big part of their recovery, and to others who say that it did nothing to help them. Be aware that it's used in many countries but is *not* legal in the United States, the European Union, Canada, Australia, and New Zealand. Patients seem to acquire it on their own and use it without medical supervision. I strongly discourage this.

Amygdalin, the active compound, is a plant substance found naturally in raw fruit seeds, particularly apricot kernels. You might be surprised to learn that apple seeds contain it. I wonder if God created these anticancer substances and put them in tiny amounts in nature to keep us healthy. I used to throw my apple core away, but now I eat the tiny seeds.

The danger comes when using high doses of the synthetic form of amygdalin, laetrile. When laetrile is broken down by the body, it forms hydrogen cyanide, which is thought to be an anticancer compound.[72] According to Ralph Moss, studies in the 1970s verified laetrile's safety and effectiveness.[73] If considering this therapy, please do further research and discuss it with your physician.

Rife therapy

Royal Rife was a medical inventor who discovered every living organism vibrates at its own unique energetic frequency. In the 1930s he measured the frequency of many microorganisms, including cancer, and was able to destroy them with targeted frequencies. Think of the opera singer who is able to hit just the right note long enough to shatter glass. Unhealthy organs put out too much or too little vibration. Stress, toxins, nutritional deficiencies, and age can alter the frequencies, causing organs to either underperform or overperform.

During the therapy, frequencies are selected to target the patient's specific diagnosis. The patient can sit comfortably on a rife mat, hold hand-held electrodes, or touch contact plates. There is no sensation felt during the session. A session can last an hour or more, and the rife machine may utilize different frequencies during the session.

Supportive oligonucleotide technique (SOT)

SOT is similar to a technique called antisense that has been used for many years, but there are differences between traditional antisense and SOT.

SOT is not a genetic therapy, nor does it involve chemotherapy. RGCC-Labs uses the mRNA (messenger RNA) of the patient's CTCs/CSCs, acquired from a blood sample and occasionally from biopsies of a tumor, to make the SOT. The SOT identifies certain gene expression patterns as targets for the therapy. SOT has the ability to induce cell death in CTCs, CSCs, and tumors. It is also able to cross the blood-brain barrier. Each dose of SOT remains active in the patient's bloodstream for approximately fourteen to sixteen weeks. The mRNA has "a stealth like ability that keeps the body from recognizing and destroying it." Chemotherapy and radiation should be avoided with SOT, as it will decrease its efficacy.[74]

Umbilical cord blood stem cell therapy

Have you ever heard of doctors asking a new mother if she would like to store her baby's cord blood? Well, there's a reason for that. Studies published on PubMed and ClinicalTrials.gov have documented the healing and regenerative power of the stem cells in umbilical cord blood. It's important that you understand that the blood is only collected from the umbilical cord of healthy full-term babies. MD Anderson is doing work with cord blood transplants on patients with blood-borne cancers with success. At this time they are giving chemotherapy or radiation before the therapy. "In some cases, the transplant can have an added benefit," Dr. Elizabeth Shpall says. "The new blood cells also attack and destroy any cancer cells that survived the chemo and radiation."[75] If you would like more information of umbilical cord blood therapy, please contact me through my website at www.cancerfreeexperts.com.

Artesunate

Artesunate was initially developed for treating malaria. Studies report that it activates mitochondrial apoptosis/cell death by utilizing the iron inside of cancer cells, causing the cells to die.[76] In 2013 Bastyr Integrative Oncology Research Center produced its initial data, which indicated that intravenous vitamin C administered in combination with intravenous artemisinin, of which artesunate is a derivative, has a positive impact on people with advanced cancers.[77] Intravenous artesunate is frequently given just before high-dose intravenous vitamin C and shows a strong indication that these two treatments work together synergistically.

Metformin

In one of the largest studies of its kind, a team of scientists analyzed cancer risk among over eight thousand diabetics, half of whom were treated with metformin, a prescription oral diabetes medication that helps control blood sugar. Over a ten-year period they observed a 54 percent lower incidence of all cancers in metformin users compared to nonusers. Metformin is derived from the French lilac plant and has shown to be nontoxic. Many patients are taking it as part of an integrative therapy protocol.

DCA (dichloroacetate)

Research on DCA has accelerated in the last few years. It "works by turning on the natural cell suicide system (called apoptosis) which is suppressed in cancerous cells, thus allowing them to die on their own....DCA also interferes with the cancer cell's use of glucose, starving the cell of energy....The latest research shows that DCA also kills many types of cancer cells, and can boost the cancer-killing effects of radiation. The first formal human cancer research using DCA was published in May 2010. It confirmed that DCA is an effective anti-cancer drug for treating glioblastoma patients."[78]

Low-dose naltrexone

Naltrexone has been used as a treatment for addiction to opioids and also to alcohol. Dr. Bernard Bihari, a New York neurologist, discovered that low doses of naltrexone can treat various immune diseases as well as cancer. Low-dose naltrexone (LDN) works by boosting the levels of a natural opioid in the body called opioid growth factor (OGF). OGF is a naturally occurring substance in the body. Many cancers respond to the increased levels of OGF, and their growth can be stopped or slowed. Use of LDN in cancer is considered "off-label." It should be used under the supervision of a physician. It can be given orally or by IV. The main side effects from this drug are insomnia or vivid dreams. A human phase I trial was done at Penn State University.

Cryotherapy

Cryotherapy or cryoablation (freezing) "is a well-established, FDA approved, minimally invasive treatment…for fibroadenomas." However, it has recently shown success in the treatment of small breast and prostate tumors. It is an outpatient procedure that involves placing a cryoprobe at the center of a tumor. The tumor cells are killed due to direct injury from freezing. It is an appealing alternative to surgery because it is minimally invasive and does not involve general anesthesia. The dead cancer cells are absorbed by the body, and some believe that the process may stimulate immunity.[79]

Chapter 35

Closing

HAVE AN OPEN MIND TO NEW INFORMATION

THE FUTURE IS bright, and we can defeat cancer. Our current system is not designed to take into account the impact of nutrition and lifestyle—important epigenetic influences. We've been waiting for people to get really sick, and then we go down the path of a surgical and drug approach. And we wonder why we've been struggling with the war on cancer. We never addressed it very fully. We studied it as a disease caused by bad genes rather than as a metabolic and lifestyle-driven disease. Our pursuit of "the cure" over the last sixty years has left many promising roads for research, treatment, and prevention relatively untraveled.

Steve Steeves, CCN, CNT, author of *The Trinity Diet*, had this to say:

> We must stop long enough to consider if our behavior is constructive for the kingdom of God, and if what we are doing as active agents for the Lord is beneficial to our bodies, our families and our communities that depend on us. Eating mindfully and worshipfully is a discipline worth striving for.[1]

Oh, how my heart rejoiced to read his words, so eloquently and perfectly written. I've struggled for years to put the pieces together. I've watched so many precious people die while I struggled to relate to them the importance of healing the heart and the physical body, not just cutting out or poisoning the cancer.

We live in a stressful world loaded with toxins. Our food supply is highly processed and lacking the nutrients the body needs for optimal health. I believe if you implement a healthy lifestyle, you will have a much better chance of avoiding or beating cancer.

And just as important, if you've already gone the route of surgery, chemotherapy, and radiation and have been pronounced "cancer-free," I encourage you to use one or more of the tests in this book to validate it. Connect with an integrative or functional medicine physician; he or she can help you prevent cancer.

Take great care of yourself. Live purposefully, and consider your choices

261

wisely. See cancer coming early. Don't let it hang around for five or ten years before it's discovered. Find it early, when it is treatable and beatable. You may find making a positive impact on your health is hard work. I don't disagree, but you are worth the effort, and life is worth living—and boy, is it a lot more fun when you're in good health!

I've learned a great deal through my personal cancer journey. Gregg Matte of Houston's First Baptist Church summed up my purpose for writing this book when he said, "Make your misery your ministry and your test your testimony."

I have experienced misery and been tested. I pray that my resulting ministry and testimony will lighten your load and has inspired, educated, and equipped you to never fear cancer.

—JENNY HRBACEK, RN

> Do you not know that your body is a temple of the Holy Spirit within you, whom you have from God? You are not your own, for you were bought with a price. So glorify God in your body.
>
> —1 CORINTHIANS 6:19–20, ESV

Congratulations!

You now possess more knowledge than most people when it comes to preventing cancer, finding it early, and treating it with methods less apt to trigger a recurrence.

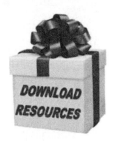

But I'm not stopping there. I have a gift for you—a treasure trove of resources at your fingertips, really helpful organizations, websites, books, and videos.

Don't just google aimlessly. Get my *free* download that will save you time and steer you in the right direction. Go to www.cancerfreeexperts .com, and click on "Free Downloads."

Take a minute and check it out today.

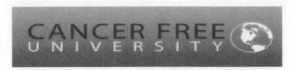

The book *Cancer-Free! Are You Sure?* and more come to life in Cancer Free University. You will hear directly from the physicians, scientists, nutritionists, and other experts. This is the best resource of its kind. New content is added frequently—all in an easy-to-learn, online, on-demand format. DVDs are available. This includes three curricula:

1. **Advanced Early-Detection Strategies and Testing Options.** Watch in-depth interviews on many of the lab tests described in this book, plus bonus interviews with Dr. Nasha Winters of Optimal Terrain Consulting and Shirley Williams, author of *Stage 4 Cancer Gone*.

2. **Treatment Options and Healing Therapies.** What are they? How do they work? Why do they work? Which ones are right for you?

3. **Powerful and Proven Prevention Strategies.** Learn about detoxification, vitamin D, water, how to make better choices in the grocery store—how you can use proven, powerful prevention to make your body healthier and live cancer-free! This includes a bonus interview on how to keep your hair during chemo.

With the purchase of your book, you're qualified for a 50 percent off scholarship. Go to www.CancerFreeUniversity.com, and enter code **Cancer50** on the payment screen. Your search for answers is over!

JOIN THE PUBLIC AWARENESS CAMPAIGN!

Share your story, encourage someone, offer
hope, and let your voice be heard at

www.NoLumpOrBump.com.

Email your cancer story, and upload videos and photos.

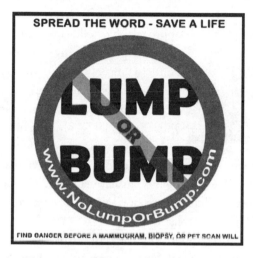

It has often been said the United States does not have a health care system;
we have a disease-management system focused on expensive drugs and
invasive surgeries. Through public awareness let's ask that the system do
more to promote health. Let's make the insurance industry aware of the
state-of-the-art cancer tests and healing therapies that we all deserve—
and aware that we want our medical plans to cover our use of them.

JENNY HRBACEK, RN

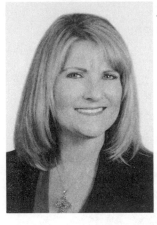

Jenny Hrbacek (her-bah-check) set out on a life-changing journey when she was diagnosed with breast cancer in 2009. Today she has launched a national campaign to change the way cancer is detected. Her inspirational approach has educated and equipped hundreds of people to live cancer-free. She moderates Cancer Free University, an online, on-demand resource with over seventy-five world-class experts, scientists, physicians, and researchers—all in an affordable, easy-to-learn, easy-to-use platform that provides lifesaving information. She presents information on viable options to chemotherapy, aggressive treatments, invasive surgery, and options that can free you from fear. What do you do? Where do you go? Whom do you listen to? That's why she created CFU.

Jenny is a featured guest on the fall 2018 television show *God's Medicine*. In 2016 she began doing segments on Doug Kaufmann's TV show, *Know the Cause*. Jenny also appears in Ty Bollinger's *The Truth About Cancer—A Global Quest* and in the Cancer Answers Global Summit. She has presented at the Academy of Comprehensive Integrative Medicine, The Tripping Over the Truth Metabolism and Cancer Retreat, the International Organization of Integrative Cancer Physicians Public Day conferences, and the Cancer Control Society conference.

Jenny is an advisory board member of BeatCancer.org, a general advisory board member of Best Answer for Cancer Foundation, and an advisory board member of Wellness Outreach Worldwide Church.

Notes

INTRODUCTION

1.   "100 Years of Diabetes Access," Diabetes Patient Advocacy Coalition, accessed May 7, 2018, http://diabetespac.org/access-action-center/about -diabetesaccessmatters/history-of-diabetesaccessmatters/.

2.   "The Genetics of Cancer," National Cancer Institute, updated October 12, 2017, www.cancer.gov/about-cancer/causes-prevention/genetics.

3.   Kathryn M. Wilson, Edward L. Giovannucci, and Lorelei A. Mucci, "Lifestyle and Dietary Factors in the Prevention of Lethal Prostate Cancer," *Asian Journal of Andrology* 14, no. 3 (May 2012): 365–374, www.ncbi .nlm.nih.gov/pmc/articles/PMC3720164/.

4.   Jim Moselhy et al., "Natural Products That Target Stem Cells," *Anticancer Research* 35, no. 11 (November 2015): 5773–88.

5.   "Cancer Stat Fact Sheets: Cancer of Any Site," National Cancer Institute, accessed May 4, 2018, https://seer.cancer.gov/statfacts/html/all.html.

6.   "Cancer Statistics," National Cancer Institute, updated March 22, 2017, www.cancer.gov/about-cancer/understanding/statistics.

7.   Tim Hume and Jen Christensen, "WHO: Imminent Global Cancer 'Disaster' Reflects Aging, Lifestyle Factors," CNN.com, updated February 4, 2014, www.cnn.com/2014/02/04/health/who-world-cancer-report/index.html.

8.   "Metastatic Cancer," National Cancer Institute, updated February 6, 2017, www.cancer.gov/types/metastatic-cancer.

9.   "Economic Impact of Cancer," American Cancer Society, accessed June 5, 2018, www.cancer.org/cancer/cancer-basics/economic-impact-of-cancer.html.

10.   "Predicting Cancer Immunotherapy Response With Tumor Mutational Burden (TMB)," accessed May 7, 2018, https://raportuldegarda.ro/wp-content/ uploads/resurse/Infografic-TMB.pdf.

CHAPTER 1: MY STORY

1.   Bernard Fisher, "Twenty-Year Follow-up of a Randomized Trial Comparing Total Mastectomy, Lumpectomy, and Lumpectomy Plus Irradiation for the Treatment of Invasive Breast Cancer," *New England Journal of Medicine* 347, no. 16 (October 17, 2002), www.nejm.org/doi/full/10.1056/NEJMoa022152.

2.   "Sentinel Lymph Node Biopsy for Early-Stage Breast Cancer," American Society of Clinical Oncology, December 12, 2016, www.cancer.net /research-and-advocacy/asco-care-and-treatment-recommendations-patients /sentinel-lymph-node-biopsy-early-stage-breast-cancer; "Extensive Lymph Node Removal Doesn't Improve Survival in Some Women With Early-Stage Breast Cancer," National Cancer Institute, October 10, 2017, www.cancer.gov /news-events/cancer-currents-blog/2017/breast-cancer-lymph-node-removal.

3.   "What is the CELLSEARCH Circulating Tumor Cell (CTC) Test?," Menarini Silicon Biosystems Inc., accessed May 7, 2018, www .cellsearchctc.com/about-cellsearch/what-is-cellsearch-ctc-test, emphasis added.

4.   Yan Ma et al., "High-Dose Parenteral Ascorbate Enhanced Chemosensitivity of Ovarian Cancer and Reduced Toxicity of Chemotherapy," *Science Translational Medicine* 6, no. 222 (February 5, 2014), http://stm.sciencemag.org/content/6/222/222ra18.full?sid=1d159157-365e-44ca-b234-effd97db5ff3.

5.   M. S. Wicha, S. Liu, and G. Dontu, "Cancer Stem Cells: An Old Idea—A Paradigm Shift," *Cancer Research* 66, no. 4 (February 15, 2006).

6.   Soonmyung Paik et al., "A Multigene Assay to Predict Recurrence of Tamoxifen-Treated, Node-Negative Breast Cancer," *New England Journal of Medicine* 351, no. 27 (December 30, 2004): 2817–2826.

7.   "NOLVADEX (Tamoxifen Citrate) TABLETS," FDA, August 27, 2004, www.accessdata.fda.gov/drugsatfda_docs/label/2005/17970s053lbl.pdf.

8.   "IARC Monographs Volume 112: Evaluation of Five Organophosphate Insecticides and Herbicides," International Agency for Research on Cancer, March 20, 2015, www.iarc.fr/en/media-centre/iarcnews/pdf/MonographVolume112.pdf.

CHAPTER 2: WHAT IS CANCER?

1.   "Cancer Stem Cell Program," Stanford Medicine, accessed May 7, 2018, http://med.stanford.edu/cancer/research/research-programs/stemcell.html.

2.   Patrick O. Brown and Chana Palmer, "The Preclinical Natural History of Serous Ovarian Cancer: Defining the Target for Early Detection," *PLoS Med* 6, no. 7 (July 2009): e1000114, https://doi.org/10.1371/journal.pmed.1000114.

3.   "Signs and Symptoms of Cancer: What Are Signs and Symptoms?," American Cancer Society, accessed May 1, 2018, www.cancer.org/cancer/cancerbasics/signs-and-symptoms-of-cancer.

4.   Otto Warburg, *The Metabolism of Tumours: Investigations From the Kaiser Wilhelm Institute for Biology*, trans. F. Dickens (London: Constable & Co. Ltd., 1930), 56 (out of print). Ref: *Hoppe-Seyler's Zeitschr Physiol Chem.* 1910 66, 305; Brian Scott Peskin in *Glycolysis*, Paul N. Lithaw, ed., (Hauppauge, NY: Nova Science Publishers Inc., 2009), accessed May 2, 2018, http://brianpeskin.com/pdf/publications/Glycolysis-chap.pdf.

5.   H. Lu, R. A. Forbes, and A. Verma, "Hypoxia-Inducible Factor 1 Activation by Aerobic Glycolysis Implicates the Warburg Effect in Carcinogenesis," *Journal of Biological Chemistry* 277, no. 26 (June 28, 2002): 23111–23115.

6.   Reginald H. Garrett and Charles M. Grisham, *Biochemistry* 5th edition (Boston: Cengage Learning, 2011).

7.   "Ketogenic Diet and Its Role in Cancer Treatment (A Special Interview With Dr. Thomas Seyfried)," Joseph Mercola, accessed May 1, 2018, http://mercola.fileburst.com/PDF/ExpertInterviewTranscripts/Interview-Thomas Seyfried.pdf.

8.   Thomas N. Seyfried, *Cancer as a Metabolic Disease: On the Origin, Management, and Prevention of Cancer* (Hoboken, NJ: Wiley, 2012).

9.   Thomas N. Seyfried et al., "Cancer as a Metabolic Disease: Implications for Novel Therapeutics," *Carcinogenesis* 35 no. 3 (March 2014): 515–527, www.ncbi.nlm.nih.gov/pmc/articles/PMC3941741/.

10.   M. Schmidt et al., "Effects of a Ketogenic Diet on the Quality of Life in 16 Patients With Advanced Cancer: A Pilot Trial," *Nutrition & Metabolism* 8, no. 1 (July 27, 2011): 54, www.ncbi.nlm.nih.gov/pubmed/21794124; T. N. Seyfried et al., "Is the Restricted Ketogenic Diet a Viable Alternative to the Standard of Care for Managing Malignant Brain Cancer?," *Epilepsy Research* 100, no. 3 (July 2012): 310–326.

11.   "Ketogenic Diet and Its Role in Cancer Treatment (A Special Interview With Dr. Thomas Seyfried)," Joseph Mercola.

12.   Yasumasa Kato et al., "Acidic Extracellular Microenvironment and Cancer," *Cancer Cell International* 13 (2013): 89, www.ncbi.nlm.nih.gov/pmc/articles/PMC3849184/.

13.   "Cancer and Lactic Acid Cycle," MistyBlue Cancer Care Foundation, accessed May 7, 2018, www.mistybluecancercare.org/uploads/2/4/5/9/2459046/cancer_and_lactic_acid_cycle.pdf; John Brennan, "What Happens to Lactic Acid After Exercise?," Leaf Group Ltd., September 11, 2017, www.livestrong.com/article/544580-what-happens-to-lactic-acid-after-exercise/.

14.   Matthias Rath, *Cellular Health Series: Cancer* (Santa Clara, CA: MR Publishing Inc., 2002), 18–20.

15.   Julita A. Teodorczyk-Injeyan et al., "Interleukin 2-Regulated In Vitro Antibody Production Following a Single Spinal Manipulative Treatment in Normal Subjects," *Chiropractic & Osteopathy* 18 (2010): 26, accessed May 2, 2018, www.ncbi.nlm.nih.gov/pmc/articles/PMC2945351/.

16.   J. E. Rossouw et al., "Risks and Benefits of Estrogen Plus Progestin in Healthy Postmenopausal Women: Principal Results From the Women's Health Initiative Randomized Controlled Trial," *Journal of the American Medical Association* 288, no. 3 (July 17, 2002): 321–333, www.ncbi.nlm.nih.gov/pubmed/12117397.

17.   Françoise Clavel-Chapelon, "Cohort Profile: The French E3N Cohort Study," *International Journal of Epidemiology* 44, no. 3 (June 1, 2015): 801–809, https://academic.oup.com/ije/article/44/3/801/629731; V. Beral et al., "Breast Cancer and Hormone-Replacement Therapy in the Million Women Study," *The Lancet* 362, no. 9382 (August 9, 2003): 419–427, www.ncbi.nlm.nih.gov/pubmed/12927427.

18.   R. T. Chlebowski et al., "Breast Cancer After Use of Estrogen Plus Progestin in Postmenopausal Women," *New England Journal of Medicine* 360, no. 6 (February 5, 2009): 573–587, www.ncbi.nlm.nih.gov/pubmed/19196674.

19.   Chlebowski et al., "Breast Cancer After Use of Estrogen Plus Progestin in Postmenopausal Women."

20.   Janet M. Gray et al., "State of the Evidence 2017: An Update on the Connection Between Breast Cancer and the Environment," *Environmental Health* 16 (2017): 94, www.ncbi.nlm.nih.gov/pmc/articles/PMC5581466/.

21.   "Key Statistics for Ovarian Cancer," American Cancer Society, last revised January 5, 2018, www.cancer.org/cancer/ovarian-cancer/about/key-statistics.html; "Key Statistics for Prostate Cancer," American Cancer Society, last revised January 4, 2018, www.cancer.org/cancer/prostate-cancer/about/

key-statistics.html; "U.S. Breast Cancer Statistics," Breastcancer.org, last modified January 8, 2018, www.breastcancer.org/symptoms/understand_bc
/statistics.

22.   "Melatonin," Milton S. Hershey Medical Center, accessed May 7, 2018,
http://pennstatehershey.adam.com/content.aspx?productId=107&pid=33
&gid=000315; Alice Park, "Working the Night Shift Could Raise Your Cancer
Risk," *Time*, January 8, 2018, http://time.com/5093052/
working-night-shift-risk-cancer/.

23.   Eileen M. Lynch, "Melatonin and Cancer Treatment," *Life Extension
Magazine* January 2004.

24.   Raphael d'Angelo, "Parasites and Cancer—the Connection," ParaWellness Research, accessed May 2, 2018, http://parawellnessresearch.com/articles/
parasites-and-cancer-the-connection/.

25.   Bruce Fife, *The Coconut Oil Miracle* (New York: Avery, 2013), 66–82.

26.   "Aflatoxins: Occurrence and Health Risks," Cornell University, updated
September 10, 2015, www.ansci.cornell.edu/plants/toxicagents/aflatoxin/
aflatoxin.html.

27.   M. Peraica et al., "Toxic Effects of Mycotoxins in Humans," *Bulletin of
the World Health Organization* 77, no. 9 (1999): 754–766, https://www.ncbi
.nlm.nih.gov/pmc/articles/PMC2557730/.

28.   Doug A. Kaufmann et al., *The Germ That Causes Cancer* (Rockwall,
TX: Mediatriton Inc., 2005).

29.   Antoine Béchamp, *The Blood and Its Third Element* (n.p.: Review Press,
2002).

30.   Bernard Jensen and Mark Anderson, *Empty Harvest: Understanding
the Link Between Our Food, Our Immunity and Our Planet* (New York: Avery,
1990).

31.   Alan Cantwell Jr., *The Cancer Microbe* (Los Angeles: Aries Rising Press,
1990).

32.   Edward L. Giovannucci, "Obesity, Insulin Resistance, and Cancer Risk,"
Cancer Prevention, Spring 2005, Issue 5, accessed May 2, 2018, https://web.
archive.org/web/20050505234906/www.nypcancerprevention.com/issue/5/con/
features/pre_ear-2.shtml.

33.   S. Thongprakaisang et al., "Glyphosate Induces Human Breast Cancer
Cells Growth Via Estrogen Receptors," *Food and Chemical Toxicology* 59 (September 2013): 129–136, accessed May 2, 2018, http://www.ncbi. nlm.nih.gov/
pubmed/23756170.

34.   Tom Polansek, "EPA Says Glyphosate, a Key Ingredient in Monsanto's
Roundup, not Likely to Be Carcinogenic to People," *St. Louis Post-Dispatch*,
December 20, 2017, http://www.stltoday.com/business/local/epa-says-glypho-
sate-a-key-ingredient-in-monsanto-s-roundup/article_6efd908d-d3b8-5a4b-
81f1-841631f28cda.html; "IARC Monograph on Glyphosate," International
Agency for Research on Cancer, January 3, 2018, https://www.iarc.fr/en/media-
centre/iarcnews/2016/glyphosate_IARC2016.php.

35. Joseph Mercola, "Monsanto Is Inside Everything," Dr. Joseph Mercola, March 22, 2016, http://articles.mercola.com/sites/articles/archive/2016/03/22/ monsanto-glyphosate.aspx.

36. James Braly and Ron Hoggan, *Dangerous Grains* (New York: Avery, 2002).

37. Gerard J. Tortora and Bryan Derrickson, *Essentials of Anatomy and Physiology*, ninth edition (Hoboken, NY: John Wiley & Sons, 2013), 71.

38. "Oncogenes, Tumor Suppressor Genes, and Cancer," American Cancer Society, https://updoc.tips/download/free-pdf-ebook-onco-tsg-cancer.

39. "Oncogenes and Tumor Suppressor Genes," American Cancer Society, last revised June 25, 2014, https://www.cancer.org/cancer/cancer-causes/ genetics/genes-and-cancer/oncogenes-tumor-suppressor-genes.html.

40. A. Roman and B. Tombarkiewicz, "Prolonged Weakening of the Geomagnetic Field Affects the Immune System of Rats," *Bioelectromagnetics* 1 (January 30, 2009): 21–22.

41. "The Human Body in Space," NASA, updated August 2, 2001, https://www.nasa.gov/hrp/bodyinspace; "Gravity Hurts (So Good)," NASA, updated December 20, 2017, https://science.nasa.gov/science-news/science-at -nasa/2001/ast02aug_1.

42. Garry F. Gordon, MD, DO, MD(H), "Why People Seldom Get Heart Cancer," *Green Living AZ*, June 1, 2011, https://greenlivingaz.com/why-few -people-seldom-get-heart-cancer/.

43. "Psychological Stress and Cancer," National Cancer Institute, reviewed December 10, 2012, https://www.cancer.gov/about-cancer/coping/feelings/ stress-fact-sheet.

44. Chris C. Wolford et al., "Transcription Factor ATF3 Links Host Adaptive Response to Breast Cancer Metastasis," *Journal of Clinical Investigation* 123, no. 7 (July 1, 2013): 2893–2906.

45. Catharine Paddock, "Stress Fuels Cancer Spread by Triggering Master Gene," Medical News Today, August 27, 2013, https://www.medicalnewstoday .com/articles/265254.php.

CHAPTER 3: STATISTICS—MISCONCEPTIONS OF REALITY

1. "Understanding Statistics Used to Guide Prognosis and Evaluate Treatment," American Society of Clinical Oncology, accessed May 2, 2018, www .cancer.net/all-about-cancer/newly-diagnosed/understanding-statistics-used- guide-prognosis-and-evaluate-treatment.

2. L. D. Dorresteijn et al., "Increased Risk of Ischemic Stroke After Radiotherapy on the Neck in Patients Younger Than 60 Years," *Journal of Clinical Oncology* 20, no. 1 (January 1, 2002): 282–288.

3. Gina Kolata, "Advances Elusive in the Drive to Cure Cancer," *New York Times*, April 23, 2009, https://www.nytimes.com/2009/04/24/health/ policy/24cancer.html.

4. "Key Statistics for Childhood Cancers," American Cancer Society, accessed May 2, 2018, https://www.cancer.org/cancer/cancer-in-children/key -statistics.html.

5.   *Reducing Environmental Cancer Risk: What We Can Do Now*, National Cancer Institute, accessed May 2, 2018, http://deainfo.nci.nih.gov/advisory/pcp/annualReports/pcp08-09rpt/PCP_Report_08-09_508.pdf.

6.   R. Mukhopadhyay et al., "Promotion of Variant Human Mammary Epithelial Cell Outgrowth by Ionizing Radiation: An Agent-Based Model Supported by In Vitro Studies," *Breast Cancer Research* 12, no. 1 (February 2010): R11, accessed May 3, 2018, https://www.ncbi.nlm.nih.gov/pubmed/20146798.

7.   "Study Raises New Concerns About Radiation and Breast Cancer," Berkeley Lab, updated May 13, 2010, http://newscenter.lbl.gov/2010/05/13/new-concerns-about-radiation-and-breast-cancer/.

8.   M. von Euler-Chelpin, M. Kuchiki, and I. Vejborg, "Increased Risk of Breast Cancer in Women With False-Positive Test: The Role of Misclassification," *Cancer Epidemiology* 38, no. 5 (October 2014): 619–622; Ronnie Cohen, "Mammography False Alarms Linked With Later Tumor Risk," Reuters, August 22, 2014, https://www.reuters.com/article/us-mammograms-false-positives/mammography-false-alarms-linked-with-later-tumor-risk-idUSKBN0GM1YU20140822.

9.   A. B. Miller et al., "Twenty-Five-Year Follow-Up for Breast Cancer Incidence and Mortality of the Canadian National Breast Screening Study: Randomised Screening Trial," *British Medical Journal* 348 (February 11, 2014): g366.

10.   Gina Kolata, "Vast Study Casts Doubts on Value of Mammograms," *New York Times*, February 11, 2014, https://www.nytimes.com/2014/02/12/health/study-adds-new-doubts-about-value-of-mammograms.html.

11.   Archie Bleyer and H. Gilbert Welch, "Effect of Three Decades of Screening Mammography on Breast-Cancer Incidence," *New England Journal of Medicine* 367, no. 21 (2012): 1998–2005.

12.   Miller et al., "Twenty-Five-Year Follow-Up for Breast Cancer Incidence and Mortality of the Canadian National Breast Screening Study: Randomised Screening Trial."

13.   Mette L. Lousdal et al., "Trends in Breast Cancer Stage Distribution Before, During and After Introduction of a Screening Programme in Norway," *European Journal of Public Health* 24, no. 6 (December 1, 2014): 1017–1022, https://academic.oup.com/eurpub/article/24/6/1017/608007.

14.   N. Biller-Andorno and Peter Jüni, "Abolishing Mammography Screening Programs? A View From the Swiss Medical Board," *New England Journal of Medicine* 370 (May 22, 2014): 1965–1967.

15.   "Colorectal Cancer Screening (PDQ)," National Cancer Institute, updated February 23, 2018, www.cancer.gov/cancertopics/pdq/screening/colorectal/HealthProfessional/page3.

16.   D. X. Yang et al., "Estimating the Magnitude of Colorectal Cancers Prevented During the Era of Screening: 1976 to 2009," *Cancer* 120, no. 18 (September 15, 2014): 2893–2901, https://www.ncbi.nlm.nih.gov/pubmed/24894740.

17.   Elisabeth Rosenthal, "The $2.7 Trillion Medical Bill: Colonoscopies Explain Why U.S. Leads the World in Health Expenditures," *New York Times*,

June 1, 2013, http://www.nytimes.com/2013/06/02/health/colonoscopies
-explain-why-us-leads-the-world-in-health-expenditures.html?pagewanted=all.

18. "Key Statistics for Small Intestine Cancer," American Cancer Society, last revised February 8, 2018, https://www.cancer.org/cancer/small-intestine-cancer/about/what-is-key-statistics.html.

19. Robert Preidt, "BRCA Breast Cancer Gene Doesn't Affect Patient Survival: Study," U.S. News and World Report, January 12, 2018, https://health.usnews.com/health-care/articles/2018-01-12/brca-breast-cancer-gene-doesnt-affect-patient-survival-study.

20. "BRCA Mutations: Cancer Risk and Genetic Testing," National Cancer Institute, accessed May 4, 2018, www.cancer.gov/cancertopics/factsheet/Risk/BRCA.

21. W. Park et al., "New Perspectives of Curcumin in Cancer Prevention," *Cancer Prevention Research* 6, no. 5 (May 2013): 387–400.

22. Liesbeth Bergmann et al., "Risk and Prognosis of Endometrial Cancer After Tamoxifen for Breast Cancer," *The Lancet* 356, no. 9233 (September 9, 2000): 881–887, http://www.thelancet.com/journals/lancet/article/PIIS0140-6736(00)02677-5/fulltext?code=lancet-site; Clemens Tempfer and Ernst Kubista, "Tamoxifen and Risk of Endometrial Cancer," *The Lancet* 357, no. 9249 (January 6, 2001): 65, http://www.thelancet.com/journals/lancet/article/PIIS0140-6736(00)03579-0/fulltext.

23. O. Lavie et al., "The Risk of Developing Uterine Sarcoma After Tamoxifen Use," *International Journal of Gynecological Cancer* 18, no. 2 (March/April 2008): 352–356, https://www.ncbi.nlm.nih.gov/pubmed/18334013.

24. A. Gennari et al., "HER2 Status and Efficacy of Adjuvant Anthracyclines in Early Breast Cancer: A Pooled Analysis of Randomized Trials," *Journal of the National Cancer Institute* 100, no. 1 (January 2, 2008): 14–20, https://www.ncbi.nlm.nih.gov/pubmed/18159072.

25. S. M. Swain, F. S. Whaley, and M. S. Ewer, "Congestive Heart Failure in Patients Treated With Doxorubicin: A Retrospective Analysis of Three Trials," *Cancer* 97, no. 11 (June 1, 2003): 2869–2879.

26. Katie Thomas, "Breaking the Seal on Drug Research," *New York Times*, June 29, 2013, https://www.nytimes.com/2013/06/30/business/breaking-the-seal-on-drug-research.html.

27. "Structure/Function Claims," FDA, updated December 14, 2017, https://www.fda.gov/Food/LabelingNutrition/ucm2006881.htm.

28. "FDA Warns Companies to Stop Marketing Fruit Products With Unproven Disease Treatment and Prevention Claims," FDA, October 24, 2005, http://web.archive.org/web/20051026040129/www.fda.gov/bbs/topics/news/2005/new01246.html; "Inspections, Compliance, Enforcement, and Criminal Investigations," Department of Health and Human Resources, updated July 8, 2009, http://wayback.archive-it.org/7993/20161023105704/http://www.fda.gov/ICECI/EnforcementActions/WarningLetters/2005/ucm075618.htm.

29. J. M. Tall et al., "Tart Cherry Anthocyanins Suppress Inflammation-Induced Pain Behavior in Rat," *Behavioural Brain Research* 153, no. 1 (August 12, 2004): 181–188, https://www.ncbi.nlm.nih.gov/pubmed/15219719.

30. "Anti-Cancer Food List," American Cancer Society, June 14, 2011, https://csn.cancer.org/node/220591.

31. *Healing Cancer From Inside Out*, directed by Mike Anderson (RaveDiet.com, 2008), DVD.

CHAPTER 4: CONVENTIONAL TREATMENTS AND TESTING

1. "How Does Chemotherapy Affect the Risk of Second Cancers?," American Cancer Society, last revised February 16, 2017, https://www.cancer.org/treatment/treatments-and-side-effects/physical-side-effects/second-cancers-in-adults/chemotherapy.html; "How Does Radiation Therapy Affect the Risk of Second Cancers?," American Cancer Society, last revised December 11, 2014, https://www.cancer.org/treatment/treatments-and-side-effects/physical-side-effects/second-cancers-in-adults/radiation-therapy.html.

2. U. Rüther, C. Nunnensiek, and H. J. Schmoll, eds., *Secondary Neoplasias Following Chemotherapy, Radiotherapy, and Immunosuppression* (Basel, Switzerland: Karger, 2000), https://www.karger.com/Article/Pdf/60441.

3. Sayer Ji, "25 Cancer Stem Cell Killing Foods Smarter Than Chemo & Radiation," GreenMedInfo LLC, May 7, 2018, http://www.greenmedinfo.com/blog/25-cancer-stem-cell-killing-foods-smarter-chemo-radiation.

4. Chris Elkins, "How Much Cancer Costs," Drugwatch.com, updated April 18, 2018, https://www.drugwatch.com/2015/10/07/cost-of-cancer/.

5. Heather Woolwine, "Study: Drug Given Routinely During Cancer Treatment Overused, Ineffective," University of Nebraska Medical Center, March 21, 2013, http://app1.unmc.edu/publicaffairs/todaysite/sitefiles/today_full.cfm?match=10663.

6. Alvin Munene, "Study Has Shown Chemotherapy Can Backfire and Make Cancer Worse," Sanvada.com, January 10, 2017, https://sanvada.com/2017/01/10/study-has-shown-chemotherapy-can-backfire-and-make-cancer-worse/.

7. "FDA News Release: FDA Commissioner Announces Avastin Decision," FDA, updated March 12, 2014, https://wayback.archive-it.org/7993/20170112232043/http://www.fda.gov/NewsEvents/Newsroom/PressAnnouncements/ucm280536.htm.

8. T. H. Connor, B. A. MacKenzie, D. G. DeBord, D. B. Trout, and J. P. O'Callaghan, *NIOSH List of Antineoplastic and Other Hazardous Drugs in Healthcare Settings, 2016* (Cincinnati, OH: U.S. Department of Health and Human Services, 2016), accessed May 8, 2018, https://www.cdc.gov/niosh/docs/2016-161/pdfs/2016-161.pdf.

9. Camille Abboud, "The Price of Drugs for Chronic Myeloid Leukemia (CML), Reflection of the Unsustainable Cancer Drug Prices: Perspective of CML Experts," *Blood* 121, no. 22 (May 30, 2013), https://www.ncbi.nlm.nih.gov/pmc/articles/PMC4190613/.

10.   Anjali Shukla, "Cancer Drugs Are Less Affordable in Low-Income Countries, Despite the Lower Retail Prices, According to a Study Released at the Annual Meeting of American Society of Clinical Oncology (ASCO)," Pharmafile, July 6, 2016, http://www.pharmafile.com/news/504979/drug -pricing-cancer-drugs-cost-most-us-most-unaffordable-india-china-study.

11.   G. Faguet, *The War on Cancer: An Anatomy of Failure, a Blueprint for the Future* (Dordrecht, Netherlands: Springer, 2006), https://www.amazon. com/War-Cancer-Anatomy-Failure-Blueprint/dp/1402086202/ref=asap_ bc?ie=UTF8.

12.   G. Morgan, R. Ward, and M. Barton, "The Contribution of Cytotoxic Chemotherapy to 5-Year Survival in Adult Malignancies," *Clinical Oncology: A Journal of the Royal College of Radiologists* 16, no. 8 (December 2004), https:// www.ncbi.nlm.nih.gov/pubmed/15630849.

13.   "Cancer," National Institute of Health, updated March 29, 2013, https://report.nih.gov/NIHfactsheets/ViewFactSheet.aspx?csid=75.

14.   Clifton Leaf, "Why We Are Losing the War on Cancer (and How to Win It)," *Fortune* 149, no. 6 (March 22, 2004): 76–82, 84–86, 88.

15.   K. M. Adams, M. Kohlmeier, and S. H. Zeisel, "Nutrition Education in U.S. Medical Schools: Latest Update of a National Survey," *Academic Medicine* 85, no. 9 (September 2010): 1537–1542, https://www.ncbi.nlm.nih.gov/ pubmed/20736683.

16.   See, for example, "Conflicts of Interest in Clinical Trial Recruitment and Enrollment: A Call for Increased Oversight," The Center for Health & Pharmaceutical Law & Policy at Seton Hall Law School, November 2009, https://law.shu.edu/Health-Law/upload/health_center_whitepaper_nov2009. pdf; B. Lo and M. J. Field, eds., *Conflict of Interest in Medical Research, Education, and Practice* (Washington, DC: National Academies Press, 2009), https:// www.ncbi.nlm.nih.gov/books/NBK22944/; Charles Ornstein and Eric Sagara, "How Much Are Drug Companies Paying Your Doctor?," *Scientific American,* September 30, 2014, https://www.scientificamerican.com/article/how-much -are-drug-companies-paying-your-doctor/.

17.   Rehema Ellis, "Cancer Docs Profit From Chemotherapy Drugs-Situation Begs the Ethical Question: Are They Overprescribing?," *NBC Nightly News,* September 21, 2006, http://www.nbcnews.com/id/14944098/ns/nbc_ nightly_news_with_brian_williams/t/cancer-docs-profit-chemotherapy-drugs/#. WpQZwujwYdU.

18.   See, for example, "Stage I Uterine Cancer," Texas Oncology, accessed May 8, 2018, https://www.texasoncology.com/types-of-cancer/uterine-cancer/ stage-i-uterine-cancer; Jeffrey C. Liu et al., "Early Oral Tongue Cancer Initially Managed With Surgery Alone: Treatment of Recurrence," *World Journal of Otorhinolaryngology—Head and Neck Surgery* 2, no. 4 (December 2016): 193– 197, https://www.sciencedirect.com/science/article/pii/S2095881116300026; David Cunningham et al., "Perioperative Chemotherapy Versus Surgery Alone for Resectable Gastroesophageal Cancer," *New England Journal of Medicine* 355 (2006): 11–20, http://www.nejm.org/doi/full/10.1056/NEJMoa055531; H. Aoyama et al., "Stereotactic Radiosurgery Plus Whole-Brain Radiation

Therapy vs Stereotactic Radiosurgery Alone for Treatment of Brain Metastases: A Randomized Controlled Trial," *Journal of the American Medical Association* 295, no. 21 (June 7, 2006): 2483–2491, https://www.ncbi.nlm.nih.gov/pubmed/16757720.

19.   Robert J. Gillies, "Causes and Effects of Heterogeneous Perfusion in Tumors," *Neoplasia* 1, no. 3 (August 1999): 197–207, https://www.ncbi.nlm.nih.gov/pmc/articles/PMC1508079/.

20.   Ji, "25 Cancer Stem Cell Killing Foods Smarter Than Chemo & Radiation."

21.   "Risk of Tumor Cell Seeding Through Biopsy and Aspiration Cytology," *Journal of International Society of Preventive and Community Dentistry* 4, no. 1 (January–April 2014): 5–11, https://www.ncbi.nlm.nih.gov/pmc/articles/PMC4015162/; Steven Nemeroff, "Preventing Surgery-Induced Cancer Metastasis," *Life Extension*, December 2009, http://www.lifeextension.com/Magazine/2009/12/Preventing-Surgery-Induced-Cancer-Metastasis/Page-01.

22.   Vincent Ansanelli., "The Ansanelli Co2 Laser Technique," Laser Breast Cancer Surgery, accessed May 8, 2018, https://laserbreastcancersurgery.com/.

23.   Genevieve Housman et al., "Drug Resistance in Cancer: An Overview," *Cancers* 6, no. 3 (September 2014): 1769–1792, https://www.ncbi.nlm.nih.gov/pmc/articles/PMC4190567/.

24.   "TP53 Gene," US Department of Health and Human Services, accessed May 8, 2018, https://ghr.nlm.nih.gov/gene/TP53#.

25.   A. Reles et al., "Correlation of p53 Mutations With Resistance to Platinum-Based Chemotherapy and Shortened Survival in Ovarian Cancer," *Clinical Cancer Research* 7, no. 10 (October 2001): 2984–2997, https://www.ncbi.nlm.nih.gov/pubmed/11595686; Thierry Soussi, "p53 Mutations and Resistance to Chemotherapy: A Stab in the Back for p73," *Cancer Cell* 3, no. 4 (April 2003): 303–305, https://www.sciencedirect.com/science/article/pii/S1535610803000813; L. Breen et al., "Investigation of the Role of p53 in Chemotherapy Resistance of Lung Cancer Cell Lines," *Anticancer Research* 27, no. 3A (May–June 2007): 1361–1364, https://www.ncbi.nlm.nih.gov/pubmed/17593631.

26.   C. S. Moreno et al., "Evidence That p53-Mediated Cell-Cycle-Arrest Inhibits Chemotherapeutic Treatment of Ovarian Carcinomas," *PLOS ONE* 2, no. 5 (May 2007): e441, https://doi.org/10.1371/journal.pone.0000441.

27.   Alexandra Sifferlin, "How Chemotherapy May Trigger Tumors' Resistance," Time Inc., August 7, 2012, http://healthland.time.com/2012/08/07/how-chemotherapy-may-trigger-tumors-resistance/.

28.   Y. Sun et al., "Treatment-Induced Damage to the Tumor Microenvironment Promotes Prostate Cancer Therapy Resistance Through WNT16B," *Nature Medicine* 18 (August 5, 2012): 1359–1368, https://www.nature.com/articles/nm.2890.

29.   M. S. Wicha, S. Liu, and G. Dontu, "Cancer Stem Cells: An Old Idea—a Paradigm Shift," *Cancer Research* 66, no. 4 (February 15, 2006): 1883-1890; discussion 1895–1896.

30.   Bill Henderson and Carlos M. Garcia, *Cancer-Free: Your Guide to Gentle, Non-toxic Healing*, 4th ed. (St. Petersburg, FL: Booklocker.com Inc., 2011), 89.

31.   "How Does Chemotherapy Affect the Risk of Second Cancers?," American Cancer Society.

32.   John Ng and Igor Shuryak, "Minimizing Second Cancer Risk Following Radiotherapy: Current Perspectives," *Cancer Management and Research* 7 (2015): 1–11, https://www.ncbi.nlm.nih.gov/pmc/articles/PMC4274043/.

33.   "Radiation Therapy for Cancer," National Cancer Institute, accessed May 4, 2018, https://www.cancer.gov/about-cancer/treatment/types/radiation-therapy/radiation-fact-sheet.

34.   Dr. Sean Devlin in interview with the author, April 2016.

35.   Dr. Sean Devlin in interview with the author, April 2016; Punit Kaur et al., "Combined Hyperthermia and Radiotherapy for the Treatment of Cancer," *Cancers* 3, no. 4 (December 2011): 3799–3823, https://www.ncbi.nlm.nih.gov/pmc/articles/PMC3763397/; J. van der Zee, "Heating the Patient: A Promising Approach?," *Annals of Oncology* 13, no. 8 (August 1, 2002): 1173–1184, https://academic.oup.com/annonc/article/13/8/1173/143799#1146293.

36.   Mary Brophy Marcus, "How a New Kind of Treatment Kicked Jimmy Carter's Cancer," CBS Interactive Inc., December 7, 2015, https://www.cbsnews.com/news/how-a-new-therapy-kicked-carters-cancer/.

37.   "Managing Cancer as a Chronic Illness," American Cancer Society, last revised February 12, 2016, www.cancer.org/treatment/survivorshipduringandaftertreatment/when-cancer-doesnt-go-away.

38.   Lale Kostakoglu, Harry Agress, and Stanley J. Goldsmith, "Clinical Role of FDG PET in Evaluation of Cancer Patients," *RadioGraphics* 23, no. 2 (March–April 2003): 315–340.

39.   "The Surprising Dangers of CT Scans and X-rays," *Consumer Reports*, March 2015, www.consumerreports.org/cro/magazine/2015/01/the-surprising-dangers-of-ct-sans-and-x-rays/index.htm.

40.   "Certain Type of PET Scan Detects Recurrence Better Than Traditional Tests," Breastcancer.org, April 1, 2016, http://www.breastcancer.org/research-news/certain-pet-scan-detects-recurrence-better.

41.   "Tumor Markers," National Cancer Institute, accessed May 4, 2018, https://www.cancer.gov/about-cancer/diagnosis-staging/diagnosis/tumor-markers-fact-sheet.

42.   "Tumor Markers," National Cancer Institute.

43.   "Tumor Markers," National Cancer Institute.

44.   "Biopsy," American Society of Clinical Oncology, accessed May 8, 2018, https://www.cancer.net/navigating-cancer-care/diagnosing-cancer/tests-and-procedures/biopsy.

45.   M. N. Hasen et al., "Manipulation of the Primary Breast Tumor and the Incidence of Sentinel Node Metastases From Invasive Breast Cancer," *Archives of Surgery* 139, no. 6 (June 2004): 634–639; discussion 639–640, https://www.ncbi.nlm.nih.gov/pubmed/15197090; M. S. Metcalfe et al., "Useless and Dangerous—Fine Needle Aspiration of Hepatic

Colorectal Metastases," *BMJ* 328 (2004): 507–508, http://www.bmj.com/content/328/7438/507; C. R. Loughran and C. R. Keeling, "Seeding of Tumour Cells Following Breast Biopsy: A Literature Review," *British Journal of Radiology* 84, no. 1006 (October 2011): 869–974, https://www.ncbi.nlm.nih.gov/pubmed/21933978.

46.   Ralph Moss, "Are Needle Biopsies Safe?," accessed May 4, 2018, http://chetday.com/needlebiopsy.htm.

47.   Daniel Haley, *Politics in Healing: The Suppression and Manipulation of American Medicine* (South Lake Tahoe, CA: BioMed Publishing Group, 2000), https://books.google.com/books/about/Politics_in_Healing.html?id=AwXtPgAACAAJ.

48.   Devra Davis, "Off Target in the War on Cancer," *Washington Post*, November 4, 2007, http://www.washingtonpost.com/wp-dyn/content/article/2007/11/02/AR2007110201648.html.

49.   "Cancer and the Environment," U.S. Department of Health and Human Services, accessed May 8, 2018, https://www.niehs.nih.gov/health/materials/cancer_and_the_environment_508.pdf.

50.   Davis, "Off Target in the War on Cancer."

51.   "Cancer Stat Fact Sheets: Cancer of Any Site," National Cancer Institute, accessed May 4, 2018, https://seer.cancer.gov/statfacts/html/all.html.

52.   Kathleen T. Ruddy, "Setting the Agenda for the PURE CURE," Breast Health and Healing Foundation, November 21, 2011, http://www.breasthealthandhealing.org/setting-the-agenda-for-the-pure-cure/.

53.   Juliet Eilperin, "Compound in Teflon a 'Likely Carcinogen,'" *Washington Post*, June 29, 2005, http://www.washingtonpost.com/wp-dyn/content/article/2005/06/28/AR2005062801458.html?noredirect=on.

CHAPTER 5: CHEMOSENSITIVITY, GENOMIC, AND NATURAL-AGENT SENSITIVITY TESTING OVERVIEW

1.   "NCI Dictionary of Cancer Terms," National Cancer Institute, s.v. *chemosensitivity assay*, accessed May 4, 2018, www.cancer.gov/dictionary?cdrid=45990.

2.   "Biomedicine And Health: The Germ Theory of Disease," Encyclopedia.com, accessed May 4, 2018, https://www.encyclopedia.com/science/science-magazines/biomedicine-and-health-germ-theory-disease.

3.   Suzanne Somers, *Knockout: Interviews With Doctors Who Are Curing Cancer and How to Prevent Getting It in the First Place* (New York: Three Rivers Press, 2009): 127.

4.   Suzanne Somers, "Chemosensitivity Tests—Why Does Big Pharma Know About Them and WE Don't?," *Gretchen Jones "Love My Hormones"* (blog), January 10, 2010, http://lovemyhormones.blogspot.com/2010/01/chemosensitivity-tests-why-does-big.html.

5.   "High-Dose Vitamin C (PDQ®)—Health Professional Version," National Cancer Institute, updated December 13, 2017, https://www.cancer.gov/about-cancer/treatment/cam/hp/vitamin-c-pdq#section/_14.

6. "Angiogenesis," The Angiogenesis Foundation, accessed May 8, 2018, https://angio.org/learn/angiogenesis/.

7. Ji, "25 Cancer Stem Cell Killing Foods Smarter Than Chemo & Radiation."

8. Sayer Ji, "Better Than Chemo: Turmeric Kills Cancer Not Patients," Wake Up World, accessed May 8, 2018, https://wakeup-world.com/2015/10/23/better-than-chemo-turmeric-kills-cancer-not-patients/.

9. Om Prakash et al., "Anticancer Potential of Plants and Natural Products: A Review," *American Journal of Pharmacological Sciences* 1, no. 6 (2013): 104–115, http://pubs.sciepub.com/ajps/1/6/1/.

10. Mike Adams, "Science Proves That Garlic Kills Cancer Cells," Natural News, January 17, 2004, https://www.naturalnews.com/000146.html#.

11. Alanna Ketler, "5 Ayurvedic Herbs That Have Been Shown To Destroy Cancer Cells," Collective Evolution, November 5, 2014, http://www.collective-evolution.com/2014/11/05/5-ayurvedic-herbs-that-have-been-shown-to-destroy-cancer-cells/.

CHAPTER 6: AMAS TEST

1. "AMAS Test for Cancer," Oncolab, accessed May 8, 2018, http://www.oncolabinc.com/AMASbrochure.pdf.

2. "Oncolab Incorporated Company Profile," BioPortfolio, accessed May 8, 2018, https://www.bioportfolio.com/corporate/company/18831/Oncolab-Incorporated.html.

3. "AMAS Test for Cancer," Oncolab.

4. "Information for Doctors," Oncolab, accessed May 8, 2018, http://www.oncolabinc.com/doctors.html.

5. "Information for Patients," Oncolab, accessed May 8, 2018, http://www.oncolabinc.com/patients.php.

6. "Information for Patients," Oncolab.

7. "Information for Patients," Oncolab.

CHAPTER 7: BIOCEPT

1. "A Simple Blood Test Can Tell You What's Happening With Your Cancer. Now.," Biocept Inc., accessed May 8, 2018, https://biocept.com/patients/; "About Liquid Biopsies," Biocept Inc., accessed May 8, 2018, https://biocept.com/patients/liquid-biopsy-faq.

2. "About Liquid Biopsies," Biocept Inc.

3. Vassilios Alexiadis, Tim Watanaskul, Vahid Zarrabi, Veena Singh, and Lyle Arnold, "High Sensitivity Detection of Rare EGFR Mutations With ctDNA Using Target-Selector TM Assays," Biocept Inc., accessed May 8, 2018, http://1dzi041pbrf98jfu01xrpf3k-wpengine.netdna-ssl.com/wp-content/uploads/2014/10/High-Sensitivity-Detection-of-Rare-EGFR-Mutations-with-ctDNA-using-Target-Selector-Assays.pdf; Farideh Z. Bischoff, Tony J. Pircher, Tam Pham, Karina Wong, Stephen D. Mikolajczyk, Philip D. Cotter, and Julie Ann Mayer, "Redefining CTCs: Detection of Additional Circulating Tumor Cells Using an Antibody Capture Cocktail and HER2 FISH," Biocept Inc.,

accessed May 8, 2018, http://1dzi041pbrf98jfu01xrpf3k-wpengine.netdna-ssl
.com/wp-content/uploads/2014/10/Redefining-CTCs-Detection-of-additional
-circulating-tumor-cells-using-an-antibody-capture-cocktail-and-HER2-FISH
-ASCO-2011.pdf.

    4. "Billing Policy," Biocept Inc., accessed May 8, 2018, https://biocept.com/
customer-service/billing-policy/.

CHAPTER 8: BREASTSENTRY

    1. "BreastSentry," Innovative Diagnostic Laboratory, accessed May 8, 2018,
https://www.myinnovativelab.com/breastsentry/.

    2.   Olle Melander et al., "Stable Peptide of the Endogenous Opioid
Enkephalin Precursor and Breast Cancer Risk," *Journal of Clinical Oncology* 33,
no. 24 (August 20, 2015): 2632–2638, http://ascopubs.org/doi/full/10.1200/
JCO.2014.59.7682; Olle Melander et al., "Validation of Plasma Proneurotensin
as a Novel Biomarker for the Prediction of Incident Breast Cancer," *Cancer
Epidemiology, Biomarkers & Prevention* 23, no. 8 (August 2014), http://cebp
.aacrjournals.org/content/23/8/1672.

CHAPTER 9: THE CANCER PROFILE

    1. "A Letter From Dr. Schandl," American Metabolic Laboratories,
accessed May 8, 2018, https://nebula.wsimg.com/12d49707988c4bb4db68d39
d601fa50f?AccessKeyId=491744267492FF9C7DAE&disposition=0&allowor
igin=1.

    2. "Cancer Profile," American Metabolic Laboratories, accessed June 10,
2018, https://web.archive.org/web/20170108025000/http://www
.americanmetaboliclaboratories.net:80/CA_Profile_.html.

    3. "Cancer Profile or CA Profile," American Metabolic Laboratories,
accessed June 10, 2018, https://nebula.wsimg.com/c1aa5cdf50e214ec4b43611
cb099b9b1?AccessKeyId=491744267492FF9C7DAE&disposition=0&allowor
igin=1.

    4. "Cancer Profile," American Metabolic Laboratories.

CHAPTER 10: COLOGUARD

    1. "How Effective Is Cologuard?," Cologuard, accessed June 10, 2018,
https://www.cologuardtest.com/meet-cologuard/how-effective-is-cologuard

    2. "Your Medicare Coverage," Medicare.gov, accessed June 10, 2018,
https://www.medicare.gov/coverage/colorectal-cancer-screenings
.html#collapse-5990.

    3.   CellMax-CRC (Colorectal), early-detection CTC blood test, www
.CellMaxlife.com, 650-564-3905 (US), +886 0800-555-885 (Taiwan/test kits).

CHAPTER 11: COLON HEALTH SCREENING FOR OCCULT BLOOD IN STOOL

    1.   *Colorectal Cancer: Facts & Figures 2017–2019* (Atlanta: American
Cancer Society, 2017), accessed May 4, 2018, https://www.cancer.org/content/
dam/cancer-org/research/cancer-facts-and-statistics/colorectal-cancer-facts-and-
figures/colorectal-cancer-facts-and-figures-2017-2019.pdf.

2. "Fecal Occult Blood Test," Cleveland Clinic, accessed June 10, 2018, http://www.clevelandclinic.org/health/health-info/docs/1700/1788.asp?index=7143.

Chapter 12: ColonSentry

1. "ColonSentry," Innovative Diagnostic Laboratory, accessed June 10, 2018, https://www.myinnovativelab.com/colonsentry.

Chapter 13: EarlyCDT-Lung Test

1. "Lung Nodule—Test Result Interpretation," Oncimmune, accessed June 10, 2018, http://oncimmune.com/lung-cancer-test/lung-nodule-test-result-interpretation/.

2. "How to Get EarlyCDT-Lung," Oncimmune, accessed June 10, 2018, http://oncimmune.com/lung-cancer-test/earlycdt-lung-how-it-works/.

3. "Lung Nodule—Malignancy Risk Assessment," Oncimmune, accessed June 10, 2018, http://oncimmune.com/lung-cancer-test/lung-nodule-malignancy-risk-assessment/.

4. "Lung and Bronchus Cancer," National Cancer Institute, accessed June 10, 2018, https://seer.cancer.gov/archive/csr/1975_2014/results_merged/sect_15_lung_bronchus.pdf.

5. "Cancer Stat Facts: Lung and Bronchus Cancer," National Cancer Institute, accessed June 10, 2018, https://seer.cancer.gov/statfacts/html/lungb.html.

Chapter 14: Human Chorionic Gonadotropin (HCG) Test

1. "HCG Urine Immunoassay," Navarro Medical Clinic, accessed June 10, 2018, http://www.navarromedicalclinic.com/index.php.

2. "HCG Urine Immunoassay," Navarro Medical Clinic.

3. "Ectopic Production of Human Chorionic Gonadotropin (hCG) by Neoplasms," American Cancer Society, accessed June 10, 2018, http://onlinelibrary.wiley.com/doi/10.1002/1097-0142(19800515)45:10%3C2583::AID-CNCR2820451018%3E3.0.CO;2-W/epdf.

4. "HCG Urine Immunoassay," Navarro Medical Clinic.

5. "HCG Urine Immunoassay," Navarro Medical Clinic.

6. R. R. Williams, K. R. McIntire, T. A. Waldmann et al., "Tumor-Associated Antigen Levels (Carcinoembryonic Antigen, Human Chorionic Gonadotropin, and Alpha-Fetoprotein) Antedating the Diagnosis of Cancer in the Framingham Study," *Journal of the National Cancer Institute* 58, no. 6 (June 1977): 1547–1551, https://www.ncbi.nlm.nih.gov/pubmed/68118.

7. R. R. Williams, K. R. McIntire, T. A. Waldmann et al., "Tumor-Associated Antigen Levels (Carcinoembryonic Antigen, Human Chorionic Gonadotropin, and Alpha-Fetoprotein) Antedating the Diagnosis of Cancer in the Framingham Study."

Chapter 15: IvyGene

1. "Non-invasive Cancer Testing," IvyGene, accessed June 10, 2018, https://www.ivygenelabs.com/.

2. "IvyGene Laboratory Report," IvyGene, accessed June 10, 2018, https://www.ivygenelabs.com/wp-content/uploads/2017/09/SAMPLE-IvyGene-Report-Form-PDF.pdf.

3. "IvyGene Biotechnology Frequently Asked Questions," IvyGene, accessed June 10, 2018, https://www.ivygenelabs.com/frequently-asked-questions/#1.

CHAPTER 16: NAGALASE TEST

1. "Nagalase in Blood," Health Diagnostics and Research Institute, accessed June 10, 2018, http://www.hdri-usa.com/tests/nagalase/.

2. "Nagalase in Blood," Health Diagnostics and Research Institute.

3. "Nagalase in Blood," Health Diagnostics and Research Institute.

4. "OncoImmunology," US National Library of Medicine, August 1, 2013, https://www.ncbi.nlm.nih.gov/pmc/articles/PMC3812199/.

5. "Metabolic Modulation, Immunotherapy, and Metronomic Chemotherapy," LifeExtension Foundation, accessed June 10, 2018, http://www.lifeextensionfoundation.org/funding_01.html.

6. "Another Alternative Autism Treatment," TheAutismDoctor.com, accessed June 10, 2018, http://www.theautismdoctor.com/another-alternative-autism-treatment/.

7. "Nagalase in Blood," Health Diagnostics and Research Institute.

8. Timothy J. Smith, "Nagalase: Friend and Foe?," The GcMAF Book, 2010, https://web.archive.org/web/20140903100355/http://gcmaf.timsmithmd.com/book/chapter/52; "Nagalase in Blood," Health Diagnostics and Research Institute; "Nagalase-Test," Office Prof. Michael Kramer, MD, accessed June 11, 2018, https://nagalase-test.de/en/questions-and-answers/.

CHAPTER 17: OralID

1. "OralID," Forward Science, accessed June 10, 2018, https://forwardscience.com/oralid.

2. "Accuracy of Dentists in the Clinical Diagnosis of Oral Lesions," US National Library of Medicine, accessed June 10, 2018, https://www.ncbi.nlm.nih.gov/pubmed/21716985.

3. "Cancer Stat Facts: Oral Cavity and Pharynx Cancer," National Cancer Institute, accessed June 10, 2018, https://seer.cancer.gov/statfacts/html/oralcav.html.

4. Jerry E. Bouquot, Patricia Suarez, and Nadarajah Vigneswaran, "Oral Precancer and Early Cancer Detection in the Dental Office—Review of New Technologies," The Journal of Implant and Advanced Clinical Dentistry 2, no. 3 (2010): 47-63; Nadarajah Vigneswaran, Sheila Koh, and Ann Gillenwater, "Incidental Detection of an Occult Oral Malignancy With Autofluorescence Imaging: A Case Report," Head and Neck Oncology 1 (2009): 37, https://doi.org/10.1186/1758-3284-1-37.

Chapter 18: Papanicolaou (Pap) and Human Papillomavirus (HPV)

1. "Cancer Stat Facts: Cervical Cancer," National Cancer Institute, accessed June 10, 2018, https://seer.cancer.gov/statfacts/html/cervix.html.

2. "Pap and HPV Testing," National Cancer Institute, accessed June 10, 2018, https://www.cancer.gov/types/cervical/pap-hpv-testing-fact-sheet.

3. "Pap and HPV Testing," National Cancer Institute.

4. "Pap and HPV Testing," National Cancer Institute.

5. "Pap and HPV Testing," National Cancer Institute.

6. "What to Do After an Abnormal Pap Test," Everyday Health, accessed June 10, 2018, https://www.everydayhealth.com/cervical-cancer/what-to-do-after-abnormal-pap-test.aspx.

7. "The Bethesda System," Signature Medical Group, accessed June 10, 2018, http://www.aaobgyn.org/health-library/hw-view.php?DOCHWID=hw26851.

8. "What to Do After an Abnormal Pap Test," Everyday Health.

9. "What to Do After an Abnormal Pap Test," Everyday Health.

10. "What to Do After an Abnormal Pap Test," Everyday Health.

11. "In-Depth Patient Education Reports," University of Maryland Medical Center, accessed June 10, 2018, https://www.umms.org/ummc/patients-visitors/health-library/in-depth-patient-education-reports.

12. "Genetics of Colorectal Cancer (PDQ®)—Health Professional Version," National Cancer Institute, accessed June 11, 2018, https://www.cancer.gov/types/colorectal/hp/colorectal-genetics-pdq; "Cervical Cancer—Patient Version," National Cancer Institute, accessed June 11, 2018, https://www.cancer.gov/types/cervical; "Pap and HPV Testing," National Cancer Institute; "In-Depth Patient Education Reports," University of Maryland Medical Center; "National Breast and Cervical Cancer Early Detection Program (NBCCEDP)," Centers for Disease Control and Prevention, accessed June 11, 2018, https://www.cdc.gov/cancer/nbccedp/.

Chapter 19: Prostate Health Index

1. "Prostate Health Index (PHI)," Innovative Diagnostic Laboratory, accessed June 11, 2018, https://www.myinnovativelab.com/prostate-cancer/.

2. "Prostate Health Index (PHI)," Innovative Diagnostic Laboratory.

3. "Prostate Health Index (PHI)," Innovative Diagnostic Laboratory.

4. W. J. Catalona et al., "A Multicenter Study of [-2]Pro-Prostate Specific Antigen Combined With Prostate Specific Antigen and Free Prostate Specific Antigen for Prostate Cancer Detection...," abstract, *Journal of Urology* 185, no. 5 (May 2011): 1650–1655, https://www.ncbi.nlm.nih.gov/pubmed/21419439; Stacy Loeb et al., "The Prostate Health Index Selectively Identifies Clinically Significant Prostate Cancer," abstract, *Journal of Urology* 193, no. 4 (April 2015): 1163–1169, https://www.jurology.com/article/S0022-5347(14)04900-3/abstract; Ya-Qiang Huang et al., "Clinical Performance of Serum [-2]Propsa Derivatives, %P2psa and PHI, in the Detection and Management of Prostate Cancer," abstract, *American Journal of Clinical and Experimental Urology* 2, no.

5 (December 25, 2014): 343–350, https://www.ncbi.nlm.nih.gov/pmc/articles/
PMC4297331/.

    5.   CellMax-Prostate, early-detection CTC blood test, www.CellMaxlife
.com, 650-564-3905 (US), +886 0800-555-885 (Taiwan/test kits).

Chapter 20: Research Genetic Cancer Center Lab Tests

    1.   "Why We Recommend and Use 'The R.G.C.C. Cancer Test,'" RGCC,
accessed June 11, 2018, http://www.rgccusa.com/files/9614/1342/6446/
Reasons-We-Use-The-RGCC-Cancer-Test.pdf.

    2.   "Tests / aCGH R.G.C.C.," RGCC, accessed June 11, 2018, https://
rgcc-group.com/?page=test_aCGH-new.

    3.   "Tests / Oncocount R.G.C.C.," RGCC, accessed June 11, 2018, https://
rgcc-group.com/?page=test_oncocount_rgcc-new; "Oncocount R.G.C.C.,"
RGCC—Research Genetic Cancer Centre S.A., accessed June 11, 2018,
https://rgcc-group.com/assets/PDF/Test.SamplesOfTheReport/
OncocountRGCC/Oncocount.pdf.

    4.   "Tests / Oncotrace R.G.C.C.," RGCC, accessed June 11, 2018, https://
rgcc-group.com/?page=test_oncotrace_rgcc-demo; "Oncotrace R.G.C.C.,"
RGCC—Research Genetic Cancer Centre S.A., accessed June 11, 2018,
https://rgcc-group.com/assets/PDF/Test.SamplesOfTheReport/
OncotraceRGCC/Oncotrace.pdf.

    5.   "Tests / Oncotrail R.G.C.C.," RGCC, accessed June 11, 2018, https://
rgcc-group.com/?page=test_oncotrail_rgcc-new.

    6.   "Tests / Onconomics," RGCC, accessed June 11, 2018, https://
rgcc-group.com/?page=test_onconomics-new.

    7.   "Tests / Onconomics," RGCC; "Onconomics," RGCC—Research
Genetic Cancer Centre S.A., accessed June 11, 2018, https://rgcc-group.com/
assets/PDF/Test.SamplesOfTheReport/OnconomicsPlus/
Chemoagents-patient's-name.pdf.

    8.   "Tests / Onconomics Plus," RGCC, accessed June 11, 2018, https://
rgcc-group.com/?page=test_onconomics_plus-new; "Onconomics," RGCC—
Research Genetic Cancer Centre S.A., RGCC, https://rgcc-group.com/assets/
PDF/Test.SamplesOfTheReport/OnconomicsPlus/Chemoagents-patient's
-name.pdf.

    9.   "Tests / Onconomics Extracts," RGCC, accessed June 11, 2018, https://
rgcc-group.com/?page=test_onconomics_extracts-new.

    10.   "Tests / Onconomics Extracts," RGCC; "Onconomics Extracts,"
RGCC—Research Genetic Cancer Centre S.A., https://rgcc-group.com/assets/
PDF/Test.SamplesOfTheReport/OnconomicsExtracts/Natural%20Sub-
stances-patient's-name.pdf.

    11.   "Tests / Immune-Frame," RGCC, accessed June 11, 2018, https://
rgcc-group.com/?page=test_immune-frame-new.

    12.   "Tests / Metastat," RGCC, accessed June 11, 2018, https://rgcc-group
.com/?page=test_metastat-new.

    13.   "Tests / ChemoSNiP," RGCC, accessed June 11, 2018, https://
rgcc-group.com/?page=test_chemosnip-new.

14. "Why We Recommend and Use 'The R.G.C.C. Cancer Test,'" RGCC.

Chapter 21: Thymidine Kinase Test

1. "TK1," Red Drop, accessed June 11, 2018, https://pdfs.semanticscholar
.org/27eb/5dd42de4b3ca5b4d923ac71ed098ba31a00a.pdf.

Chapter 22: Videssa® Breast Test

1. "The Insider's Guide to Videssa Breast," Videssa Breast, accessed June
11, 2018, http://cdn2.hubspot.net/hubfs/1781856/PDFs/Downloadable
_Content/eBooks/Videssa_Breast_Overview_eBook.pdf?__hssc=1702931
83.16.1521059381451&__hstc=170293183.fa5db842b24ebaed8c780f5d51
506f97.1521059381451.1521059381451.1521059381451.1&__hsfp=633398250
&hsCtaTracking=b468ef83-f7e0-45e8-8a30-b77eda627d2d%7Cc769138a
-d20a-4af2-b1c5-1d940d1b578b.

2. "Clinically Proven Results," Provista, accessed June 11, 2018, https://
www.provistadx.com/clinical-results.

Chapter 23: Biofocus® Tests

1. "Molecular Oncology," Biofocus, accessed June 11, 2018, http://www
.biofocus.de/media/files/downloads/101_bf-111-brochure-m-oncology.pdf.

Chapter 24: CELLSEARCH

1. "What is the CELLSEARCH® Circulating Tumor Cell (CTC) Test?,"
CELLSEARCH, accessed June 11, 2018, https://www.cellsearchctc.com/
about-cellsearch/what-is-cellsearch-ctc-test.

2. "How are the Results Interpreted and What Do They Mean?," CELL-
SEARCH, accessed June 11, 2018, https://www.cellsearchctc.com/clinical
-applications/interpretation-of-results.

3. "How are the Results Interpreted and What Do They Mean?," CELL-
SEARCH.

4. Maintrac (CTC count and drug analysis), www.maintrac.de, phone:
0921/850200.

Chapter 25: Caris Molecular Intelligence

1. "Demonstrated Utility—Improved Clinical Outcomes," Caris Molecular
Intelligence, accessed June 11, 2018, https://www.carismolecularintelligence
.com/clinical-utility-tumor-profiling/; D. Spetzler, et al., "Multi-Platform
Molecular Profiling of 1,180 Patients Increases Median Overall Survival and
Influences Treatment Decision in 53% of Cases," *European Journal of Cancer*,
Volume 51, S44 (September 2015).

2. "Demonstrated Utility—Improved Clinical Outcomes," Caris Molecular
Intelligence; D. Spetzler et al., "Multi-Platform Molecular Profiling of 1,180
Patients Increases Median Overall Survival and Influences Treatment Decision
in 53% of Cases," *European Journal of Cancer* 51, S44 (September 2015).

3. "How Tumor Profiling Works," Caris Molecular Intelligence, accessed June 11, 2018, https://www.carismolecularintelligence.com/tumor-profiling -works/.

CHAPTER 26: FOUNDATIONONE

1. "What is FoundationOneHeme?," Foundation Medicine, accessed June 11, 2018, https://www.foundationmedicine.com/genomic-testing/foundation -one-heme.

2. "What is FoundationACT?," Foundation Medicine, accessed June 11, 2018, https://www.foundationmedicine.com/genomic-testing/foundation-act.

3. "What is FoundationOne CDx?," Foundation Medicine, accessed June 11, 2018, https://www.foundationmedicine.com/genomic-testing/foundation -one-cdx.

4. "Foundation Medicine Announces New Data Using Next-Generation Sequencing to Detect Cancer-Related Mutations Not Identified by Conventional Methods," Business Wire, accessed June 11, 2018, https://www .businesswire.com/news/home/20120602005008/en/Foundation-Medicine -Announces-New-Data-Next-Generation-Sequencing.

5. Jaime Rosenberg, "First-of-a-Kind Companion Test for Cancer Gene Profiling Gets FDA Approval," *The American Journal of Managed Care* (December 4, 2017), http://www.ajmc.com/newsroom/firstofakind-companion -test-for-cancer-gene-profiling-gets-fda-approval.

6. Among those companies: Admera Health LLC, LiquidGx™, www .AdmeraHealth.com, 908-222-0533; Guardant Health LLC, Guardant360 (73 Genes), www.guardanthealth.com/, 855-698-8887; and Invitae Corporation©, Invitae Multi-Cancer Panel (84 Genes), www.Invitae.com, 800-436- 3037. (When results are negative, Invitae offers expanded testing at no charge for ninety days after original test.)

CHAPTER 27: NAGOURNEY CANCER INSTITUTE

1. "How We Test Your Cancer," Nagourney Cancer Institute, accessed June 11, 2018, https://www.nagourneycancerinstitute.com/functional-profiling.

2. "How We Test Your Cancer," Nagourney Cancer Institute.

3. "EVA-PCD Functional Analysis," Nagourney Cancer Institute, accessed June 11, 2018, https://cdn2.hubspot.net/hubfs/571280/edited_Specimen _Processing-NCI.pdf?t=1520552725768.

4. "Personal Cancer Testing and Consultations," Nagourney Cancer Institute, accessed June 11, 2018, https://www.nagourneycancerinstitute.com/ cancer-consultations-and-testing.

5. "Personal Cancer Testing and Consultations," Nagourney Cancer Institute.

CHAPTER 30: CONNECTING WITH AN INTEGRATIVE PHYSICIAN

1. "About," Best Answer for Cancer, accessed June 11, 2018, https:// bestanswerforcancer.org/about/.

2. "About Us," Society for Integrative Oncology, accessed June 11, 2018, https://integrativeonc.org/about-us/about-sio.

3. "About Us," Naturopathic Physicians: Natural Medicine. Real Solutions., accessed June 11, 2018, https://www.naturopathic.org/about.

4. "Vision and Mission," OncANP, accessed June 11, 2018, https://oncanp .org/vision-and-mission/.

5. "The Mission of the ACIM," ACIM Connect, accessed June 11, 2018, https://www.acimconnect.com/our-mission.

CHAPTER 31: FUNCTIONAL TESTING OVERVIEW

1. C. de Martel et al., "Global Burden of Cancers Attributable to Infections in 2008: A Review and Synthetic Analysis," *The Lancet Oncology* 13, no. 6 (June 2012): 607–615, https://www.ncbi.nlm.nih.gov/pubmed/22575588.

CHAPTER 32: LOW-DOSE APPROACH TO CHEMOTHERAPY

1. "IPT/IPTLD Treatment," Best Answer for Cancer, accessed June 11, 2018, https://bestanswerforcancer.org/patients/iptiptld-cancer-treatment/.

2. Nadine Rudiger et al., "Chemosensitivity Testing of Circulating Epithelial Tumor Cells (CETC) in Vitro: Correlation to in Vivo Sensitivity and Clinical Outcome," *Journal of Cancer Therapy* 4, no. 2 (April 2013): 597–605; G. I. Lau G, W. T. Loo, and L. W. Chow, "Neoadjuvant Chemotherapy for Breast Cancer Determined by Chemosensitivity Assay Achieves Better Tumor Response," *Biomedicine & Pharmacotherapy* 61, no. 9 (October 2007): 562–565, https://www.ncbi.nlm.nih.gov/pubmed/17913448.

3. "Complementary Cancer Therapies," Best Answer for Cancer, accessed June 11, 2018, https://bestanswerforcancer.org/patients/resources/ complementary-cancer-therapies/.

4. Steven G. Ayre, MD, "The Physiology and Clinical Pharmacology of Insulin in its Application in Insulin Potentiation Therapy," The Ayre Clinic for Contemporary Medicine, accessed June 11, 2018, http://contemporarymedicine .net/the-physiology-and-clinical-pharmacology-of-insulin-in-its-application-in -insulin-potentiation-therapy/.

5. Oliver Alabaster, Barbara K. Vonderhaar, and Samir M. Shafie, "Metabolic Modification by Insulin Enhances Methotrexate Cytotoxicity in MCF-7 Human Breast Cells." *European Journal of Cancer and Clinical Oncology* 17, no. 11 (1981): 1223–1228.

6. C. Damyanov et al., "Low Dose Chemotherapy in Combination With Insulin for the Treatment of Advanced Metastatic Tumors. Preliminary Experience," *Journal of BUON* 14, no. 4 (October–December 2009): 711–715, www .ncbi.nlm.nih.gov/pubmed/20148468, http://studyres.com/doc/2707742/low -dose-chemotherapy-in-combination-with-insulin-for-the.

7. Christo Damyanov et al., "Insulin Potentiation Therapy in the Treatment of Malignant Neoplastic Diseases: A Three Year Study," *Journal of Cancer Science & Therapy* 4 (April 2012): 088–091.

8. "Battling Cancers With a Well-Functioning Immune System," Integrative Medicine of New York, accessed June 11, 2018, www.linchitzmedical wellness.com/cancer-treatment-options.

9. "Whole Being Healing," Best Answer for Cancer, accessed June 11, 2018, https://bestanswerforcancer.org/patients/resources/whole-being-healing/.

10. "About," Best Answer for Cancer.

CHAPTER 33: CANCER—BEAT IT, DON'T FEED IT

1. *Arizona Republic*, February 14, 2014, www.newspapers.com/ newspage/120435786/.

2. Q. Yang et al., "Added Sugar Intake and Cardiovascular Diseases Mortality Among US Adults," *Journal of the American Medical Association Internal Medicine* 174, no. 4 (April 2014): 516–524.

3. Nanci Hellmich, "Cancer to Skyrocket Worldwide, Study Says: WHO Report Faults Smoking, Obesity, Rise in Population," *Arizona Republic*, February 15, 2014, https://www.newspapers.com/newspage/120436626/; Tim Hume and Jen Christensen, "WHO: Imminent Global Cancer 'Disaster' Reflects Aging, Lifestyle Factors," CNN, February 4, 2014, www.cnn.com /2014/02/04/health/who-world-cancer-report/index.html.

4. "World Cancer Day 2014," American Cancer Society, accessed January 27, 2014, www.cancer.org/cancer/news/world-cancer-day-2014.

5. *Merriam-Webster*, s.v. "food," accessed June 11, 2018, https://www .merriam-webster.com/dictionary/food.

6. Albert Sanchez et al., "Role of Sugars in Human Neutrophilic Phagocytosis," *American Journal of Clinical Nutrition* 26, no. 11 (November 1, 1973): 1180–1184.

7. Stephanie Strom, "U.S. Cuts Estimate of Sugar Intake," *New York Times*, October 26, 2012, https://www.nytimes.com/2012/10/27/business/ us-cuts-estimate-of-sugar-intake-of-typical-american.html; "Sugar: The Bitter Truth," Kolp Institute, November 4, 2012, http://kolpinstitute.org/facts -about-sugar/.

8. "The FDA Takes Step to Remove Artificial Trans Fats in Processed Foods," Centers for Disease Control and Prevention, June 16, 2015, http:// content.govdelivery.com/accounts/USCDC/bulletins/10a0af6.

9. David A. Kessler, *The End of Overeating: Taking Control of the Insatiable American Appetite* (New York: Rodale, 2009), 14.

10. *Dietary Guidelines for the Brazilian Population* (Brasília, Brazil: Ministry of Health of Brazil, 2014), accessed June 11, 2018, https://www .foodpolitics.com/wp-content/uploads/Brazilian-Dietary-Guidelines-2014.pdf.

11. Sarah Boseley, "Mexico Enacts Soda Tax in Effort to Combat World's Highest Obesity Rate," Guardian News and Media Limited, January 16, 2014, https://www.theguardian.com/world/2014/jan/16/mexico-soda-tax-sugar -obesity-health.

12. Amy Guthrie, "Health Battle Over Soda Flares in Mexico," *Wall Street Journal*, August 29, 2013, https://www.wsj.com/articles/health-battle-over -soda-flares-in-mexico-1377735538.

13.   Ellen Davis, *Fight Cancer With a Ketogenic Diet* (N.p.: Gutsy Badger Publishing, 2013), 6, accessed June 11, 2018, https://www.amazon.com/Fight-Cancer-Ketogenic-Diet-Third/dp/1943721033.

14.   "Chef Rachel Albert Writes on the Benefits of A Ketogenic Diet, Part 1," The Healthy Cooking Coach, accessed June 11, 2018, http://www.thehealthycookingcoach.com/chef-rachel-albert-writes-on-the-benefits-of-a-ketogenic-diet-part-1/.

15.   "Chef Rachel Albert Writes on the Benefits of A Ketogenic Diet, Part 1," The Healthy Cooking Coach.

16.   Weston A. Price, *Nutrition and Physical Degeneration* (Australia: Project Gutenberg, 2012), accessed June 11, 2018, http://gutenberg.net.au/ebooks02/0200251h.html.

CHAPTER 34: THE TOOLBOX

1.   Ellen R. Copson et al., "Germline BRCA Mutation and Outcome in Young-Onset Breast Cancer (POSH): A Prospective Cohort Study," *The Lancet*, accessed June 11, 2018, http://www.thelancet.com/pdfs/journals/lanonc/PIIS1470-2045(17)30891-4.pdf.

2.   Navneet Singh et al., "A Comparative Study of Fluoride Ingestion Levels, Serum Thyroid Hormone and TSH Level Derangements, Dental Fluorosis Status Among School Children From Endemic And Non-Endemic Fluorosis Areas," *SpringerPlus* 3 (January 3, 2014): 7, www.ncbi.nlm.nih.gov/pmc/articles/PMC3890436.

3.   See, for example: "Environmental Exposure to Xenoestrogens and Oestrogen Related Cancers: Reproductive System, Breast, Lung, Kidney, Pancreas, and Brain," Environmental Health, accessed June 11, 2018, https://ehjournal.biomedcentral.com/articles/10.1186/1476-069X-11-S1-S8; "The Estrogen Hypothesis of Obesity," *PLOS ONE* (June 10, 2014), http://journals.plos.org/plosone/article?id=10.1371/journal.pone.0099776.

4.   Mary Rodavich, MS, RD, LDN, "CPE Monthly: Skin Cancer and Nutrition," *Today's Dietitian* 17, no. 2 (February 2015): 50, http://www.todaysdietitian.com/newarchives/021115p50.shtml.

5.   Cedric Garland et al., "The Role of Vitamin D in Cancer Prevention," *American Journal of Public Health* 96, no. 2 (February 2006): 252–261.

6.   Laura Vuolo et al., "Vitamin D and Cancer," *Frontiers in Endocrinology* 3 (February 20, 2012): 58.

7.   "Natural Products That Target Cancer Stem Cells," US National Library of Medicine, accessed June 11, 2018, https://www.ncbi.nlm.nih.gov/pubmed/26503998; Ji, "25 Cancer Stem Cell Killing Foods Smarter Than Chemo & Radiation."

8.   International Agency for Research on Cancer, World Health Organization, "Some Organophosphate Insecticides and Herbicides," vol. 112 (2017), 398, http://monographs.iarc.fr/ENG/Monographs/vol112/mono112.pdf.

9.   William Davis, *Wheat Belly: Lose the Wheat, Lose the Weight, and Find Your Path Back to Health* (New York: Rodale Books, 2011), https://www

.amazon.com/Wheat-Belly-Lose-Weight-Health/dp/1609611543/ref=tmm
_hrd_swatch_0?_encoding=UTF8&qid=&sr=.

10.   William B. Hobbins, MD, and Wendy Sellens, L.Ac., *Breast Cancer Boot Camp: Dr. Hobbins's Breast Thermography Revolution* (Mustang, OK: Tate Publishing, 2013), 92–99, https://www.amazon.com/Breast-Cancer-Boot -William-Hobbins/dp/1625637993.

11.   Hobbins and Sellens, *Breast Cancer Boot Camp*, 61, 98, 163; C. Duffy, K. Perez, and A. Partridge, "Implications of Phytoestrogen Intake for Breast Cancer," *CA: A Cancer Journal for Clinicians* 57, no. 5 (September–October 2007): 260–277.

12.   Hobbins and Sellens, *Breast Cancer Boot Camp*, 40.

13.   J. A. Stephenson et al., "Tumour Angiogenesis: A Growth Area—From John Hunter to Judah Folkman and Beyond," *Journal of Cancer Research* (2013), https://www.hindawi.com/journals/jcr/2013/895019/.

14.   H. C. Lai, N. P. Singh NP, and T. Sadaki, "Development of Artemis-inin Compounds for Cancer Treatment," *Investigational New Drugs* 31, no. 1 (February 2013): 230–246.

15.   Robert Jay Rowen, "Artemisinin: From Malaria to Cancer Treatment," *Townsend Letter*, December 2002.

16.   N. Widodo, "Selective Killing of Cancer Cells by Leaf Extract of Ashwagandha: Components, Activity and Pathway Analyses," US National Library of Medicine, January 10, 2008, https://www.ncbi.nlm.nih.gov/ pubmed/18191020; Babli Halder, Shruti Singh, and Suman S. Thakur, "*Withania somnifera* Root Extract Has Potent Cytotoxic Effect Against Human Malignant Melanoma Cells," US National Library of Medicine, September 3, 2015, https://www.ncbi.nlm.nih.gov/pmc/articles/PMC4559428/.

17.   Wen Tan et al., "Berberine Hydrochloride: Anticancer Activity and Nanoparticulate Delivery System," *International Journal of Nanomedicine* 6 (August 24, 2011): 1773–1777; "Berberine," WebMD, accessed May 7, 2018, https://www.webmd.com/vitamins-supplements/ingredientmono-1126 -BERBERINE.aspx.

18.   Jun Yin, Huili Xing, and Jianping Ye, "Efficacy of Berberine in Patients with Type 2 Diabetes," US National Library of Medicine, May 1, 2009, https:// www.ncbi.nlm.nih.gov/pmc/articles/PMC2410097/.

19.   Petr Sima, Luca Vannucci, and Vaclav Vetvicka, "Effects of Glucan on Bone Marrow," US National Library of Medicine, February 2, 2014, https:// www.ncbi.nlm.nih.gov/pmc/articles/PMC4202472/.

20.   Douglas A. Wyatt, "Leaky Gut Syndrome: A Modern Epidemic With an Ancient Solution?," *Townsend Letter*, June 2014, http://jeffreydachmd .com/wp-content/uploads/2015/06/Leaky-Gut-Syndrome-Modern-Epidemic -Douglas-Wyatt-Townsend-Letter-2014.pdf.

21.   D. Karunagaran, R. Rashmi, and T. R. Kumar, "Induction of Apop-tosis by Curcumin and Its Implications for Cancer Therapy," *Current Cancer Drug Targets* 5, no. 2 (March 2005): 117–129.

22. James Howenstine, MD, "Use of Cesium Chloride to Cure Malignancies," NewsWithViews.com, June 29, 2004, http://www.newswithviews.com/Howenstine/james14.htm.

23. Nicholas Gonzalez, MD, "The Gonzalez Therapy: A Look Back, And an Update," Dr-Gonzalez.com, accessed June 11, 2018, http://www.dr-gonzalez.com/totalhealth_6_04.htm; N. J. Gonzalez and L. L. Isaacs, "Evaluation of Pancreatic Proteolytic Enzyme Treatment of Adenocarcinoma of the Pancreas, With Nutrition and Detoxification Support," US National Library of Medicine, 1999, https://www.ncbi.nlm.nih.gov/pubmed/10368805?dopt=Abstract.

24. Jim Moselhy et al., "Natural Products That Target Cancer Stem Cells," *Anticancer Research* 35, no. 11 (November 2015), http://ar.iiarjournals.org/content/35/11/5773.long.

25. Bagora Bayala et al., "Anticancer Activity of Essential Oils and Their Chemical Components—A Review," US National Library of Medicine, November 19, 2014, https://www.ncbi.nlm.nih.gov/pmc/articles/PMC4266698/.

26. Y. Zu et al., "Activities of Ten Essential Oils Towards Propionibacterium Acnes and PC-3, A-549 and MCF-7 Cancer Cells," *Molecules* 15, no. 5 (April 30, 2010): 3200–3210.

27. Anasuya Ray, Smreti Vasudevan, and Suparna Sengupta, "6-Shogaol Inhibits Breast Cancer Cells and Stem Cell-Like Spheroids by Modulation of Notch Signaling Pathway and Induction of Autophagic Cell Death," *PLOS ONE* (September 10, 2015), http://journals.plos.org/plosone/article?id=10.1371/journal.pone.0137614; Sayer Ji, "Ginger: 10,000x Stronger Than Chemo (Taxol) In Cancer Research Model," GreenMedInfo.com, September 23, 2015, http://www.greenmedinfo.com/blog/ginger-10000x-stronger-chemo-taxol-cancer-research-model-1; S. Wang, C. Zhang, G. Yang, and Y. Yang, "Biological Properties of 6-Gingerol: a Brief Review," US National Library of Medicine, July 2014, https://www.ncbi.nlm.nih.gov/pubmed/25230520.

28. "Haelan 951 Info Sheet—A Fermented, Organic, Non-GMO Soy Product," Haelan 951, accessed June 12, 2018, https://haelan951.com/wp-content/uploads/2018/01/Mechanisms-of-Action-Haelan-951.pdf.

29. David Williams, "Honokiol: The Swiss Army Plant," Foundation for Alternative and Integrative Medicine, accessed June 12, 2018, http://www.faim.org/honokiol-the-swiss-army-plant.

30. See, for example, Arumugam Nagalingam et al., "Honokiol Activates AMP-Activated Protein Kinase in Breast Cancer Cells Via an LKB1-Dependent Pathway and Inhibits Breast Carcinogenesis," US National Library of Medicine, February 21, 2012, https://www.ncbi.nlm.nih.gov/pmc/articles/PMC3496153/.

31. Williams, "Honokiol: The Swiss Army Plant."

32. Isaac Eliaz, "Honokiol Research Review: A Promising Extract With Multiple Applications," *Natural Medicine Journal* 5, no. 3 (July 2013), https://www.naturalmedicinejournal.com/journal/2013-07/honokiol-research-review.

33.   Jonathan Wright, MD, and Lane Lenard, PhD, *Why Stomach Acid Is Good for You: Natural Relief from Heartburn, Indigestion, Reflux and GERD* (Washington, DC: M. Evans & Company, 2001), https://www.amazon.com/Why-Stomach-Acid-Good-You/dp/0871319314/.

34.   Nurul Husna Shafie et al., "Pro-Apoptotic Effect of Rice Bran Inositol Hexaphosphate (IP6) on HT-29 Colorectal Cancer Cells," *International Journal of Molecular Sciences* 14, no. 12 (December 2013): 23545–23558, https://www.ncbi.nlm.nih.gov/pmc/articles/PMC3876062/; Mallikarjuna Gu, "Inositol Hexaphosphate Down-Regulates Both Constitutive and Ligand-Induced Mitogenic and Cell Survival Signaling, and Causes Caspase-Mediated Apoptotic Death of Human Prostate Carcinoma PC-3 Cells," *Molecular Carcinogenesis* 4, no. 9 (January 2010): 1–12, https://www.ncbi.nlm.nih.gov/pmc/articles/PMC2798913/.

35.   B. A. Eskin, "Iodine and Mammary Cancer," *Advances in Experimental Medicine and Biology* 91 (1977): 293–304.

36.   Nancy Piccone, "The Silent Epidemic of Iodine Deficiency," Life Extension, October 2011, http://www.lifeextension.com/magazine/2011/10/The-Silent-Epidemic-of-Iodine-Deficiency/Page-01.

37.   "Prostate Cancer, Nutrition, and Dietary Supplements: Q&A About Lycopene," National Cancer Institute, updated October 31, 2017, www.cancer.gov/cancertopics/pdq/cam/prostatesupplements/Patient/page4.

38.   Kun Liao et al., "Parthenolide Inhibits Cancer Stem-Like Side Population of Nasopharyngeal Carcinoma Cells via Suppression of the NF-κB/COX-2 Pathway," Theranostics, accessed June 12, 2018, http://www.thno.org/v05p0302.htm.

39.   V. Coothankandaswamy et al., "The Alternative Medicine Pawpaw and Its Acetogenin Constituents Suppress Tumor Angiogenesis Via the HIF-1/VEGF Pathway," *Journal of Natural Products* 73, no. 5 (May 28, 2010): 956–961.

40.   "What is Poly-MVA?," Poly-MVA, accessed June 12, 2018, https://polymva.com/faqs/.

41.   "PolyMVA," Poly-MVA, accessed June 12, 2018, https://polymva.com/about/.

42.   "Poly-MVA Introduction," Poly-MVA, accessed June 12, 2018, http://www.polymva4doctors.com/polymva_introduction.html.

43.   "PolyMVA," Poly-MVA.

44.   Paul S. Anderson, NMD, "Lipoic Acid Mineral Complex Introduction and Protocols," Poly-MVA, accessed June 12, 2018, http://www.polymva4doctors.com/pdfs/LAMC-Complete-FINAL-2015.pdf.

45.   "PolyMVA," Poly-MVA.

46.   "Poly-MVA Breakthrough for Doctors and Patients," Poly-MVA, accessed June 12, 2018, http://www.polymva4doctors.com/pdfs/Poly-MVA-Breakthrough-FINAL-Feb-2015.pdf.

47.   "Poly-MVA Breakthrough for Doctors and Patients," Poly-MVA; "PolyMVA Survivors," PolymvaSurvivors.com, accessed June 12, 2018, http://www.polymvasurvivors.com/scientific_research.html.

48. "Poly-MVA Breakthrough for Doctors and Patients," Poly-MVA; F. J. Antonawich et al., "Regulation of Ischemic Cell Death by the Lipoic Acid-Palladium Complex, Poly MVA, in Gerbils," US National Library of Medicine, September 2004, https://www.ncbi.nlm.nih.gov/pubmed/15296831.

49. "Poly-MVA Breakthrough for Doctors and Patients," Poly-MVA.

50. "Poly-MVA Breakthrough for Doctors and Patients," Poly-MVA.

51. Lich Thi Nguyen et al., "Quercetin Induces Apoptosis and Cell Cycle Arrest in Triple-Negative Breast Cancer Cells Through Modulation of Foxo3a Activity," US National Library of Medicine, February 21, 2017, https://www.ncbi.nlm.nih.gov/pmc/articles/PMC5343054/; Senping Cheng et al., "Clinical Cancer Research," American Association for Cancer Research, December 2010, http://clincancerres.aacrjournals.org/content/16/23/5679.

52. G. A. Potter and M. D. Burke, "Salvestrols—Natural Products With Tumour Selective Activity," *Journal of Orthomolecular Medicine* 21, no. 1 (2006), http://orthomolecular.org/library/jom/2006/pdf/2006-v21n01-p34.pdf.

53. G. I. Murray et al., "Tumor-Specific Expression of Cytochrome P450 CYP1B1," *Cancer Research* 57, no. 14 (July 15, 1997): 3026–3031.

54. Brian A Schaefer, *Salvestrols: Nature's Defence Against Cancer: Linking Diet and Cancer* (Victoria, BC: Clinical Intelligence Corp., 2012).

55. "Milk Thistle (PDQ)—Health Professional Version," National Cancer Institute, updated June 19, 2017, https://www.cancer.gov/about-cancer/treatment/cam/hp/milk-thistle-pdq.

56. Carlo Selmi et al., "The Effects of Spirulina on Anemia and Immune Function in Senior Citizens," *Cellular & Molecular Immunology* 8, no. 3 (May 2011): 248–254, https://doi.org/10.1038/cmi.2010.76; Hiromi Okuyama et al., "*Spirulina* Lipopolysaccharides Inhibit Tumor Growth in a Toll-Like Receptor 4-Dependent Manner by Altering the Cytokine Milieu From Interleukin-17/Interleukin-23 to Interferon-γ," *Oncology Reports* 37, no. 2 (February 2017): 684–694, https://doi.org/10.3892/or.2017.5346.

57. R. Koníčková et al., "Anti-Cancer Effects of Blue-Green Alga Spirulina Platensis, a Natural Source of Bilirubin-Like Tetrapyrrolic Compounds," *Annals of Hepatology* 13, no. 2 (March–April 2014): 273–283.

58. "Vitamin C: Fact Sheet for Health Professionals," National Institutes of Health, updated March 2, 2018, https://ods.od.nih.gov/factsheets/VitaminC-HealthProfessional.

59. Orthomolecular Medicine News Service, "Intravenous Vitamin C Is Selectively Toxic to Cancer Cells," news release, September 22, 2005, http://orthomolecular.org/resources/omns/v01n09.shtml.

60. "Childhood Lead Poisoning," World Health Organization, 2010, http://www.who.int/ceh/publications/leadguidance.pdf.

61. Walter Blumer and Elmer Cranton, "Ninety Percent Reduction in Cancer Mortality After Chelation Therapy With EDTA," *Journal of Advancement in Medicine* 2, no. 1–2 (Spring/Summer 1989).

62. "Photodynamic Therapy," American Cancer Society, revised March 18, 2015, https://www.cancer.org/treatment/treatments-and-side-effects/treatment-types/photodynamic-therapy.html.

63. "Photodynamic Therapy," American Cancer Society.

64. "Complementary Cancer Therapies," Best Answer for Cancer Foundation, accessed June 12, 2018, https://bestanswerforcancer.org/patients/resources/complementary-cancer-therapies/.

65. "Complementary Cancer Therapies," Best Answer for Cancer Foundation.

66. "Complementary Therapies," EuroMed Foundation, accessed June 12, 2018, https://euromedfoundation.com/procedures/treatment-methods/complementary-therapies.

67. E. J. Lim et al., "Methylsulfonylmethane Suppresses Breast Cancer Growth by Down-Regulating STAT3 and STAT5b Pathways," *PLOS One* 7, no. 4 (2012), https://doi.org/10.1371/journal.pone.0033361.

68. M. A. Franco-Molina et al., "Antitumor Activity of Colloidal Silver on MCF-7 Human Breast Cancer Cells," *Journal of Experimental Clinical Cancer Research* 29 (November 2010): 148.

69. "Marijuana and Cancer," American Cancer Society, revised March 16, 2017, https://www.cancer.org/treatment/treatments-and-side-effects/complementary-and-alternative-medicine/marijuana-and-cancer.html; M. Solinas et al., "Cannabidiol Inhibits Angiogenesis by Multiple Mechanisms," *British Journal of Pharmacology* 167, no. 6 (November 2012): 1218–1231, https://doi.org/10.1111/j.1476-5381.2012.02050.x; G. Velasco, C. Sánchez, and M. Guzmán, "Anticancer Mechanisms of Cannabinoids," *Current Oncology* 23, supplement 2 (March 2016): S23–S32, https://doi.org/10.3747/co.23.3080.

70. Sang Ho Choi, Su Yun Lyu, and Won Bong Park, "Mistletoe Lectin Induces Apoptosis and Telomerase Inhibition in Human A253 Cancer Cells Through Dephosphorylation of Akt," *Archives of Pharmacal Research* 27, no. 1 (January 2004): 68–76, https://link.springer.com/article/10.1007%2FBF02980049; "Mistletoe Extracts (PDQ)—Patient Version," National Cancer Institute, updated April 12, 2018, https://www.cancer.gov/about-cancer/treatment/cam/patient/mistletoe-pdq#section/all.

71. "Mistletoe Extracts (PDQ)," National Cancer Institute.

72. "Laetrile/Amygdalin (PDQ)—Patient Version," National Cancer Institute, updated April 5, 2018, https://www.cancer.gov/about-cancer/treatment/cam/patient/laetrile-pdq.

73. Ralph Moss, "Why We Are Losing the War on Cancer," *Consumer Health* 13, no. 5 (June 1990), www.consumerhealth.org/articles/display.cfm?ID=19990831140122.

74. "S.O.T. for Cancer Support," Center for New Medicine, 2014, http://cfnmedicine.com/wp-content/uploads/2014/11/SOT-Handout.pdf.

75. Ronda Wendler, "After a Stem Cell Transplant, Professor Returns to the Classroom," *Conquest* (Fall 2016), https://www.mdanderson.org/publications/conquest/fall-2016/transplanted-strength.html.

76. Jong-Lyel Roh et al., "Nrf2 Inhibition Reverses the Resistance of Cisplatin-Resistant Head and Neck Cancer Cells to Artesunate-Induced Ferroptosis," *Redox Biology* 11 (April 2017): 254–262, https://doi.org/10.1016/j.redox.2016.12.010.

77.   Bastyr University, "Integrative Oncology Study Draws Attention for Promising Results," news release, December 4, 2013, https://bastyr.edu/news/general-news-home-page/2013/12/integrative-oncology-study-draws-attention-promising-results.

78.   "DCA (Dichloroacetate) Frequently Asked Questions," Medicor Cancer Centres, updated April 1, 2017, http://medicorcancer.com/dca-dichloroacetate-frequently-asked-questions/; see also E. D. Michelakis et al., "Metabolic Modulation of Glioblastoma With Dichloroacetate," *Science Translational Medicine* 2, no. 31 (May 12, 2010): 31–34, https://doi.org/10.1126/scitranslmed.3000677.

79.   G. Klevos et al., "Cryoablation of Benign and Malignant Breast Tumors," *Interventional Oncology 360* 4, no. 6 (2016): E95–E100, https://www.interventionaloncology360.com/article/cryoablation-benign-and-malignant-breast-tumors; "Cryoablation (Freezing)," Robert G. Pugach, MD, accessed June 12, 2018, https://www.pacificcoasturology.com/cryoablation-freezing/.

CHAPTER 35: CLOSING

1.   Steve Steeves, *The Trinity Diet* (Magnolia, TX: Lucid Books, 2013), 10.

Index